Professional Practice in
Public Health

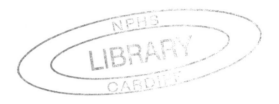

Professional Practice in Public Health

Edited by Jill Stewart and Yvonne Cornish

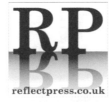

reflectpress.co.uk

This book is dedicated to
Cian, Sean and both our Bens.

Contents

Part Three: ENVIRONMENTAL HEALTH IN
PUBLIC HEALTH

Abbreviations

AQMA	Air Quality Management Area
ARCP	Annual Review of Competence Progression
A&E	Accident and Emergency
BBC	British Broadcasting Corporation
BBV	Blood-Borne Virus
BERR	(Department for) Business, Enterprise and Regulatory Reform
BHF	British Heart Foundation
BME	Black and Minority Ethnic
BSc	Bachelor of Science (degree)
BRE	Building Research Establishment
BSE	Bovine Spongiform Encephalopathy
BSHF	Building and Social Housing Foundation
CAA	Comprehensive Area Assessment
CCDC	Consultant in Communicable Disease Control
CCT	Certificate of Completion of Training
CDH	Community Development for Health
CDSC	Communicable Disease Surveillance Centre
CHD	Coronary Heart Disease
CHDW	Community Health Development Worker
CIEH	Chartered Institute of Environmental Health
CIH	Chartered Institute of Housing
nvCJD	New variant Creutzfeldt-Jakob disease
CMO	Chief Medical Officer
CMO	Context-Mechanism-Outcome (in HIA)
COI	Central Office of Information
COSPH	Comparison of Santé/Public Health
CPA	Comprehensive Performance Assessment
CPD	Continuing Professional Development
CS	Community Strategy
CSO	Civil Society Organisation
CQC	Care Quality Commission
CVD	Cardio Vascular Disease
CWRWC	Christian World Reform World Committee
DALYs	Disability-Adjusted Life Years
DCLG	Department for Communities and Local Government
DECC	Department for Energy and Climate Change
DEFRA	Department of Environment, Food and Rural Affairs
DETR	Department of the Environment, Transport and the Regions

DFID	Department for International Development
DfEE	Department for Education and Employment
DfT	Department for Transport
DoH	Department of Health
DPH	Director of Public Health
DTI	Department of Trade and Industry
DTLR	Department of Transport, Local Government and the Regions
DWP	Department for Work and Pensions
EBP	Evidence-Based Practice
EC	European Commission
EHCS	English House Condition Survey
EHO	Environmental Health Officer
EHP	Environmental Health Practitioner
EPS	Electronic Prescription Service
ESRC	Economic and Social Research Council
EU	European Union
FAO	Food and Agriculture Organisation
FPH	Faculty of Public Health
FSA	Food Standards Agency
GCSE	General Certificate of School Education
GDP	Gross Domestic Product
GIS	Geographical Information System
GLA	Greater London Authority
GLA	Gangmasters Licensing Authority
GMC	General Medical Council
GP	General Practitioner
HA	Health Authority
HDA	Health Development Agency (now subsumed into NICE)
HEA	Health Education Authority
HFEA	Human Fertilisation and Embryology Authority
HHSRS	Housing Health and Safety Rating System
HIA	Health Impact Assessment
HIV/AIDS	Human Immuno-deficiency Virus/AIDS
HM	Her Majesty
HMO	House in Multiple Occupation
HMSO	Her Majesty's Stationary Office
HNA	Health Needs Assessment
HPA	Health Protection Agency
HPT	Health Persuasion Techniques
HPU	Heath Protection Unit
HSE	Health and Safety Executive
HV	Health Visitor
ICD	International Classification of Disease
IDeA	Improvement and Development Agency
IFED	International Federation of Environmental Health
IFF	International Faculty Forum (of IFED)
IIA	Integrated Impact Assessment
IMD	Index of Multiple Deprivation

IPC	International Planning Committee
IPCC	Intergovernmental Panel on Climate Change
IPO	Initial Public Offering
JRF	Joseph Rowntree Foundation
JRT	Joseph Rowntree Trust
JSNA	Joint Strategic Needs Assessment
LA	Local Authority
LAA	Local Area Agreement
LACORS	Local Authority Coordinators of Regulatory Services
LAH	Legislation for Health
LHB	Local Health Board (Wales)
LHC	London Health Commission
LSP	Local Strategic Partnership
MFPH	Member of the Faculty of Public Health
MMR	Measles Mumps and Rubella (vaccine)
MP	Member of Parliament
MRSA	Methocillin resistant staphylococcus aureus
MSc	Master of Science (degree)
MTAS	Medical Training Application System
NAM	National AIDS Manual
NGO	Non Governmental Organisation
NHMRC	National Health and Medical Research Council
NHS	National Health Service
NHS CRS	NHS Care Records Service
NICE	National Institute for Health and Clinical Excellence
NMC	Nursing and Midwifery Council
NO_x	Oxides of nitrogen
NPHLP	National Public Health Leadership Programme
ODPM	Office of the Deputy Prime Minister
ONS	Office for National Statistics
OSPHE	Observed Structured Public Health Examination
PAH	Polycyclic aromatic hydrocarbons
PCH	Personal Counselling for Health
PCT	Primary Care Trust
PDPH	Regional Directors of Public Health
PESTLE	Political, Economic, Social, Technological, Legal, Environmental
PhD	Doctorate of Philosophy
PHLS	Public Health Laboratory Service
PHO	Public Health Observatory
PHORCaST	Public Health Online Resource for Career and Skills Training
PHRU	Public Health Resource Unit
PM_{10} $PM_{2.5}$	Particulate matter
PSA	Public Service Agreement
RCT	Randomised Control Trial
RIA	Regulatory Impact Assessment
RITA	Record of In-Training Assessment
RoSPA	Royal Society for the Prevention of Accidents
RSPH	Royal Society for Public Health

SARS	Severe Acute Respiratory Syndrome
SEA	Strategic Environmental Assessment
SEU	Social Exclusion Unit
SIT	Specific Impact Tests
StHA	Strategic Health Authority
STI	Sexually Transmitted Infection
StR	Specialist Trainee
TB	Tuberculosis
TPB	Theory of Planned Behaviour
TUC	Trades Union Congress
UN	United Nations
UK	United Kingdom
UKPHA	United Kingdom Public Health Association
UKPHR	United Kingdom Public Health Register
USA	United States of America
UV	Ultra Violet
WHO	World Health Organisation
WI	Women's Institute

Acknowledgements

First and foremost we owe a debt of gratitude to Judith Harvey for very positively agreeing to publish our book and for her continued advice, support and encouragement throughout its development. We are also grateful to the reviewers for their very helpful advice and suggestions and for acknowledging the importance of environmental health and the need for such a text.

We are extremely grateful to the chapter authors who have been so willing to share their knowledge and professional practice in writing for this book, which would simply not have been possible without them. Their biographical details indicate their dedication and ongoing commitment to future developments in environmental and public health. We have been immensely impressed with their professionalism and knowledge shown and thank them for working to such a tight timescale so effectively.

We are grateful to Dr Stephen Battersby, CIEH President, for writing the Foreword.

The editors, authors and publisher would like to thank the following people and organisations for permission to reproduce their material in this book. Every attempt has been made to seek permission for the copyright material that has been used. However, if we have inadvertently used copyright material without permission/acknowledgement, we apologise and we will make the necessary correction at the first opportunity. We list the specific chapters and acknowledgments in order below.

Chapter 5: Organisation and delivery of the public health agenda

- Rachel Flowers, Consultant in Public Health, for her contribution on defining public health partnerships.
- Ian Gray for the PHORCaST figure, an illustration prepared as part of the PHORCaST Project Board.

Chapter 6: Environment, health and sustainability

Nottingham Health and Environment Partnership and Sussex-air Air Quality Partnership for permission to use their material in case studies.

Chapter 7: Meeting the challenges of poverty, inequality and social exclusion

The English Collective of Prostitutes.

Chapter 8: Health promotion: a multi-causal approach

We are grateful to the editor for permission to reproduce: Thomas, S. and Stewart, J. (2005) 'Optimising health promotion activities', *Journal of Community Nursing*, 19 (1): 9–12.

Chapter 9: Health protection

Mike Studden of the Health Protection Agency's Environmental Health and Risk Assessment Unit, Stonehouse, Gloucestershire.

Chapter 10: Health needs assessment

- Dr Jayshree Pillaye for permission to adapt her work on teenage pregnancy in the London Borough of Brent from the abridged version of her report submitted for the Part II Examination for Membership for the Faculty of Public Health Medicine.
- David Wainwright for permission to adapt his work on participative HNA.

Chapter 11: Health impact assessment

- Dr Alex Scott-Samuel for permission to use the Merseyside HIA model diagram.
- Professor Sarah Curtis and Ben Cave for permission to adapt the CMO model diagram.
- Elsevier Social Science and Medicine for permission to reproduce the diagram in Dunn and Hayes (2000) 'Social inequality, population health, and housing: a study of two Vancouver neighbourhoods'.
- Paul Plant and Nannerl Herriot for permission to use the HIA on the draft London Plan and the follow-up included in the sustainability appraisal.
- Professor Geoff Green for permission to use the Sheffield HIA on housing policy.

- Belfast Healthy Cities for permission to use their Community Health Impact Assessment Pilot Project Report.

Chapter 17: Globalisation and public health

Charles Oham for his contribution on fair trade in food.

Chapter 18: Environmental health practice

We would like to offer a particular thanks to Ian Gray for his hard work and enthusiasm for both chapters he co-authored, but also more widely for his general enthusiasm for this text.
The CIEH for the diagram of EH 2012 and the curriculum 'daisy'.

Chapter 20: The challenges for health and community in the private housing sector

London Boroughs of Islington and Newham for permission to use the respective case studies.

Contributors

Allan McNaught BSc (Hons), MPhil, PhD, FRSM, MInstL&M

Following a degree at London Southbank, Allan entered the NHS Management Training Scheme and subsequently worked in a variety of general management jobs in the London and Essex area. After five years teaching at Southbank, he then worked internationally on major aid-funded health reform projects and as a health management consultant with a private health economics practice, based in Washington DC. His advanced studies have been principally in the area of health policy, implementation and management, and he has a major interest in black and minority ethnic (BME) health care, and the role of the voluntary and community sector in health care. Allan is Head of the Health Development Department and Enterprise Lead for the School of Health and Social Care, University of Greenwich.

Anne Gill SRN, DipN (Lond), Cert Ed, BSc (Hons) MSc

Anne Gill has a nursing background and has worked in Australia, Germany, Scotland and England. She has been involved in continuing professional development for health and social care workers since 1984. A more recent but related interest is in flexible learning for mature students utilising e.learning and blended learning. She is currently programme leader for a Foundation Degree in Care Management involving e.learning plus flexible attendance. She was also part of a team that developed a programme of clinical supervision workshops that is being used by NHS Trusts throughout south-east England. Anne is currently a Senior Lecturer at the University of Greenwich.

Anneyce Knight MSc, PGCE, BA (Hons), RN

Anneyce Knight previously worked as a nurse in a variety of clinical settings before taking up her current position as Senior Lecturer at the University of Greenwich. She is Programme Leader for BScHealth/ Combined Studies and European Lead for the School of Health and

Social Care. She teaches students across a range of programmes, both undergraduate and postgraduate. She was recently UK project lead for a part-funded European Interreg IIIA project, Health Interreg Santé. This project facilitated the cross-Channel mobility of health professionals and students between Kent and Nord-Pas de Calais and led to the exchange of best practice while promoting networks between individuals and institutions in the Euro-region. She has lectured in France and the Czech Republic. Her research interests include health inequalities, particularly in the area of cancer and palliative care.

Benjamin (Ben) Bruneau, BA (Hons), MSc, M Inst M, RN, RMN, RNT, DNT, PhD

Ben works in the Health Development Department of the School of Health and Social Care of the University of Greenwich. He is presently Programme Leader for the BSc Honours Complementary Therapies Programmes. Prior to moving to this position, he worked as Programme Leader for the BSc Honours Health Programme, as Assistant Director for Research for the School, and, prior to that, for a number of years, he was a teacher of nurses in a primary care setting. Ben is an active researcher. His research is mainly in the area of personality and stress, and in particular the role played by the individual when coping with their stress. He also has interests and experience in research approaches and in new technologies that facilitate methods of studying relationships among psychological constructs.

Carlos Moreno-Leguizamon BA, MA, PhD

Carlos Moreno-Leguizamon has a social sciences background – medical anthropology and health communication – and has worked in Colombia, the USA, India, Ghana, Tanzania, Kenya and the UK. Professionally he combines two key areas of experience: on the one hand, programme design, implementation and evaluation of health, cultural and environmental projects from the grass-roots level to the macro institutional level and, on the other, teaching and researching health, culture and medical systems. In particular, his research has related to the discourse analysis of illegal drug use, development and environment issues and, above all, health-illness in three medical traditions – Ayurveda, Biomedicine and Indigenous Medicine from Colombia. Currently, as Senior Lecturer and Programme Leader for MSc Research at the School of Health and Social Care at the University of Greenwich, he is involved in the implementation of action research projects on Black Minority and Ethnic health issues in the south-east of England as well as in the teaching of culture competency and equality and diversity issues to health and social care students.

Charles Oham MBA

After his graduation from MOCA (now Imo State Polytechnic), Charles was actively involved in business start-up and enterprise in Nigeria, West Africa. On returning to the UK, he became actively involved in the development of community businesses and private public partnership intervention at a grassroots level. He was appointed to the board of an EU-funded Objective 2 Pathway Programme for Edmonton in 1997 to develop programmes and projects that mitigated deprivation, social exclusion and economic decline in the area. Charles has worked in various capacities – as an Associate Lecturer at the Open University, and an Innovations Services Coordinator for a multi-million pound EU-funded project at the University of East London. He has accumulated several years' experience managing non-profit organisations and small and medium enterprises (SMEs). Charles is actively involved in social entrepreneurial activity, community development and social enterprise in East London, Essex, Kent and Norfolk. His research interests include business sustainability, business development, faith-based management, strategy and innovation within the context of the third sector and emerging economies. He is a Senior Lecturer in Social Enterprise in the School of Health and Social Care at the University of Greenwich.

Clarence Spigner, MPH, DrPH (USA)

Clarence Spigner's background is in medical sociology, anthropology and public health. While a pre-doctoral fellow he worked as a health planner for the National Health Service in 1982. He wrote his doctoral dissertation on race, ethnicity and health in the UK and the USA. Spigner's areas of expertise in the health of the public encompass race and ethnic relations, health promotion, programme evaluation and health planning. His publications include knowledge and perceptions about organ donation and transplantation, tobacco-related behaviour, the intersection of popular culture on perceptions and behaviour, and the African Diaspora. He has a visiting professor appointment at the University of Greenwich (UK) and is currently an associate professor at the University of Washington (USA).

Evelyn Gloyn BSc, MSc, Chartered EHP

Evelyn Gloyn has worked in environmental health for nearly 25 years; in private sector housing, food safety and health and safety. She has pioneered local environmental health and public health policy, developing strategies on food matters and health inequalities. She worked with the Chartered Institute of Environmental Health (CIEH) and Primary Care

Trusts on the development of public health practitioners, and attained an MSc in Public Health and Urban Renewal at Queen Mary University of London and City University where she guest lectures on environmental health. At the fifth Warwick Healthy Housing Conference (2008), she presented a paper on overcrowding and health using health impact assessment techniques. Evelyn is currently working in neighbourhood governance, in a role to engage people in local democracy.

Ian Gray FCIEH, ATSI, Chartered EHP, MBE

Ian is a Chartered Environmental Health Practitioner (EHP) and principal policy officer for health development at the CIEH. Ian is a well-known campaigner for public health, and a strong advocate for the role of environmental health practitioners in improving health. He previously had a long career in local government in East London, where he managed both regulatory services and health promotion staff. In 2002 he led the joint project with the former Health Development Agency, which both critically examined current environmental health practice and set out the vision for future development. The publication of *Environmental Health 2012 – A key partner in delivering the public health agenda* has been highly influential in shaping modern training and practice.

His main area of work is in developing the environmental health practitioner role within the wider public health workforce. This includes the development of skills, competences and career pathways including registration as public health practitioners, which will become available in 2009. Most recently he had a lead role in the development and implementation of the smoke-free legislation, which is widely acknowledged as a landmark in public health history. Ian was awarded an MBE in 2009 in recognition of his contribution to public health.

Jill Stewart BSc (Hons), MSc, PhD, PGCE (PCET), MCIEH, FRSPH, FRGS, ACIH

Jill Stewart worked as an Environmental Health Officer in local government specialising in private sector housing for several years before taking up her current position as Senior Lecturer at the University of Greenwich's School of Health and Social Care, where she is currently involved in teaching housing and public health students at undergraduate and postgraduate levels. As departmental Research Lead, her interests particularly include the interfaces of public health and housing and the effectiveness of contemporary practitioner interventions. She is currently involved in an initiative to promote, develop and use housing and health evidence in practice online, one of the key recommendations of her PhD. Her publications include books, contributions to books and over 35 peer reviewed and professional papers, and she has made various presentations to a variety of local, national and international audiences.

Lynne Jump RGN BSc (Hons) MA ODE

Lynne undertook initial nurse training before specialising in intensive care nursing in London, gaining experience in cardiothoracic and neurological intensive care. Her first sister's post was as a QARNN at Royal Naval Hospital Haslar, experiencing general surgery, general medicine and coronary care. The Falklands war caused a shortage of nurse teachers in the Royal Navy, which led Lynne to undertake a teacher's qualification at Ipswich College before graduate and postgraduate study and she is currently studying for a professional Doctorate in Education while concurrently working at the University of Greenwich. Her main teaching interests include human life sciences, research methods, academic skills and teaching and learning and she is particularly interested in electronic learning using virtual learning environments. She is programme leader for the MA Professional Practice in Health and Social Care that is delivered for the most part online. Lynne's research interests are also related to e.learning, particularly regarding collaborative learning among adult learners and health information systems.

Mandy Mitchelmore RGN, BA (Hons), MSc (Nursing), MSc (Research), PGD Ed

Mandy Mitchelmore has a nursing background and has worked in a joint appointment between the University of Greenwich and an NHS Trust for a number of years. She has also worked at a senior level in an acute NHS Trust before moving to work full time at the university, leading on Ethics. Mandy has also taught on the pre-registration curriculum for all branches of nursing and midwifery on subjects such as academic skills, values and evidence-based practice. She is currently the Programme Leader for adult nursing within a joint pre-registration interprofessional learning curriculum with Christ Church Canterbury University.

Nargis Kayani BSc. MCIEH

Nargis Kayani is a corporate member of the CIEH and has worked for several London local authorities. Since 2003, Nargis has been a senior consultant at Sanctum Consultants providing environmental and public health consultancy services, to a diverse group of public and private sector clients. Nargis is committed to providing solutions for low income and vulnerable groups in relation to housing and noise issues and is the founder of Noisedirect, the National Noise Advice Line. Nargis has lectured in food and health, presented at national conferences, and writes a regular public health column for the CIEH's monthly professional journal.

Paul Mishkin, BSc (Hons), PgDip Public Health Practice, MCIEH

Paul Mishkin qualified as an Environmental Health Officer in 1999. He has focused on the housing aspect of environmental health work since 2001, working in various local authorities in and around London. He has been keen to work with other practitioners and was seconded to Islington PCT for six months where he completed a Health Impact Assessment on the local private sector housing strategy. His project for a Post-Graduate Diploma in Public Health Practice related to tackling childhood accidents in private rented housing. Paul is currently a Senior Environmental Health Officer in the London Borough of Islington and sits on a number of Steering Groups relating to Housing and Health, such as the National HMO Network and Energy Efficiency Partnership for Homes, Private Sector Sub Group.

Rachel Flowers BSc (Hons), PGDip, MSc, FCIEH, FFPH, Chartered EHP

Rachel works as a Consultant in Public Health in Newham PCT (the 'East End' of London). She has the lead role for her PCT in cardiovascular disease. This means providing the public health inputs for the commissioning of all prevention, primary care, community and acute care services for diabetes, cardiac conditions, hypertension and stroke and vascular risk assessments. Prior to moving to the NHS in 2002, Rachel worked in local government for over 20 years in both environmental health and health promotion roles. She has extensive experience of delivering health improvements at both regional and national levels, including membership of the Social Exclusion Unit Policy Action Team. Rachel is known as being passionate about public health and reducing health inequalities. She is currently vice chair of the UK Public Health Association, vice chair of the Policy Development Board of the CIEH, a visiting lecturer for several universities and an assessor for the UK Register for Public Health Specialists.

Russell Moffatt BSc (Hons), MPH, MCIEH

Russell is an Environmental Health Practitioner with experience in both housing and public health fields. He achieved his bachelor honours degree in Environmental Health at Greenwich University in 2002 and completed his Masters in Public Health at King's College, London in 2006. Russell has worked for a number of London boroughs as an environmental health officer specialising in housing and regeneration. He now leads a team of practitioners dealing with empty residential properties in Newham, London. Newham has pioneered the systematic use of Compulsory Purchase powers to tackle vacant property and land.

Stuart Lines BSc (Hons), MSc, PGCE, FFPH, FCIEH

Stuart Lines has a background in teaching and environmental health and has worked for local authorities in London and Hertfordshire. He was part of one of the first national cohorts of trainees from a background other than medicine to be admitted to a public health training programme in 2001 and was the first EHP to qualify as a Consultant in Public Health via the formal training route. Since qualifying, Stuart has worked in a Primary Care Trust in East London and is currently working as a Consultant in Public Health for NHS Luton. He maintains an interest in teaching and is in the process of becoming a trainer in public health.

Suri Thomas RGN, HV, BA (Hons) MSc, CertEd

Suri worked as a health visitor before becoming Principal Lecturer at the University of Greenwich where she is currently Programme Leader for the BSc (Hons) Public Health. She is a Personal Tutor Group leader for the adult branch of nursing and course leader across a range of health and health promotion courses. Based on her health visiting experience, she is a community link teacher for nursing and midwifery students. Suri has taught in the Czech Republic as part of the Erasmus project and has participated in the European Interreg IIIA project, Health Interreg Santé, a project which included facilitating the cross-Channel mobility of health professionals between Kent and Nord-Pas de Calais, helping to build networks and leading to the exchange of best practice in the Euro-region.

Swatee Patel GDipMaths, MSc, Chartered Stat

Swatee is a medical statistician and has worked at St George's Medical School, London and St Thomas' Medical School, London before joining the University of Greenwich as a Lecturer in Statistics. She was one of the first academics at the university to be awarded a Principal Lecturer post for excellence in teaching in 1997. She has taught statistics in all subject areas, including psychology, business, chemistry, biology, environmental health, public health, and osteopathy. She teaches statistics at all levels, including undergraduate, MSc and PhD. Swatee carries out medical statistical consultancy work for doctors at local NHS Trusts. Her current collaborative research is on the epidemiology of asthma in children, with the Department of Epidemiology and Community Health at Imperial College, London.

Tony Lewis PGDip, BSc, MCIEH, Chartered EHP

Tony is a Chartered EHP and has worked as Principal Education Officer at CIEH since 2002. He has been responsible for the design and introduction of the 2003 Curriculum for Environmental Health, which marked a shift away from pure knowledge to a curriculum delivering a mix of knowledge, skills and competencies. More recently, Tony was one of the architects of the radical 2007 curriculum for environmental health that permits the development of specialists on graduation. Tony currently represents CIEH on the HSE's Long Term Training Needs Board that is developing the competence framework for health and safety regulators, and he is also a member of the national steering group developing National Occupational Standards for Health Protection. He currently contributes to the LLM in Environmental Health Law at the University of Surrey. Prior to joining CIEH, Tony taught environmental health and public health at Nottingham Trent University, at the School of Public Health Medicine at Nottingham University, and contributed to the Master of Studies programme at the Homerton School of Health Sciences at Cambridge University.

Ven Veeramah RMN, Dip (Lond), Cert Ed, BSc (Hons), MSc, PhD

Ven Veeramah has a background in mental nursing. He has been involved in the education of nurses and other health care professionals since 1987. His main interest is in research and evidence-based practice and he has been involved in several research projects. He was until recently the Programme Leader for the MSc in Health Research at the School of Health and Social Care. Ven is currently a Principal Lecturer at the University of Greenwich and teaches research methods and supervises research projects at both undergraduate and post-graduate levels.

Veronica Habgood BSc, MSc, MCIEH

Following a degree in Environmental Science, Veronica Habgood worked for a number of years as an environmental health officer in Suffolk and London, concurrently undertaking further study in environmental protection. She has worked at the University of Greenwich since 1989, lecturing primarily in environmental protection, public health and the environment-health interface and is a contributor to a number of established publications. Veronica is currently the Director of Learning and Quality in the School of Health and Social Care at the University of Greenwich, and a corporate member of the CIEH.

Yvonne Cornish BA (Hons), MSc, PhD, FFPH

Yvonne Cornish's public health career started in 1990 at the Public Health Department of Brighton District Health Authority, before moving to North West Thames Regional Health Authority to work in an inter-regional role for the Regional Directors of Public Health Group. This was followed by an academic post at the South East Institute of Public Health, focusing largely on the development of multi-disciplinary public health practice. During this time, she helped set up the Multi-disciplinary Public Health Forum, was co-opted onto the Chief Medical Officer's Project to Strengthen the Public Health Function, and became one of the first Specialist Visitors for the Faculty of Public Health Training Scheme. She was made an Honorary Member of the Faculty of Public Health in 1999 and a Fellow in 2006. As a public health academic, she has undertaken applied research and consultancy for NHS public health departments, evaluated public health programmes and initiatives, and developed, taught and examined public health courses at undergraduate and postgraduate level. She currently provides academic and professional leadership in public health across the School of Health and Social Care at the University of Greenwich.

Foreword

I am delighted to have been invited to write the Foreword to this book on professional practice in public health, which includes contributions from a number of distinguished environmental health practitioners.

The work of environmental health practitioners (EHPs) and other public health workers, regardless of their employment, is (or should be) aimed ultimately at reducing inequalities in health. This requires that they avoid operating narrowly as mere 'regulators' or 'compliance auditors'. This may be difficult with the 'better regulation' agenda and increasing pressure on resources. However, it cannot be assumed that legislation and its enforcement will inevitably deliver better public health or address inequalities. Nor will it address inequity in health. EHPs may not have seen themselves as helping to deliver social justice in health but that is what they need to do. The community advocacy role is also an essential part of the EHP's work. For those working in local government, the failure to act as a public health and community advocate may at least explain why environmental health work has not always been appreciated adequately.

The WHO Commission on Social Determinants of Health has argued the need for action on the social determinants of health so as to attain greater health equity. The social gradient points to health inequalities as a consequence of the unequal distribution of resources, so government action is required but EHPs can also contribute. As Professor Marmot who chaired the WHO Commission has argued, we should look at the 'causes of the causes'. Why, for example, are there inequalities in smoking and obesity, which are clearly potent causes of ill health? The answer is that the causes lie in the circumstances in which people are born, grow, live, work and age. It is also argued that the social gradient reflects the degree of control people have over these circumstances – control over their own lives. If this approach is accepted, it is not difficult to see how living in poor quality housing in degraded environments and in low-wage but highly demanding employment can have adverse health effects, including on mental health.

This book addresses some key issues for public health practitioners including EHPs and their development as part of the public health workforce. Without doubt there is great potential for EHPs to work with partners to contribute more effectively to public health and deliver interventions to secure improved health and wellbeing. Such interventions have to be based on evidence, including from the assessment and evaluation of the impact of activities already taken on health equity. This book will help EHPs' development and also encourage them to demonstrate to their employers how they can better contribute to the health and wellbeing of communities. It is my hope that this book will also help EHPs and other workers to better act as advocates and articulate needs in the cause of improved public health. At this time of economic woe, good professional practice in public health is needed more than ever.

Dr Stephen Battersby
President, Chartered Institute of Environmental Health

Chapter 1

Introduction

Jill Stewart, Yvonne Cornish and Lynne Jump

WHAT IS PROFESSIONAL PRACTICE IN PUBLIC HEALTH?

Public health is essentially about improving health and addressing inequalities and is most commonly defined as: 'the science and art of preventing disease, prolonging life and promoting health through organised efforts and informed choices of society, organisations, public and private, communities and individuals' (Acheson, 1988; as amended by Wanless, 2004). The original Acheson definition was extended by Wanless to encompass the emphasis on both personal and community responsibility for health and a recognition of the wide range of statutory and non-statutory organisations that have a role to play. Indeed the Faculty of Public Health tells us that public health:

- is population-based;
- emphasises collective responsibility for health, its protection and disease prevention;
- recognises the key role of the state, with recognition of the socio-economic determinants of health and disease; and
- emphasises partnership working.

(Faculty of Public Health website: **www.fph.org.uk**, (accessed 9 July 2009)

Defining public health professionalism

A key message that underpins the definition of public health by Acheson and Wanless is that of an emerging new professional community that is made up of a whole population, collections of health professionals and the state – all working in partnership. While this is useful in some contexts, the sheer complexity of the statement does lead to difficulties when attempting to define what is meant by a 'public health professional' – which we refer to in this book using the more extensive terminology of 'public health practitioner'.

Attempting to define the term 'professional' (or 'professionalism') can be complicated. Firstly what is it about 'being professional' that is determined by the quality of what that person does, and of the conduct, demeanour and standards that guide what they do (Hargreaves, 2000)? 'Being a professional' is determined by how the professional feels that they are seen through other people's eyes, in terms of their status, standing, regard and levels of professional reward (Hargreaves, 2000).

Professionalism has been traditionally determined by a set of characteristics that professions such as law and medicine were seen to embody. Such characteristics emerge from what is considered to be the 'trait' approach (Hall and Marsh, 2000) and are founded in earlier descriptions of professionalism by Millerson (1964) and Goode (1960) based on two core characteristics of any professional; that of:

- a lengthy period of training in a specific body of knowledge; and
- a strong service orientation.

Over time these two characteristics have been added to, to include the assumption that there is a community of interest that, in the context of an appropriate code of ethics, determines the skills, knowledge and conduct of that group resulting in professional autonomy and a substantial level of control within that professional community (Hall and Marsh, 2000).

For public health practice, the combination of a core set of occupational competences that are explicitly related to 'improving health' and an academic framework that spans both undergraduate and postgraduate provision contribute to a strong argument for the applicability of this definition to public health. There are, however, other definitions of professionalism that relate more to levels of expertise (Mezirow, 1991; Benner, 1984; Schon, 1987) and the way that professionals constantly make sense or meaning of their experience. Reflection, critical thinking and value systems are central to these definitions. While there are requirements for expertise and competence (Southon and Braithwaite, 1998), there are also high levels of uncertainty and complexity.

There is an additional complexity when defining professionalism for those people who work within public health practice and Hanlon (1998) states that when defining professionalism there is a need to explore the relationship between the employer and the professional. Those professionals working within the service sector enjoy a relationship of trust with their employers and in return the 'professional employee' responds with an ability to perform to an expected standard.

Hargreaves (2000) argues that the postmodern age of professionalism is driven by economics, which includes policies that are driven by a 'market orientated' ethos of practice, and information technology and the internet. Within any professional setting Hargreaves (2000) argues that this entails dealing with centrally controlled and frequently changing standards and targets but ever-tightening regulations, controls and complexity at a local level. It also means that public health professionals will encounter a variety of partnerships as more and more social groups voice their views and exert their influence on important public health issues. Learning to work in partnership will be a key competence in order to be a public health professional and, as Hargreaves (2000) states, the solution to postmodern professionalism is that of 'collegial professionalism' as a basis for strength.

THE DETERMINANTS OF HEALTH AND INEQUALITIES IN HEALTH

Our ideas about what determines health and disease have altered radically over time. There has been a changing pattern of disease (the epidemiological transmission) from infections to chronic disease. We now know that there are multiple causes of disease, that we can act collectively rather than individually and that we need to focus on prevention, not treatment. How we understand the causes of disease informs the strategies we develop and implement in public health.

Many factors affect health and health inequality and it is estimated that more than 70 per cent of all health determinants lie outside the scope of the NHS, and are due to demographic, socio-economic and environmental conditions (US Office of Disease Prevention, 1996). In turn, many of these health determinants are beyond the control of the individual and communities they affect and have negative impacts on health and well being. Determinants of health are summarised in Table 1.1 below.

Age, sex and hereditary factors.	Biological factors – fixed.
Individual lifestyle factors.	Family structure and functioning; risk taking behaviour; diet; smoking; drug and alcohol misuse (coping mechanism/stress); exercise; recreation; means of transport.
Social and community networks.	Social capital and support; social enterprise; culture; peer pressure; discrimination; spiritual participation; anomie.
Living and working conditions, including public services.	Education (all levels); agriculture and food production; work environment and occupation type; income; unemployment; water and sanitation; housing. Availability of and access (including disabled access) to public services, including health care; baby and child care; social services; leisure services; other health agencies and services.
Socio-economic-environmental factors, including public policy.	Air quality; water; noise; smell; visual amenity; public safety; shops – access, quality, value for money; communications – rail, road; land use; refuse disposal; energy; environmental amenity. Economic, social, environmental and health priorities, policies, programmes and projects at national, regional and local level.

Table 1.1 Determinants of health (adapted from Dahlgren and Whitehead, 1991 and Scott-Samuel *et al.*, 2001)

Yvette Cooper, Parliamentary Under Secretary for Public Health (2002), asked: 'What greater inequality can there be than to die younger and to suffer more illness throughout your life as a result of where you live, what job you do and how much your parents earned?' (cited in NHS Trent Regional Office and Sheffield Hallam University, 2002). Her colleague, Dawn Primarolo, (at the time of writing) Public Health Minister, said: 'Where people live shapes how they feel about themselves and their general health even before you factor in exercise, drugs and alcohol' (cited in Carlisle, 2008).

The 1980 Black Report favoured a materialist explanation of health determination. More recent work has focused on social class and the importance of other factors such as gender. Psychosocial explanations have also been demonstrated and that it is necessary to tackle relative poverty and inequality and build social capital (Wilkinson, 1996; Blane,

Brunner and Wilkinson, 1996). However, despite this research and knowledge, the health divide continues to widen even though we are generally better off (Marmot and Wilkinson, 2006).

Mortality and morbidity are closely related to relative (rather than absolute) income and health is 'extraordinarily sensitive' to socio-economic circumstances. The psychosocial effects of social position account for the larger part of health inequalities, bringing substantial implications for public policy (Wilkinson, 1997). Better integration in a network of social relations is known to benefit health. We need increased cohesion in society through economic integration, reduced unemployment, material security and narrower income differences. Community infrastructure and social capital are seen as key to affecting environmental, behavioural and lifestyle determinants (Marmot and Wilkinson, 2006).

The Acheson Report (1998) revived interest in health inequalities. It had three main recommendations, which were firstly, that all policies likely to have an impact on health should be evaluated in terms of their impact on health inequalities; secondly, that high priority should be given to families with children; and thirdly that further steps should be taken to reduce income inequalities and improve living standards in poor households. The report argued that a socio-environmental approach was necessary as:

- most diseases and long-term conditions are multi-causal;
- health is strongly influenced by the physical (material) and social environments in which we live; and
- risk conditions in these environments damage health both directly and indirectly.

Various policy documents have called for a wider understanding of health, better and more coordinated public health function, partnership working, community development and public involvement, a more capable and increased public health workforce and increased health protection (for example, DoH, 2001a). In tackling health inequalities across social groups and in improving health and quality of life for all, we need to improve social, economic and physical environments and to secure good health for the whole population. There is a need for a 'fully engaged scenario' focusing on prevention, the wider determinants of health and cost-effective action to improve health and reduce inequalities (Wanless, 2001 and 2004). Wanless (2004) focused on the need for sustainable, evidence-based and cost-effective action to bring about long-term health impacts. An emphasis of recent papers has been on enabling healthier lifestyles through increased information, advice and support in areas such as smoking, sexual health, drinking and mental wellbeing (DoH, 1998a; DoH, 1999a; DoH, 2004).

Evidence-based health promotion and health investment should be asking: What determines a population's health and the most effective and efficient interventions to protect and improve it. Achievements of health outcomes should be focused on the determinants of health (Marmot and Wilkinson, 2006) (see Box 1.1).

Box 1.1 Public health: the key principles

- Taking a proactive and not reactive approach.
- Focusing on determinants of health locally.
- Identifying health inequalities in the population/community.
- Sourcing appropriate, relevant evidence (data, case studies, etc. if available).
- Suitably qualified and skilled practitioners applying partnership-based, evidenced interventions.
- Working closely with those affected to help enable sustainable solutions.
- Continually adding to, reviewing and evaluating the evidence base.

PARTNERSHIPS FOR PUBLIC HEALTH

Public health partnership frameworks are about improving health and reducing inequalities, particularly through strengthened NHS and local authority public health roles. The organisational structure is now well established, but there are still factors requiring attention, including shared priorities and objectives and there are still challenging issues to reconcile across the various partnerships, including capacity, organisational change and differing performance management regimes.

As a result, there has been a continued focus on organisational change, most particularly in developing new strategic partnerships to take the public health agenda forward. Alongside this has been an emphasis on evidence-based policies and finding new ways of tackling determinants of health. The Health Development Agency (HDA) (now under the auspices of the National Institute of Health and Clinical Excellence) (NICE) was established in 2000 in part to assess the effectiveness of interventions. Health Needs Assessment and Health Impact Assessments have become of increasing importance in all stages of policy, but remain discretionary.

There has been a myriad of partnerships to take the public health agenda forward. Local Strategic Partnerships (LSPs) are non-statutory and bring together public, private, business, voluntary and community initiatives and services to support one another and operate at local level. Their main objectives are to help sustainable growth, encourage social, physical and economic regeneration in deprived areas, meet local need, give local communities more influence over decision making in their neighbourhoods and encourage non-governmental sectors to take a more active role, and they are pivotal to finding new joined-up ways of tackling local priorities including crime, employment, health and housing. Community strategies also emphasise the needs and role of the community and seek to enhance quality of life. Local Area Agreements (LAAs) establish priorities agreed between central government and a local area (the local authority and LSP) and other local key partners to simplify some central funding, help join up public services more effectively and allow greater flexibility and reduced bureaucracy for local solutions to local circumstances to enhance local areas.

Joint Strategic Needs Assessments (JSNAs) are a new process requirement for Primary Care Trusts (PCTs) and local authorities to establish the current and future health and wellbeing needs of their population, leading to improved outcomes and reductions in health inequalities.

Internationally, the WHO Commission on the Social Determinants of Health (2008) emphasised the importance of social justice and how people live and how this affects their health, pointing to the need for an integrated global approach to health and recommending improvements to daily life. Domestically, the recent Darzi Review, *High Quality Care for All Next Stage Review Final Report* (Professor the Lord Darzi of Denham, 2008), requires that every PCT commissions comprehensive wellbeing and prevention services in partnership with local authorities to meet local and personalised need. Darzi recommended a focus on tackling obesity, reducing alcohol harm, treating drug addiction, reducing smoking rates and improving sexual and mental health, and further suggested a coalition for better health between government, private and third sector organisations to improve health outcomes.

ENVIRONMENTAL HEALTH IN PUBLIC HEALTH

Environmental health is a major part of public health, with a focus on the determinants of health and appropriate interventions to alleviate negative health impacts and promote positive impacts. Environmental health has traditionally operated from within local government, but environmental health practitioners (EHPs) are increasingly thinking beyond local government and work in partnerships to prevent and control the factors (i.e. 'environmental stressors') that have an adverse effect on the health of the public. These are factors such as inequalities and sustainable development, and EHPs recognise the challenges coming from globalisation, technology, energy usage and waste, residential and transport changes and inequalities (MacArthur, 1998).

Environmental health has a unique role in maintaining health rather than curing illness and its role has increasingly extended into 'wellbeing'. However, continued work needs to be done to move away from the enforcement-led agenda, and to prioritise interventions where they will have most impact. Nevertheless, EHPs increasingly have a role to play in the public health agenda as key partners in protecting and improving the health and quality of life of individuals and communities by reducing health inequalities; working directly with communities and applying expert interventions in identifying, controlling and preventing current and future risks; and playing a leading role in the new strategies at all levels (Burke, *et al.*, 2002).

REFLECTIVE PRACTICE IN PUBLIC HEALTH

There is an emphasis throughout this practice-based text on reflective practice with experience and learning as an essential part. This book provides an interactive approach that includes (real and hypothetical) case studies, activities and reflection points so that readers are encouraged to engage with the theory, practice, knowledge and skills that may be useful in building professional portfolios. Overall, the book seeks to help raise the professional stakes in delivering effective public health interventions that both improve health and tackle health inequalities where they are at their most acute.

A SYNOPSIS OF THE BOOK

The book is structured in three major parts. Part One provides a theoretical and organisational overview and its chapters are as follows:

Chapter 2: Theory, research and practice in public health;

Chapter 3: Equality, equity, diversity and culture;

Chapter 4: Developing and implementing policy;

Chapter 5: Organisation and delivery of the public health agenda.

Part Two is concerned with the background, policy and processes in public health. The chapters are ordered as follows:

Chapter 6: Environment, health and sustainability;

Chapter 7: Meeting the challenges of poverty, inequality and social exclusion;

Chapter 8: Health promotion: a multi-causal approach;

Chapter 9: Health protection;

Chapter 10: Health needs assessment;

Chapter 11: Health impact assessment;

Chapter 12: Leadership in community health development;

Chapter 13: Information technology and public health (ehealth);

Chapter 14: Social capital, social enterprise and community development;

Chapter 15: Ethics in public health;

Chapter 16: Evidence-based practice;

Chapter 17: Globalisation and public health.

Part Three emphasises the importance of environmental health in public health. Its chapters largely explore the potential of EHPs and their partners to contribute more effectively to public health in delivering evidence-based interventions in improving health. The chapters are specifically concerned with:

Chapter 18: Environmental health practice;

Chapter 19: Food, health and wellbeing;

Chapter 20: The challenges for health and community in the private housing sector.

Conclusions are drawn in Chapter 21.

Useful websites

Faculty of Public Health: **www.fph.org.uk** (accessed 9 July 2009).

UK Public Health Association: **www.ukpha.org.uk** (accessed 9 July 2009).
A multi-disciplinary organisation committed to improving public health.

Part One: Theoretical and Organisational Overview

Chapter 2

Theory, research and practice in public health

Carlos Moreno-Leguizamon and Clarence Spigner

This chapter informs later chapters by exploring theory, research and practice, identifying some significant historical events and the contribution of sociology, anthropology and psychology to the discipline of public health.

Learning outcomes

In this chapter you will learn how to:

- identify the key paradigms of knowledge that underpin the theory, research and practice in public health;

- appraise significant historical events associated with the consolidation of public health as a discipline;

- discuss key contributions of sociology, anthropology and psychology to the making of the public health discipline.

INTRODUCTION

Professional Practice in Public Health is designed to provide students and professionals in the field with a comprehensive and contemporary overview of the public health discipline. Hence, this chapter addresses various key epistemological, historical and disciplinary events that underpin the theory, research and practice in public health. It is a strong conviction of the authors of this chapter that contemporary students and professionals of public health need to understand where thinking and practice in this field comes from, as well as understanding some of the historical and cultural events that shape it. If students and professionals in this field want to be critical thinkers and doers, they have to understand that public health, in as much as it is a borrower of theory and method from many disciplines, is clearly not a neutral field. On the contrary, public health functions are shaped by a disciplinary, political, cultural, social, economic, historical and epistemological context. This therefore makes this field a complex one, made out of many dimensions and not just the scientific evidence-based field that seems to be the dominant force in all health matters right now. In fact, as Crawshaw (2007b: 136) quoting Wall states, the latter 'evidence-based discourse has attained considerable power, perhaps largely because it fits more easily with the biomedical approach . . .'. Thus, this chapter, in interweaving and addressing key historical, epistemological and multi-disciplinary issues in public health, expects that students and professionals will be able to appreciate what lies underneath any public health theory, so that later, when researching and practising in this field, they are able to be more critical.

THEORY, RESEARCH AND PRACTICE IN PUBLIC HEALTH

Theory, research and practice are three major components inherent in the art and science of preventing and controlling disease and early death. A holistic concept of health is employed here (see also Chapter 10 on health needs assessment, which defines health). It is also important to point out that while, ideally, there should be a complete integration of biomedicine and public health, the reality is that biomedicine tends to be more concerned with the health of the individual and public health is more focused on the health of the entire community. Also, while biomedicine tends to work more with a model of natural science, public health is more eclectic and combines a natural/social science approach. Medicine deals with treatment and public health with prevention.

Historically, public health dates back to antiquity (before the advent of nineteenth-century biomedicine) when recognition of polluted water and disposal of waste linked to the health of human societies. Hence, the use of deductive reasoning and recognition of causal links to the public's health have tended to be Eurocentric from the very beginning. For instance, Nuland observed in *Doctors: the Illustrated History of Medical Pioneers*:

> The Greeks were the first to believe that the universe functions by rational, reasonable rules. They gave us the concept of cause and effect and thereby laid the ground work for science. Even before Aristotle, there was Hippocrates. (Nuland, 2008: 14)

The ancient Greeks established many public health techniques which, as an echo of the past into the present, tended to benefit mainly the wealthy. Hygeia, from where the term hygiene derives, was the Greek goddess of health and the daughter of Asclepius, the god of medicine. The Roman physician of Greek origin, Galen, reportedly born six centuries before Hippocrates, produced theories that continue to have major influence on Western medicine. The Greek Hippocrates (460–377 BC), deemed the 'Father of Medicine', employed deductive reasoning and uncovered links between ecology and diseases. Today, most public health organisations within nations reflect varying abilities to protect and promote the health of their populations.

In public health theory, research and practice come together as a consequence of the very nature of the profession. Thus, theory is defined mainly as the use of acquired evidence that supports an idea which stems from the application of logic and the rules of investigatory procedure that predict or explain the phenomena of interest. Similarly, knowledge systematisation and organisation or, in other words, research, is not pursued simply for the sake of knowledge but because it has almost always to be applied (practised) and disseminated for the sake of the public's wellbeing. Meanwhile, practice means the practical application of evidence from which theory derives as well as the dissemination of knowledge. Something that, however, is key to address from the outset in this chapter is that theory in public health, the basis of research and practice, is not a value-free and neutral matter. Watts' *Epidemics and History: Disease, Power and Imperialism* (1997) for example, states that 'Theory (is) based on Europeans' ideas that their own past established rules applicable always and everywhere' (1997: xiv). However, the nature of the world is changing, and we are living in a global and multicultural world. These facts demand that the traditional understanding of theory, research and practice in public health has to be different and more inclusive.

The development of theory

As contemporarily practised the public health profession grew from the application of scientific thought with theories constructed with a positivist Eurocentric worldview and multi-disciplinary and ideological endeavours (Crawshaw, 2007a; Scriven, 2007; Chilton 2004; Donaldson, 2001). For example, common in almost every public health or medical textbook are the historical accounts of the eighteenth century English surgeon Sir Percival Pott (1714–88) who in 1775, through deductive reasoning, linked the disease of scrotal cancer infecting the British working class to the prominent occupation of chimney sweeping. Also, in 1855, British physician Sir John Snow (1813–58) is known to have employed deductive reasoning to trace the source of the water-borne cholera germ in a public pump to stem the tide of that disease in London.

The fundamental basis of the modern public health movement was likely to have been initiated by social reformer Edwin Chadwick's (1800–90) efforts to reform the English Poor Laws in favour of the indigent. Chadwick wrote *The Sanitary Conditions of the Labouring Population* in 1842, which related Britain's terrible sanitary conditions to the public's dismal health. In conjunction, German social scientist Friedrich Engels (1820–95), in his 1845 book *The Condition of the Working Class in England*, described the deplorable circumstances which workers were forced to endure. Empirical studies such as Seebohm Rowntree's *Poverty: A Study of Town Life* (1901) and Charles Booth's *Life and Labour of the People of London* (1903) documented poverty in the towns of York and London with Rowntree (1901) providing a measurement for poverty for the first time. Other writers such as Pember Reeves (1913) and Spring Rice (1939) documented the experiences of working families and women's lives. German medical scientist Robert Koch (1842–1910) employed the scientific tradition to discover the living organism that caused cholera, bringing to an end the false belief that bad health was caused by foul smells (miasma). Koch introduced the germ theory of disease (Wolinsky, 1988).

Contemporarily, although the public health profession continues to be mainly governed and reinforced by positivist Eurocentric theories and ideologies, the epistemological debate on how we know what we know, mainly during the twentieth century, came to challenge this pervasive paradigm. The search for a non-positivist epistemology in social sciences by theorists under the influence of phenomenology, social constructionism, critical theory or postmodernism, as well as the influence of contemporary quotidian life in the constitution of social reality, are two of the most significant considerations affecting the traditional way of theorising, researching and practising social sciences in general and public health in particular. Aspects as diverse as the subject-object relationship when theorising and researching, the impact of culture, the meaning of knowledge, and interdisciplinarity are among some of the elements to understand in this epistemological debate.

Box 2.1's figure and list of details related to each paradigm of knowledge, attempts to summarise each one of the underpinning assumptions. As stated earlier the understanding of where any theory and research approach comes from in the public health field should contribute to making students and practitioners more critical. Currently, as mentioned by Hunter (2007: 17), the 'blurring of the public private boundary in areas like health in the interest of abandoning ideology and supporting what works may, however, unwittingly, be making the job of public health increasingly problematic'. It is against the backdrop stated by Hunter that we consider it important to address the various differences in approaches to theory, research and practice in public health.

Box 2.1 Basic scheme of the characteristics of epistemology

How we know what we know

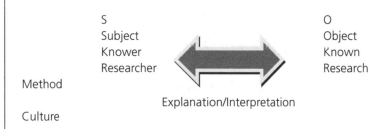

S		O
Subject		Object
Knower		Known
Researcher		Research

Method

Explanation/Interpretation

Culture

Figure 2.1 Basic scheme of the characteristics of epistemology

Positivism – underpinning assumptions in public health would comprise the following.

- Neutral valuation or objectivity is a must in the subject-object dyad. This means that the relation with the other, while one is getting to know him or her through one's research, must be without any kind of 'contaminated' or subjective view.

- Natural sciences and social sciences are treated as one. Methodological monism according to Von Wright as quoted by Jones-Devitt and Smith (2007).
- The role of scientific knowledge is mainly to explain by establishing cause-effect relations and general laws (Jones-Devitt and Smith, 2007).

Phenomenology – underpinning assumptions in public health would comprise the following.

- If language is a medium that stands between us and the world, we can avoid the true-false differences that language imposes on us and, instead, obtain knowledge or representations by contact with reality in a more direct way than through emphasis on method. Thus, another subject or an object is as we perceive them in our human consciousness. Neither the subject nor the object exists independently of our consciousness.
- Phenomena can only be studied or researched subjectively, since the constitution of reality is inter-subjective.
- Natural sciences and social sciences are different and they only make interpretations.

Social Constructionism – underpinning assumptions in public health would comprise the following.

- People create knowledge and meaning from their experiences in order to function pragmatically in life.
- The subject or the object is very much a construction of the subject.
- Phenomena in the world can be fruitfully conceptualised many different ways, knowledge being what the person has made of the world.
- Natural sciences and social sciences are social constructions.

Critical Theory – underpinning assumptions in public health would comprise the following.

- Knowledge as a social and historic activity creates the condition of its own existence. Hence, it participates along with other dimensions of society in games of divisions, interests, politics and ideologies.
- Knowledge can never be a neutral force, much less social knowledge.
- To a certain extent subjectivism is valid.

- Although less keen on the use of the scientific method, critical theory does not exclude its use at all.

Postmodernism – underpinning assumptions in public health would comprise the following.

- A critique of that form of rationality which links reason with truth, truth with an autonomous Western male, an autonomous Western male with progress, truth and reason, and progress, truth and reason with an apolitical theory and just one reality.
- A rejection of the organic whole through science, morality and art. Also it is incredulous of meta-narratives or any grand theory that tries to explain the organic whole.
- Reality is socially constructed through language.
- A suspicion of the scientific method in as much as this looks for universal truths.

Activity 2.1 Reflective exercise: approaches in public health

Consider any matter in public health that is of interest to you. Then look in a rapid way for 10 to 15 journal abstracts that discuss the matter. Read the abstracts, keeping in mind the various principles identified above for each knowledge paradigm. Are you able to identify the epistemological approach in the abstract by the terminology used to describe the abstract?

EVENTS SHAPING THE HISTORY OF PUBLIC HEALTH

Krieger reminds us that health cannot be fully understood if viewed from an 'ahistorical' perspective (1987). History is the study of the past and it is the past that provides a pathway to chart public health's roots and subsequent development. The path has prominent Eurocentric road-signs. This path has usually been attributed to Hippocrates due to his analytical approach and his mind/body connection (our current holistic view of health). But during the era of epidemics that included the Bubonic Plague (1347–51) and what Italian scholar Petrarch (1304–74) described as the 'Dark Ages', this holistic view became lost under the dominance of the Church. French philosopher and mathematician Rene Descartes (1596–1650), who helped usher in the Enlightenment, was instrumental in reinforcing the view that while the body belonged to medicine the mind belonged to God (Wolinsky, 1988).

The 'Age of Enlightenment', the era starting roughly in the 1600s and based squarely in Europe, questioned everything, but most notably the authority of the aristocracy and the dominance of the Church.

> It was the spirit of the *Age of Enlightenment* that pervaded the atmosphere in which European and American philosophers worked during most of the eighteenth century. The thinkers of that intellectual epoch were characterized by a willingness, actually more like a crusading zeal, to question every given that had been bequeathed to them. (Nuland, 2008: 157.)

The Enlightenment is so celebrated because it brought with it the ideals of the Glorious Revolution (1688) in Britain, the *Declaration of Independence* (1776) in the US and the French Revolution (1789). This period is interestingly also referred to as the 'Age of Reason' in spite of the outrageous contradictions of industrial greed, class exploitation and oppressive colonialism and the brutality of human slavery (Hazelwood, 2004; Palmer, 1981). Such events wreaked havoc on the health of populations across cities, nations and continents. Nevertheless, Western figures such as the English lawyer Sir Thomas Moore (1478–1535) and the Utopian Robert Owen (1771–1858) dreamed of 'ideal' communities.

In the specific case of the health field, the scientific part of it arguably started when Dutchman Zacharius Jannssen (1580–1638) invented the telescope, which led to the invention of the microscope in 1590. By 1670, Dutchman and scientist Anton van Leeuwenhoek (1632–1723) refined the microscope to discover blood cells. In 1628, English physician William Harvey (1578–1657) published *An Anatomical Study of the Motion of the Heart and the Blood of Animals*, which described the heart pumping blood in the body. Even so, bloodletting as a medical practice continued in Western societies. By 1747, Scottish naval surgeon James Lind (1716–94) had published the *Treatise of the Scurvy* where he described citrus fruits as a cure for scurvy. In 1796, Edward Jenner (1749–1823), a British scientist, discovered a vaccination for smallpox. In 1867 Joseph Lister (1827–1912) published *On the Antiseptic Principle of the Practice of Surgery* which detailed the importance of surgeons and recommended that surgical instruments being clean to diminish infections. In the 1870s, French chemist Louis Pasteur (1822–95) and the previously mentioned German physician Robert Koch (1843–1910) are credited with uncovering the germ theory of disease. The prevailing health 'wisdom' before was that diseases were caused by bad smells or miasma. It is also telling that Watts (1997) observed:

> It was some time before Koch's radical ideals won general acceptance and came to influence the therapeutic doctors trained in the 'scientific truths' of the Great Traditions which held that diseases were caused by miasmas, undisciplined lifestyles, and anything other than tiny living organisms. (Watts, 1997: xii)

In one very concrete case in the public health field the development of vaccines is revealing. Vaccines, essentially a prophylactic used to prevent or treat a disease, became very prominent in the nineteenth and twentieth centuries. The discovery and use of various vaccines for immunisations marked the time when medicine and public health truly came together. Vaccines or immunisations against cholera were discovered by 1879; vaccines against anthrax in 1881; against rabies in 1882; and for typhoid fever in 1896. Around 1890, antitoxins used to develop tetanus and diphtheria vaccines were discovered. In 1897 came a vaccine against the plague. In 1897, Briton Ronald Ross (1857–1932), born in Almora, India, demonstrated how mosquitoes transmitted malaria and was awarded the Nobel Prize in 1902. In 1899, German chemist Felix Hoffman (1868–1946) developed the aspirin. Austrian biologist Karl Landsteiner (1868–1943) developed human blood-typing in 1901 and blood transfusions followed in 1907. Landsteiner received the Nobel Prize in 1930. English biochemist Frederick Gowland Hopkins (1861–1947) hypothesised the existence of vitamins. He was awarded the Nobel Prize in 1929. By 1922, insulin to treat diabetes started to be used. In 1923, vaccines for diphtheria were discovered; whooping cough in 1936; tuberculosis and tetanus in 1927; typhus in 1937; and influenza in 1945. Scottish biologist Alexander Fleming (1881–1955) discovered penicillin in 1928 and was awarded the Nobel Prize in 1945.

The American influence, long evident, became even more apparent in 1953 when American molecular biologist James D. Watson (1928) and English molecular biologist Francis Crick (1916–2004) described the DNA molecule and its relationship to heredity. With New Zealand-born British molecular biologist Maurice Wilkins (1916–2004), Watson and Crick were awarded the Nobel Prize in 1962. By 1954, American surgeon Joseph Murray (1919–) had performed the first kidney transplant. In 1957, Netherlands-born American physician Willem Kolff (1911–) implanted an artificial heart in a dog that lived for 90 minutes. Kolff is known as the 'Father of Artificial Organs'. South African surgeon Christian Barnard (1922–2001) performed the first human heart transplant in 1967. In 1955, American biologist Jonas Salk (1914–95) discovered a polio vaccine. In 1964, a vaccine for measles was discovered, followed by a vaccine for mumps in 1967; rubella in 1970; chicken pox in 1974; pneumonia in 1977; meningitis in 1978; hepatitis B in 1981; hepatitis A in 1992; and Lyme disease in 1998. By 1993, HIV, the virus that causes AIDS, was discovered.

SOCIOLOGICAL, ANTHROPOLOGICAL AND PSYCHOLOGICAL INFLUENCES IN PUBLIC HEALTH

Sociological influences

Sociology is the study of human behaviour. The study of sociology includes aspects of economics, politics and religion regarding the human condition and is therefore central to the provision of the public's health (Wolinsky, 1988). The interpretive or hermeneutics route to knowledge acquisition so inherent in public health is integral to the discipline of sociology by way of Comte's concepts of positivism. In fact, Comte coined the term sociology in *Cours de Philosophie Positive*. Comte, theoretically it must be pointed out, saw a shifting of society as it advanced through history, i.e. from God to metaphysics to positivism. Similar theories that society evolved as if it was a living organism emerged in the frameworks of thought from other major Western thinkers such as the already-mentioned Friedrich Engels, who would co-author *The Communist Manifesto* (1848) with German philosopher, political economist and sociologist Karl Marx (1818–83). English philosopher Herbert Spencer (1820–1903) and French sociologist Emile Durkheim (1858–1917) are also major figures. It is instructive that Hippocrates' own analysis of *Air, Waters and Places* foretold of methods employed by Victorian Era sociologists in descriptions of communities ravaged by the Industrial Revolution. Marx knew all too well the brutality of poverty since two of his own children died from its wretchedness. Marx's understandable outrage and pessimism was directed towards the infant monster that would grow into the privately-owned system of wealth production called capitalism. He called for political and economic revolution, which was deemed to return society to its 'natural' state. Similarly Herbert Spencer, borrowing analogies from English naturalist Charles Darwin's (1809–82) *Origin of the Species* (1859), surmised that society was governed by 'natural selection'. Known as the 'Father of Sociology', Spencer believed that those in society who could not benefit from the dictates of the Industrial Revolution were unfit (i.e. inferior) to begin with. As if applying the apocalyptic theories of English economist and demographer Thomas Malthus (1766–1834), Spencer advocated dispensing with English Poor Laws, which were the nineteenth century equivalent to social welfare today (as discussed in Chapter 7 on poverty, inequality and social exclusion). Spencer's nurturing of the industrial order and condemnation of workers unable to sustain their own state of wellbeing were a far cry from the healthy communities envisioned by Utopians such as Robert Owen (Longres, 1990).

Current theories, research and practice in public health owe much to these Victorian-era sociologists, in particular to Emile Durkheim's rigorous examination of human events surrounding social institutions such as education, crime, the labour force, religion and suicide. Such studies have shaped much of our contemporary understanding of the public's health. Durkheim established the first journal of sociology, *L'Annee Sociologique*. He formulated theories and tested hypotheses by conducting massive demographic and statistical analyses with databases to explain how social events shaped individual and social wellbeing. Durkheim's *Division of Labour in Society* (1893) and *Suicide* (1897) are seminal in describing social, economic, religious and psychological forces that shape the health of communities (Wolinsky, 1988). Durkheim provided a common bridge to other academic disciplines such as the sociological, anthropological and psychological use of positivistic and hermeneutic approaches.

By the early twentieth century, sociology became influenced by many American scholars as well. Perhaps the most influential was Talcott Parsons (1901–79) who elaborated on Durkheim's theories, particularly in his work *The Social System* (1951). Along with sociologists such as Robert K. Merton (1910–2003), who was a student of Parsons and responsible for the term 'self-fulfilling prophecy', he posited the view that sociological theories had less to do with social reform than with the sociologist simply articulating the structure of the social order. This concept was termed 'functionalism'. Other American sociologists such as C. Wright Mills (1916–62), author of such books as *The Power Elite* (1956), took major exception to Parson and Merton's theories about social order by expressing the effect of power relationships and class stratification (Longres, 1990; Tischler, Whitten and Hunter, 1986).

One significant issue that sociology has brought to the public health field is class. In the case of the UK, this is a very important issue. Class is defined as those who are grouped by a distinction based mainly on their economic position (income) in society. Health status is correlated with class structure, particularly as constructed in industrial societies.

Even in the time of Hippocrates, the wealthy benefited more with better health than the poor. Through the Dark Ages, the Victorian era and to the modern era, with the *Black Report* in England and the *Unequal Treatment* report in America, the poorer sectors have endured the worst health. Spencer blamed the impoverished people caught up in the Industrial Revolution for their own ill-health status rather than blaming the conditions that surrounded them. Current reiterations of this 'blame the victims' mentality have re-emerged as 'old wine in new bottles'. Regurgitated theories of a 'culture of poverty' (Lewis, 1961) and 'the underclass' (Auletta, 1982; Wilson, 1988) used psychological measures and perceptions to see the poor as responsible for their own plight, and therefore ill health, in a bustling society. The same epidemiological and theoretical frameworks forged in the past continue to be recast to explain modern-day inequalities in health. Thus, as Scriven (2007: 7) clearly states: 'class analysis remains an essential tool if public health practitioners are to understand the dynamic of, and solutions to, tackling health inequalities'.

Anthropological influences

Anthropology is the study of man. Anthropology has broad and historical relevance to public health because it is the study of socially acquired values, beliefs and behaviours among human collectives or cultures. Even before Hippocrates, Greek historian Herodotus (484BC–425BC), known as the 'Father of History', recorded enquiries about people. As an academic discipline, anthropology came in tandem with European colonialism and imperialism. German philosopher Johann Herder (1744–1803) and German historian and sociologist Wilhelm Dilthey (1833–1911) strove to understand not just different cultures but the inner manifestations of human behaviour. This research advocated a bottom-up approach as opposed to the top-down mentality of outsiders studying the cultures of others. This is essentially the phenomenological or hermeneutic approach. Dilthey's emphasis, as opposed to Comte's, was less on any notion of societal transitions than the need to understand the essence of human behaviours.

Watts (1997: xiii) points out that the 'full medicalisation (sic) of the west', where 'lay peoples' acceptance of the medical doctor as the front line of defense against disease', is viewed as happening during the transitional years that fell between 1880 and 1930. Watts goes on to observe: 'it coincided with the great age of European and North American Imperialism' (1997: xiii). The health of indigenous populations (and that of the imported African slaves) suffered greatly as Western germs invaded the New World (Brumwell, 2005; Sheridan, 1985). In the early twentieth century, German-American anthropologist Franz Boas (1858–1942) and Polish scholar Bronislaw Malinowski (1884–1942) advocated more emphasis be given to in-depth examinations of human behaviour (phenomenological or hermeneutics). Sensitive to the obvious Western bias and the top-down methods in the acquisition of knowledge, research and theory-building, he needed to start with such study techniques as participant-observation, in-depth interviewing (in the language of the subjects) and cultural immersion. Boas mentored such noted anthropologists as Americans Margaret Mead (1901–78) and Ruth Benedict (1887–1948) whose respective works went on to influence an international call for gender and racial equality. Anthropology's sub-fields are archaeology, ethnology and linguistics, which relate directly to public health. The careful study of a community's past architecture, landscape, ecology, diet, religion, art, language and kinship patterns can reveal valuable insights into contemporary patterns of wellbeing.

The theories and methods of sociology and anthropology came together in building an understanding about equality, equity, diversity and culture relative to the profession of public health. Perhaps most relevant is anthropology because of its emphasis on the interpretive approach (phenomenological) and the study of different cultures.

Psychological influences

Psychology, the study of the mind or the mental processes of human behaviour, is integral to public health. Psychology, also with its philosophical roots in the ancient civilisations, emerged as a discipline from the studies of history, sociology and anthropology. During the nineteenth century American sociologist Charles Horton Cooley's (1864–1929) notion of the 'looking glass self', for instance, saw the concept of self as a product of how we come to see ourselves as a consequence of how we are seen by others. American sociologist George Herbert Mead (1863–1931) blended sociology with psychology and showed how the mind and the self emerged as a result of social processes. For instance, Mead's theory of signs in the process of social communication, or what is termed symbolic interaction, is indicative in the attribution society assigns to doctors simply when physicians wear white coats. Austrian psychiatrist Sigmund Freud (1856–1939), the founder of the psychoanalytic school of psychology, delved even deeper into the influence of the unconscious mind. Freud's theories of the psyche, the id, ego and super-ego, and the psychosexual stages of human development, continue to have major influences in public health theory, research and practice (Wolinsky, 1988). The definition of health is the integration of social, physical and mental wellbeing. Psychology's emphasis on mental health does not negate the influence of social and physical determinants on the mind. Whether the individual is viewed as a product of biology or environment, or deemed a 'blank slate', inequalities and disparities in health should not be blamed on the victim. But this notion of 'free will' and individual responsibility for health or self-care diminishes the role of social determinants. While 'free will' does not belong exclusively within the domain of psychology, the public's engagement in behaviour that produces negative health is often construed at the cognitive level and thus interpreted as individual behaviour.

CONCLUSION

The public's health is assessed by accounting for demographic variation such as nationality (race, ethnicity, immigrant or refugee status, issues of discrimination), experience in early life (maternal and child), education (quality), employment (income), occupation (exposures, safety, hazards), food (diet, nutrition), water (cleanliness), shelter (residence, crowding, density, air pollution, traffic, noise), stress (life changes, discrimination), health services (access, quality, cultural competency), social support (lifestyle, friends, family) and social cohesion (social capital). These are the social determinants of health (Blum, 1981; Marmot, 2008). Medical services have a role to play, but public health is about prevention.

We have briefly articulated what we see as the core academic disciplines that are felt to be integral to a fundamental study of public health. There are also sub-fields not discussed here. For instance, biology, in our view, relates more directly to the profession of medicine. Specific biological factors relating to public health usually come under the concept of social epidemiology. Thus, biology would still entail the social factors expressed in this chapter. The decline in mortality rates throughout history had little to do with medical care and more to do with public health prevention and interventions (Blum, 1981; Marmot, 2008).

Academic training in public health can roughly be divided into two major categories. Both have strong social science orientations that are not exclusive of biological-based training: (1) bio-medical/environmental health sciences, and (2) social/administrative health sciences. Numerous programmes of study encompass these two fundamental categories. These tend to be epidemiology, biostatistics, environmental health, maternal and child health, social and behavioural sciences, health education and health promotion, health policy, health administration and management, health programme planning and health programme evaluation. New and innovative areas are constantly emerging. We recommend public health students and professionals be strongly grounded in the discussions on epistemological, historical and other related disciplines in order to be critical and properly serve our multicultural and highly globalised world.

Chapter 3

Equality, equity, diversity and culture

Carlos Moreno-Leguizamon, Clarence Spigner and Allan McNaught

This chapter explores the concepts of equality, equity, diversity and culture in the context of public health and helps inform later chapters.

Learning outcomes

In this chapter you will learn how to:

- identify the concepts of equality, equity, diversity and culture in their individual capacity as well as their interpretation and application in public heath.

- reflect on the central value of the concepts of equality, equity, diversity and culture to public health.

INTRODUCTION

The practice of public health is an organised effort to improve and protect the health of communities through processes such as sanitation, vaccinations and preventive medicine. It is dissimilar to medical care in that medicine is more focused on the individual while public health is concerned with the entire community (Blum, 1981; Schneider, 2000).

Cultural diversity is characteristic of communities and, therefore, issues of equality, equity and culture are at the core of professional practice in public health. For instance, in multicultural societies like the UK or the

USA, the expanding generations of black and brown citizens, who make familial and cultural linkages to the peoples of Africa, India, Pakistan, Sri Lanka, Bangladesh, the Caribbean and North America, must be considered (Reynolds, 2006; Spigner, 2006/7). The religion of Islam has transcended its origins in the Middle East, as has the Jewish Diaspora, and both now encompass a diversity of groups and communities throughout Europe, America and the world. The race categorisation assigned to 'Asians', for example, comprises more than 25 different and distinct ethnic groups (Zane, *et al.*, 1994). Similarly, in the USA, the term 'Latino' has been standardised, with worldwide implications (Hayes-Bautista and Chapa, 1987). Epidemiological designations are crucial for developing proper health policy, yet such demographics within a multicultural society are fraught with conceptual and methodological problems. Knowledge and application of equality, equity, diversity and culture are more salient to public health than ever before.

This chapter, with the above-mentioned complexities as a background, articulates and relates the concepts of equality, equity, disparities and cultural diversity to public health, using examples of two multicultural societies: the UK and the USA. Even though the chapter illustrates that the underlying philosophy of public health globally has always been social justice and public safety, the definitions, concepts and terminology have differed through time, place and society. Thus, being aware that postmodern society is more characterised by multiculturalism and globalisation than when the movement was founded in the nineteenth century, the chapter emphasises that equality, equity, disparities and cultural diversity are significant concepts that must be understood and applied by students and practitioners of public health.

A brief background to public health

The concept of public health dates back to antiquity, even before Hippocrates (considered to be the 'Father of Medicine' in most Western societies) and the Roman-born Greek physician Galen. The Public Health Movement that developed in the nineteenth century has remained dominated by medical ideology although, ironically, this had little to do with improving population health (Schneider, 2000). Watts' (1997) observation of history and health is significant: 'Lay people's acceptance of medical doctors as the first line of defense against disease coincided with the great age of European and North American Imperialism'. This historical view is reflected in many of our present-day health infrastructures and a continuing social hierarchy in health status and health care delivery. The advent of 'racial' categories in the eighteenth century supplemented the class inequalities already prevalent in public health systems. The ideology of humanitarianism was inherent in Charles Edward Amory Winslow's 1923 definition of public health:

> The science and art of preventing disease, prolonging life and promoting physical health efficiently through organized community efforts for the sanitation of the environment, the control of community infections, and the education of the individual in principles of personal hygiene. The organization of medical and nursing services for the early diagnosis and prevention or treatment of disease, and the development of the sound machinery which will ensure every individual in the community a standard of living adequate for the maintenance of health. (Schneider, 2000: 5)

Essentially, from the very beginning of this discipline, there was a call for health equality and health equity. This has been expanded to accommodate a culturally diverse world, as was evident from the *LaLonde Report* (1974) in Canada, *The Black Report* (1982) in the UK, and *The Future of Public Health* (1988) in the USA.

HEALTH INEQUALITY AND HEALTH INEQUITY

The concept of health inequalities is seen by Dahlgren and Whitehead (1991) as consisting in whether the health consequence was avoidable. Carter-Pokras and Baquet (2002) go further in pointing to Whitehead's definition of inequities as 'differences in health which are not only unnecessary and avoidable but, in addition, are considered unfair and unjust' (2002: 427). A difference between compared groups could be the result of a choice, such as engaging in a risky sport, where there can be no implication of unfairness. On the other hand, poor populations may have little choice about living in an unsafe and unhealthy neighbourhood and this may be viewed as an injustice (Hebert, *et al.*, 2008). Kawachi, *et al.* (2002) make distinctions between health inequality and health inequity, seeing the first concept as a measurable quantity and the second one as a political and moral commitment to social justice. Carter-Pokras and Baquet (2002: 426) observe how 'disagreements exist regarding the definition and use of concepts like "disparity," "inequality," and "inequity"' and, echoing Dahlgren and Whitehead (2002: 426), ask: 'whether a judgment of what is avoidable and unfair is included'. Braveman (2006) reports that little consensus exists in the meaning of terms such as 'health disparities', 'health inequalities', or 'health equity'. The term 'disparity' is used interchangeably with 'racial/ethnic' differences in health almost exclusively in the USA. 'Health disparities refer to the differences between morbidity, mortality, and access to health care among population groups defined by factors such as socio-economic status, gender, residence, and especially race and ethnicity' (Dressler, *et al.*, 2005). 'The term "health inequity" or "health inequality" is more commonly used outside of the United States' (Carter-Pokras and Baquet, 2002: 427) such as, for instance, in the UK. Braveman (2006) also points out that . . . '"health equity" is a term rarely encountered in the United States but more familiar to public health professionals elsewhere' (Braveman, 2006: 167).

SOCIAL JUSTICE IN PUBLIC HEALTH

Taking into account the different ways of defining public health with regard to its principles, concepts, doctrines, notions or even ideology, it is important to address some historical elements. The humanitarian ideal of social justice in public health was further encouraged during the 'Age of Enlightenment'; a period that also brought forth England's Glorious Revolution (1688), North America's *Declaration of Independence* (1776) and France's French Revolution (1798). Still, the ideals of democracy and equality coexisted with the contradicting realities of inequality and injustice (Smedley, *et al.*, 2002; Townsend, 1979).

The administration of equity through the exercise of 'money and power' (Marmot and Friel, 2008) to diminish social inequalities may, in reality, reinforce health disparities. The concept of equity is present in both economics and law and therefore tied to social justice. Darr (1991: 22) observed that 'justice is especially important for certain administrative (and clinical) decision-making, such as resource allocation'. Equal justice in all things is not an absolute, however. For instance, assuring gender equality in tobacco smoking would not be in the best interests of public health, even if it is a question of upholding women's rights, as is so vehemently advertised by the tobacco industry (Sanchez-Martinez and Ribeiro, 2008). In public health practice, concepts of equality and equity along with cultural diversity stem from a common framework and hence lead to a common destiny.

DIVERSITY, 'RACE', ETHNICITY AND CLASS

The definition of the concept of 'diversity' encapsulates the right of people to be different in any society without the socially or politically enforced imposition of superiority or inferiority upon them. The concept of racial and ethnic diversity is globally recognised, but is particularly inherent in certain Western societies, such as Europe and North America.

'Race is deemed a social construct, meaning it is whatever people say it is at a given time and place. There have been as few as three and as many as 37 different races in Western history (Cooper, 1984; Graves, 2002; Williams and Rucker, 2000). In Western societies especially, social groups have become racially defined based on superficial physical traits and attributes from birth, such as skin colour and hair. As Loomba quoting Miles states:

> Either 'black' or 'white' but never 'big-eared' and 'small eared'. The fact that only certain physical characteristics are signified to define 'races' in specific circumstances indicates that we are investigating not a given, natural division of the world's population, but the application of historically and culturally specific meaning to the totality of human physiological variation . . . 'races' are socially imagined rather than biological realities. (Loomba, 2005: 105)

Meanwhile, 'ethnicity' as a concept refers, by definition, to a social group whose individuals share a common nationality, culture, religion or set of traditions and folkways. Watt and Norton (2004) state that we all belong to an ethnic group regardless of whether it is a minority or a majority. The assumption, in a society like the UK and the USA, that this is a concept only applied to minorities is nothing other than a common ethnocentric practice, in which the culture of the major ethnic group, having the power to define and differentiate among human groups, is taken for granted and therefore regarded as the norm. Also, as Bradby and Chandola (2007) point out, if this differentiation is done in an ordered and hierarchical way then this practice becomes more an oppressive ideological act than a scientific truth. A contemporary challenge of many social health organisations is to know if they are really differentiating between 'ethnicity' and 'race' or merely replacing the first with the second. 'Race' is an ascribed trait and much more intractable than ethnicity. Demographic variables found in the collecting and analysing of epidemiological data in public health include racial identity, and this is particularly prominent in the US (Smedley *et al.*, 2006). On the other hand, collecting race-specific data is much less prominent in the UK, as the concept of 'race' and thus racial discrimination was confined more to its colonies (Goulbourne, 1998) or, until recently within the UK, to migrant populations (Bradby and Chandola, 2007). Social class is the epidemiological variable in the UK while 'race' is rising in prominence due to an increasing multicultural population (Bardsley, 2000; Castles, 1984; Goulborne, 1998). As of 2007, for instance, roughly 10 per cent of the UK population was defined as 'non-white'. Britain's all encompassing term 'ethnic minorities' has been revised to 'Black' and 'Minority Ethnic groups' (BME). The separate distinction of the 'black' social group is in response to the realities of race-based discrimination (Bardsley, 2000).

Racial and ethnic discrimination has been revealed to be a causal factor of health status in many societies. Race and ethnic discrimination is related to 'severe and early chronic disease and poor wellbeing due to inequality in jobs, education and access to health care' (Al-Osaimi, 2008). For instance, '14 years after the end of the apartheid laws in South Africa, Blacks and Coloureds are still being under-served and disadvantaged regarding health care compared to their White and Asian counterparts' (Kon and Lukan, 2008). Racial bias has been shown to be directly linked to health disparities and the evidence speaks for itself (Cobie-Smith, *et al.*, 2002; Crawley, *et al.*, 2008; Dovidio, *et al.*, 2008; Hausmann, *et al.*, 2008; Van Ryn and Burgess, 2006; Van Ryn and Fu, 2003).

Meanwhile, 'class', which is a socio-political and economic concept, defines social groups who share a common socio-economic position (i.e. occupation) resulting in similar incomes and, therefore, similar lifestyles or consumption patterns. In the UK, the effects of class on health and disease were identified systematically for the first time in the 1982 *Black Report*. As Thompson (2004) states, this report showed inequalities across the class spectrum. For example, the report revealed higher infant mortality among unskilled parents, higher use of health services among working class adults in contrast to children, as well as higher incidences of accidents and higher incidences of chronic diseases. The trend of health inequalities according to social class has not changed dramatically and is, in fact, seemingly widening due to the current economic situation.

Culture

Defined generally the concept of culture refers to the inherited, shared and learned set of guidelines through which human beings come to make sense of the world they inhabit, their behaviours and emotions. The relationship between culture and health is a significant one due to the fact that culture determines, in many ways, whether consciously or unconsciously, the beliefs, behaviour, perception, emotion and even language with which an individual will construct and explain his or her view about health and illness (Helman, 2007). Thus, as a major force shaping human reality and underpinning the concept of heath and illness, culture has a number of characteristics that various authors (Watt and Norton 2004; Holland and Hogg 2004), quoting Andrews and Boyle (1995: 10), point out as noteworthy in the context of health.

- 'It is learned from birth through the process of language acquisition and socialisation. From society's viewpoint, socialisation is the way culture is transmitted and the individual is fitted into the group's organised way of life.
- It is shared by all members of the same cultural group: in fact, it is the sharing of cultural beliefs and patterns that binds people together under one identity as a group (even though this is not always a conscious process).
- It is an adaptation to specific activities related to environmental and technological factors and the availability of natural resources.
- It is a dynamic, ever-changing process'.

However, as Helman (2007) adds, culture is part of a wider historical, social and economic context and therefore it is not the only force influencing human behaviour. In conjunction with culture, factors such as economic status, gender, education and demography would also influence personal beliefs about most health and illness issues.

In terms of culture and health inequalities, it is crucial to understand their interrelationship for various reasons. Firstly, the concept of culture, if misused, can contribute towards legitimising the exclusion of groups as when perpetuating the traditional dichotomies of majorities-minorities, mainstream-marginal groups or, in other words, the us-them, in which the minority, the marginal or 'them' are the ones identified as ethnic and needy, in contrast to the majority or mainstream groups that are taken for granted and, therefore, are considered the norm.

Secondly, as Thompson (2004) states, culture being a discriminatory concept in itself, when not used appropriately, could perpetuate racist attitudes, especially when, explicitly or implicitly, one culture claims superiority over another. Again, the use of the superior-inferior dichotomy is an ethnocentric trait, very pervasive in many societies in which, instead of considering itself different in respect to another human society, one group considers itself just superior. In this regard the history of almost all Western societies is relevant. The ethnocentric attitude (my country, my group or my team is superior) could very well happen when individuals of two different cultures communicate and one of them assumes, implicitly, that he or she comes from a superior culture or even, in the health context, when the provider of a health service assumes that its professional culture and expertise (i.e. nursing or medicine) is superior, and not different, to the one of the service user when it comes to issues of health and illness.

Lastly, many cultural assumptions, as argued by Thompson (2004), are of a discriminatory nature. As a result, on many occasions these assumptions are negative and patronising when depicting older people, women and people with a different sexual orientation or cultural background.

Addressing the disposition and attitude necessary to be aware of one's own assumptions and the assumptions of others, Jones-Devitt and Smith (2007) quoting Paul and Elder (2005), point out ten strategies that could lead to a successful performance. They are reproduced here because we found them significant for students and practitioners of public health:

- being able to identify accurately one's own assumptions and those of others;
- making assumptions that are reasonable and justifiable in the context of both situation and evidence;
- making assumptions that have widespread consistency;
- having awareness of the tendency to use stereotypes, prejudices, biases and distortions in one's own reasoning, alongside identifying the same within others' thought processes;
- being able to state accurately the assumptions and underlying inferences made by both self and others; then assessing whether the assumptions made are justifiable;
- recognising that assumptions occur primarily at unconscious and/or subconscious levels;
- recognising that the human mind seeks to hide unsustainable assumptions in order to maintain a preferred belief system or to pursue selfish objectives;
- being able to seek out such unjustifiable assumptions, hidden within these unconscious and/or subconscious levels;
- accurately identifying assumptions contained within specific subjects, disciplines and texts;
- identifying assumptions embedded in the concepts and theories selected to study.

(Jones-Devitt and Smith, 2007: 30)

Activity 3.1 Reflective exercise: differentiating between concepts

In light of the above discussions, please consider the following questions:
- could you make a rapid differentiation between the concept of equality and equity?
- could you make a rapid differentiation between the concept of 'race' and 'ethnicity'?

Activity 3.2 Reflective exercise: culture and cultural assumptions in health and illness

- Why is it important to understand the role of culture in health and illness?
- Could you list or describe the 'taken for grantedness' in any of your cultural assumptions about ethnic groups, women, older people, disabled people and people with a different sexual orientation?

SOCIAL POLICY AND EQUITY

In the context of social justice and economics (Darr, 1991) equity is employed and defined with regards to the fair distribution of resources, with 'fair' being the operative word. Equity, in conjunction with health policy, is manifested in supporting social equality or civil rights, in order to diminish health disparities occurring between the rich and the poor, the privileged and the disadvantaged, the mainstream and the marginalised, and between whites and people-of-colour (Darr, 1991; Hebert, *et al.*, 2008; Marmot and Wilkinson, 1999; Marmot and Friel, 2008). Resources are appropriately allocated (i.e. in the form of equity) under the rationale that positive health is a benefit that is to be shared by all. It is unfair (unjust) that the burdens (disease and early deaths) fall disproportionately on any one group.

Health planning scholar Henrik L. Blum (1981) defines, in part, the use of the term equity with regards to 'balancing equity' in public health planning:

> Determine who benefits and who pays in each intervention or proposed program, so that policymakers can tell when one group pays a disproportionately higher share for some basic services (for example, at present the poor spend a much higher percentage of their income for less medical care than the higher income groups). Because need, want, demand, availability and accessibility are all potentially different criteria for equity, in receiving services, equity must be defined in each given circumstance. (Blum, 1981: 307)

It was more than a quarter century ago that Blum cautioned about the disproportionate burden of inequity being carried by the poor. Recently, Arrdondo and Najera (2008), in their cross-sectional survey of patients searching for and receiving health care in public and private institutions, found that in health systems based on social security, public assistance and private institutions, the out-of-pocket costs to patients were still inequitable since most fell disproportionately upon those who were socially and economically marginalised. Such institutional discrimination is not independent of racial disparities in health (Cobie-Smith, *et al.*, 2002; Crawley, *et al.*, 2008; Van Ryn and Burgess, 2006; Van Ryn and Fu, 2003).

Medicine (i.e. treatment) and public health (i.e. prevention) focus on concepts of equity and inequity in order to discern the extent to which health care utilisation is or is not being distributed according to need, regardless of income (Bago, *et al.*, 2008). Racial minorities in particular are disproportionately more at risk for being poor due to the imposition of social inequalities (i.e. racial discrimination) and are more likely to unfairly share the burden of inequities in health, as an extensive body of the literature shows (Cobie-Smith, *et al.*, 2002; Crawley, *et al.*, 2008; Van Ryn and Burgess, 2000; Van Ryn and Fu, 2003; Dovidio, *et al.*, 2008; Hausmann, *et al.*, 2008). Inequality and inequity bring health disparities and are reflected in racial/ethnic differences, whether under a nationalised health system as in the UK (Bardsley, 2000) or a market-oriented health system as in the US (Smedley, *et al.*, 2000). For example, social groups of colour in Britain and in the US are exposed to multiple assaults on their health due to their lower class or socio-economic status, race and ethnic characteristics (often exacerbated by religious bigotry and linguistic differences). Questions arise as to whether removing financial barriers to health and medical services will ameliorate health disparities or is discrimination the overriding variable?

PRACTICE AND HEALTH POLICY

Equality and equity are not mutually exclusive concepts and both involve the social gradient (or class status). On the other hand, 'ethnicity' and 'race' can be viewed as mutually exclusive, although they are often used interchangeably depending on the time and place. Most agree that 'class' is an achieved status while 'race', though still socially defined, is ascribed and is without choice and unavoidable. In America, Barack Obama is the offspring of a white mother and a black African father and has achieved the status of the 44th President of the United States of America. He is considered to be within the racial category of African American (Obama, 2006). The Prime Minster of Britain, Gordon Brown, on the other hand, is a white male. Brown has always been accorded all the unearned privileges that come with being a white male regardless of his achieved status as Prime Minister (McIntosh, 1988).

Hebert, *et al.* (2008), in methodologically discerning the difference between racial/ethnic disparities in health and the dynamics of choice, avoidance and control, point to how health status cannot be decontextualised from history or socio-environmental determinants. The social determinants of health (Marmot and Wilkinson, 1999) comprise of: 'inalterable factors' such as 'race' and age; 'neighbourhood and environmental factors' such as housing, education and health facilities; 'informed and unconstrained choices' such as engaging in reading or exercise; 'health care systems factors' such as interacting with health providers; and 'treatment factors' such as racial bias and stereotypes. In each and every case that Hebert and colleagues reviewed, race/ethnic groups (the authors combine the two while distinguishing their differences) were seen to be at a higher risk and therefore incurred greater disparities than the white comparison group. Thus, health policies are needed to overcome discriminatory practices that lead to health disparities (Dressler, *et al.*, 2005).

Laws, in the form of health policies, can help close the unequal health gap by applying 'horizontal equity' (Meghani and Gallagher, 2008). This is when resources (power and money) are administered across the board to everyone experiencing unequal health as a result of social inequality. By everyone we mean those in the social gradient as defined by class, gender, age, residence, occupation, and race in the USA and ethnicity, disability, gender, sexual orientation, religion and age in the UK. Poverty is usually the common variable across social groups. Thus, the impoverished in society (and with globalisation, in the world) should benefit from the administration of horizontal equity in health policies.

Vertical equity would direct resources to overcome the negative impact of social inequalities with regard to 'at-risk' social groups. The most 'at-risk' social groups are those defined by their ascribed status, and experience higher rates of morbidity, mortality and less access to health care facilities due to the effects of social inequality (Dailey, 2008). Assurances of equal treatment under the law (social justice) would therefore be directly related to the needed allocation of resources (equity) that diminish the social inequalities that result in disparities in health.

CONCLUSION

It is the task of the public health professional to discern how limited resources (in the form of power and money) are to be allocated towards diminishing or eliminating health disparities and inequalities. The recognition of cultural or racial or ethnic diversity within populations is critical. Whether under the auspices of horizontal or vertical equity, social justice must be the goal. Health policies must be designed with those specific social groups who are at highest risk from unequal delivery of care in mind. We seriously believe that such groups tend to be those that are defined by their ascribed status and are unfairly discriminated against and, consequently, suffer health disparities. Thus, emphasis should be directed towards the social determinants of health (Marmot and Wilkinson, 1999) for these groups as well as for all others where inequalities and disparities are found.

Social determinants of health are interdependent and include such factors as genetic make-up, sexuality, early life experiences, social and physical environment, education, employment, lifestyle, nutrition, social exclusion and social support. Thus, health services must be considered in terms of equality, equity, diversity and culture. Most diseases, even those deemed to be race-specific, are mediated by the population's gene pool and are not independent of geographical and social interaction (Cooper, 1984). Geographical or residential factors are reflected in access to educational institutions which influence class or socio-economic status and vice-versa (Williams and Rucker, 2000). Class status is reflective in lifestyle patterns of behaviour and can influence the quality of interaction between the public patient and the health providers (Van Ryn and Fu, 2003). Such social, cultural and even political dynamics that shape aspects of social exclusion or social support (Berkman and Syme, 1979) are found where health policies and the professional practice of public health can play a decisive role.

Chapter 4

Developing and implementing policy

Jill Stewart and Yvonne Cornish

This chapter is largely concerned with the theory of public health policy processes and seeks to inform later chapters. It provides an introductory overview in thinking about power, ideology, interest and value in the policy process and sets the public health agenda within its current political ethos: the Third Way.

Learning outcomes

In this chapter you will learn how to:

- assess policy process, in particular how power flows through it;

- appreciate who has power, how this can be challenged and the role of participation in democratic processes;

- understand the challenges facing the policy processes and how actual policy may differ from original policy intent;

- evaluate the New Right and the New Left (the Third Way) in the UK and explore how and why political ideology has influenced public health.

POWER, POLICY AND THE STATE: AN INTRODUCTION

Understanding the concept of power helps to explain a society or philosophy and the scale ranges from powerful to powerless. Policy processes are bound together by the organisation of the state (or government), which is dynamic and comprises institutions, apparatuses, processes and their interrelationships. The policy environment comprises uncertainty (unpredictability, change, a lack of control and discretion), relative autonomies and potential conflict (values, interests, ideology, institution) – through which different groups trade, secure, seek or maintain power. Gaining or maintaining power involves the scope for action, the use of that scope and how it is realised, each of which are affected by the actor and others involved. This may relate to authority and influence as well as rules and resources that may be naturally occurring, acquired or conferred (see for example Giddens, 1984).

Power is a multi-layered phenomenon. It can be about actors battling over a particular issue, or a means of getting issues on to or off the agenda, or about wider social processes that allow some actors easier access. Power is played out at all stages of policy development as follows:

- the power to influence what gets on to the policy agenda;
- the power to influence what stays off the agenda; and
- the power to influence the context in which the policy agenda is embedded.

Power is also important in implementation in influencing the ways in which policy is implemented (or not implemented, or changed during implementation).

Power is important in determining how decisions are made, who decides who will get what resource and who should dictate priorities because the way in which all resources are allocated and used depends on the distribution of power – in government, in organisations and in wider society. Theories and approaches in understanding power are summarised in Table 4.1.

Theory/approach	Belief
Elite	Power is in the hands of small networks of elites who are influential because of their wealth and position.
Marxist	Power is related to the ownership of means of producing goods and services. Power is possessed, e.g. by classes, individual, politicians or state servants. Power flows from a centralised source from top to bottom, e.g. from the state, law or economy. Power is primarily repressive in its expression. It bans, prohibits and censors and it is usually backed by sanctions.
Pluralist	Power is equally distributed, but shifts between different individuals, interest groups and pressure groups over time depending on the issues. Power is exercised rather than possessed. Power is seen as coming from the bottom up – it is everywhere. Power is productive.
Structuralist	Power is distributed within organisations (such as health services), dominant groups (e.g. the medical profession), challenging groups (e.g. managers) and repressed interest groups (e.g. patients).

Table 4.1 Theories and approaches to understanding power (adapted from Jones *et al.*, 2001; Lukes, 1974; Barker, 1996; Walt, 1994)

Values, ideology and interest

Gaining and maintaining power in the policy process is influenced by values, ideology and interest (or stakeholders). Each can help to shape how decisions are made, the nature of emerging policy, how representative it is of those it seeks to serve and this can be summarised as follows.

- **Values** are about ethics, principles, holding certain beliefs, to be concerned enough about something to hold it as a personal belief and as a way of operating.
- **Ideology** can best be defined as 'the science of ideas: "idea-ology"'. While there are different perspectives on its definition, there is some consensus that it is about collective values and concerned with

the culture of a society, and of everyday thinking. It may need to be prefixed to avoid confusion, for example as a political ideology, intellectual ideology, moral ideology, etc. For ideas and beliefs to be ideological, they need to be shared by a significant number of people, to form a kind of coherently related system and connect with the notion of power within society – either as a dominant ideology or counter ideology.

- **Interest** can be defined as having a right to, a claim to, a stake in, or an ability to influence something. An interest group enables those involved to speak up for their interests.

(See, for example, Eagleton, 1991; George and Wilding, 1988; Jones, *et al.*, 2001.)

Activity 4.1 Reflective exercise: ideology in practice

The very development of the public health movement is a good example of how a predominant ideology of *laissez faire* was challenged by Victorian philanthropists and scientists who argued in favour of a new government and voluntary sector role in addressing poor living and working conditions. After the First World War, the government took a more direct role in policies affecting health, becoming a provider of public services and introducing the Welfare State after the Second World War. This continued largely unchallenged until the Thatcher government from 1979, with a rolling back of the welfare state and quasi-privatisation across many services, favouring the individual. The Labour government responded after 1997 with a renewed focus on public health, favouring communities and seeking to address wider socio-economic determinants of health.

Think about political and counter ideologies informing the development of the public health movement. Show how ideology and values have shaped policy developments, giving examples.

You may wish to refer to the following publication: Stewart, J. (2005) 'A review of UK housing policy: ideology and public health'. *Public Health*, 119 (06): 525–534.

Activity 4.2 Thinking about power

- How would you define power in one sentence?
- Is it an absolute or relative concept?
- How would you recognise power?
- What are the uses of power in the public health policy process?
- How do the apparently powerless gain power?

ORGANISATIONS AND POLICY

There has been an increasing blurring of organisational boundaries in recent years, in particular since the Thatcher government from 1979, as government organisations were required to take on new domains and objectives. There was an emphasis on the market and therefore the customer whom, it was argued, would demand increasingly customer-driven services. In addition, some of the traditional roles of the community (third, or voluntary sector) – which was seen to deliver client-focused services – were absorbed into the public sector services and the new agencies, and it was argued that this would move away from a top-down, bureaucratic public sector to a new 'customer'-driven one. Competition between services favoured by the New Right has been replaced by a working together, partnership remit. There is now more of a partnership focus, aimed at working together, rather than competing against. However, elements of the New Right remain, retaining something of a market ethos, although one which favours social responsibility and not individual profit, in particular with the emergence of new 'social enterprises', that will increasingly be incorporated into public health organisations through new commissioning roles (see Chapter 14). Organisational roles and objectives are summarised in Table 4.2.

Organisational type		
MARKET (business)	STATE (government)	COMMUNITY (third, or voluntary sector)
Accountable to shareholders.	Accountable to the electorate.	Accountable to members, donors.
Legitimised by market share.	Legitimised by the vote.	Legitimised by trust and members.
Driven by profit.	Driven by rules.	Driven by commitment.

Table 4.2 Organisational roles and objectives (see also Table 14.1)

Activity 4.3 Organisational domains

To what extent have your organisation's boundaries and objectives (market, government, third sector) become blurred in recent years? Give examples.

Activity 4.4 Organisational functions and roles

- What is the purpose of your employing organisation?
- Is it in harmony or in conflict with government policy? Give examples.
- Who influences it and has a stake in it?
- Where are its boundaries?
- Which other organisations influence it?
- What are the tensions among management, professionals, other employees?
- How does it respond to change?
- Does it achieve what it sets out to do?

UNDERSTANDING THE POLICY PROCESS

'Policy' is sometimes described as 'a slippery concept' and Cunningham, in Barker (1996: 20) suggests that: 'Policy is rather like an elephant – you recognise it when you see it, but cannot easily define it'. Policy is made up of legislation, guidelines, written documents, political decisions, statements of intent, plans, etc. and Buse *et al.* (2005) suggest that policy is a broad statement of goals, objectives and resource creating an overall framework, often expressed via documentation, but which may also remain implicit (Buse, *et al.*, 2005). In other words, according to Barker (1996: 1): 'Policies are expressed in a whole series of practices, statements, regulations and even laws which are the result of decisions about how we will do things'.

A key feature of policy is that decisions are made by those with responsibility for a given policy area (Buse, *et al.*, 2005). However, it is sometimes extremely difficult to pinpoint when a particular decision has been made or by whom. Policy is sometimes therefore described as a 'network' of decisions (and non-decisions). In summary, Barker (1996: 30) suggests that the following factors constitute a policy:

- taking decisions, producing statements;
- making plans or developing an approach;
- implementation;
- policies exist even when there has been no conscious policy-making.

Public policy refers to government policy and is about what governments decide to do (or not do) about areas under their control, including health policy and other areas that also affect health, such as education, transport and housing. Public (and private sector) policies in relation to health and health care might include reducing health inequalities, reducing smoking, obesity, teenage pregnancy, etc., increasing physical activity levels, and increasing consumption of fruit and vegetables. Policies in relation to health care might include the ways in which health services are paid for, the organisation of local health services, regulation of the pharmaceutical products and the regulation of health professionals.

Health policy is a rapidly growing area of academic study and debate because the health sector is an important part of the economy in most countries and, in many industrialised countries, health care accounts for more than 10 per cent of gross domestic product (GDP). The National Health Service (NHS) is the biggest employer in Europe and countries such as the UK have unprecedented opportunities for prevention, treatment and care. The health sector can be seen as a 'sponge' – absorbing large amounts of national resources in staff costs and the cost of new technologies and drugs. Conversely, it can be seen as an investment, as a healthy workforce is important for economic development. But it can also be seen as a 'driver' of the economy through, for example, investment/ innovation in bio-medical technology and the production and sales of pharmaceuticals.

Economic factors are always going to be significant policy drivers as are considerations of how governments decide to fund health services, how much public spending is allocated to health and health care, how this funding is divided up within the NHS and whether (or not) NHS staff can provide certain services or prescribe certain (expensive) new drugs or treatments (Baggott, 2004).

Public health practitioners need to understand the relationship between health policy and the health of the population both to better understand the policy and organisational context in which they work and so that they can work with others to tackle major health issues (e.g. obesity,

HIV/AIDS, etc). To be effective, public health professionals need to become aware of how (some) issues get on the policy agenda, how policy-makers treat evidence and why some policies get implemented while others do not.

Health policy – the policy context

Conventional accounts of health policy tend to highlight key dates, important committees, Acts of Parliament, etc. These tell us what has happened in health policy (and tend to focus on health service policy). However, they do not really help us to understand why or how policies are developed and implemented. There are different ways of thinking about policy and these include analytical approaches, looking at policy-making and policy-implementation as a process, that enable us to gain a better understanding of what factors drive the policy process, who is involved in the making and implementing of policy and how we can begin to influence the process.

External 'policy drivers' include demographic change, the changing health status of the population, political/ideological influences, economic factors, social change, cultural influences and technological advances. There is some consensus that the greatest influence is economics.

There are various 'actors' involved in the policy process – individuals, groups and organisations and policy analysts sometimes talk about 'policy communities', which may include government, politicians, civil servants, advisory committees, professional groups, consumer and voluntary groups and others, each with a differing amount of power to influence the policy process.

The ways in which policies are initiated, developed and implemented are often depicted as a four-stage model (Walt, 1994: 45):

- problem/issue identification;
- policy formulation;
- policy implementation;
- policy evaluation.

In summary, the policy process is complex and interactive with many groups and actors in the policy arena trying to influence what goes into policy (and what comes out). We cannot assume that the process ends once the policy has been agreed (even if it has been widely consulted on) and written down.

WHAT IS POLICY IMPLEMENTATION?

Implementation has been defined as 'what happens between policy expectations and (perceived) policy results' (DeLeon, 1999 in Buse, *et al.*, 2005: 121). It can be described as 'the missing link' between policy development and policy evaluation. Implementation is often seen as the role of management (see, for example, Barker, 1996).

Top-down approaches

Top-down theorists began to develop lists of 'necessary and sufficient' conditions for implementation, including clear and logically consistent objectives, adequate causal theory (i.e. valid theory as to how particular actions would lead to desired outcomes), an implementation process structured to enhance compliance by implementers (e.g. appropriate incentives and sanctions), committed and skilful implementing officials, support from interest groups and legislature, and no changes in socio-economic conditions that undermine political support or causal theory underlying the policy. Hogwood and Gunn (1984) suggest that there are pre-conditions for 'perfect implementation' as follows:

- circumstances external to the agency do not impose crippling constraints;
- adequate time and resources are available;
- the required contribution of resources is available at each stage of the implementation process;
- the policy is based on a valid theory of cause and effect;
- there is a direct cause-effect relationship;
- there is a single implementing agency;
- there are shared/agreed objectives;
- the tasks required are clearly specified;
- there is perfect communication/coordination;
- those in authority can demand perfect obedience.

However, all these approaches assumed a 'top-down' model of policy making, i.e. that there is a clear division between policy-making and implementation; that policy-making is a mostly linear, rational process (the 'stages' model); and that subordinate levels put into practice policies made at a higher level. Critics of the 'top-down' model argued that all ten conditions were unlikely to be present at the same time, and that the 'top-down' model was neither a good description of what happens in practice nor a very helpful guide to improving implementation.

Bottom-up approaches

Bottom-up approaches acknowledge that policy-making and policy implementation are much more 'messy' and iterative and that, even for centrally-defined policies, local actors (managers, administrators) have some degree of discretion. They suggest that exercising this discretion can result in redefining policy objectives. One of the most prominent examples being Lipsky (1980), who studied the behaviour of 'street level bureaucrats' – frontline staff in health and social services – in relation to their clients in the delivery of frontline services, recording the range of discretion and difference applied.

Participation in policy-making

Involving citizens in decisions affecting them is an important part of the policy process. It enables a shift from a top-down to a bottom-up approach to policy development, implementation and accountability. It provides the basis for people to influence collective action over their lives and enables a wider range of issues to be addressed so that majority and minority preferences and diversity can be more fairly balanced. The range of participation between state (or organisation) and citizen is often represented as the 'Ladder of Participation', where at the top rung there is a high level of participation and power sharing, and at the bottom rung a low level (Gaster and Taylor, 1993; Arnstein cited in Taylor, 1995) as represented in Table 4.3.

TOP – high level of participation	Power sharing and partnership.
	Some control.
MIDDLE – medium level of participation	Advisory.
	Consultation and feedback.
BOTTOM – low level of participation	Information giving only.

Table 4.3 Levels of power and participation (adapted from Arnstein cited in Taylor, 1995)

Policy implementation cannot be seen as a separate part in a sequential process as policy-making and policy implementation are part of a complex, iterative process influenced by a wide range of actors and supported, or constrained, by structural, organisational and cultural factors. Policy-making is still in progress when it is delivered (Hudson and Lowe, 2004) and the implementation phase is complex and interactive (Walt, 1994), with implementers themselves active in the process of change and innovation.

THE NEW RIGHT TO THE NEW LEFT – THE THIRD WAY: AN OVERVIEW

The New Right from 1979 brought major changes to the policy environment with a marked shift toward a neo-liberal ideology. The Welfare State was rolled back and it was argued that the individual should have choice in the services they accessed (public choice theory) as forms of quasi-privatisation introduced marketisation, competition, contracting and new forms of accountability across emerging public services subject to rapid organisational change. A range of deregulations and new agencies focused on the 'customer' who would increasingly take personal responsibility for themselves.

The Third Way (the New Left) is an international philosophy seeking to modernise the political (centre) left. The United States Democratic Leadership Council (1999: 1) argues that: 'The Third Way philosophy seeks to adapt enduring progressive values to the new challenges of the Information Age. It rests on three cornerstones: the idea that government should promote equal opportunity for all while granting special privilege for none; an ethic of mutual responsibility that equally rejects the politics of entitlement and the politics of social abandonment; and a new approach to governing that empowers citizens to act for themselves'.

Sociologist Tony Giddens sees the Third Way as a modern agenda for politics situated between socialist and neo-liberal ideologies, and he was a key adviser under Tony Blair from 1997. The Third Way responds to globalisation, changes in personal life and our relationship with nature, and seeks to have wide appeal. Giddens argues that contemporary societies are post-scarcity and post-traditional and tensions of work, family, gender and generations need to be reconciled as part of an inclusive, multicultural society through active citizenship and dialogue in cosmopolitan, pluralist policies. There is an emphasis on responding to new social identities and a need for new ways of financing government policies (Sociologyonline, undated).

The Third Way has attracted both support and criticism as it seeks to both combine ideas and offer diverse policies. The main critics have come from the traditional left, who argue that it fails to offer real political substance and that it is hard to define. Giddens however maintains that the Third Way continues to evolve and offers realistic, flexible approaches to addressing inequalities in wealth and power (London School of Economics, undated; Mann, 1999).

THE PUBLIC HEALTH POLICY ENVIRONMENT

Current policies favour sustainable, evidence-based practice over a strict ideology, arguing that this promotes better services (Hudson and Lowe, 2004), responding to an evolving labour market, new family structures and increased consumerism (Page, 2005). There has been an emphasis on involving service users in public services, with a new relationship between state, community and individual, encouraging personal responsibility and more active community involvement (Page, 2005). These changes have been felt throughout new policies in health and housing, posing new challenges for the policy process.

The policy environment comprises a complex mixture of players operating with different interests, values, power levels and professional and personal allegiances at different phases of the policy-making, implementing and evaluation (or accountability) process. While the government sets the overall agenda, what is actually delivered may be affected through these stages as policy-making is essentially interactive. This is because there are so many different organisations and people involved in the policy process, so the original intention may be diluted by time, bureaucracy, rules and discretion (Baldwin, 1995), professional involvement, affiliation, change and uncertainty (Hill, 1997; Walt, 1994).

There has been a theoretical emphasis on local strategy with devolved decision-making based on local evidence, which has given rise to some tensions across partner organisations, and implementation has been affected by lack of resources, with managers balancing rules and discretion within budgets (Hill, 1997). Although Primary Care Trusts (PCTs) carry overall control for health improvement, they are not responsible for local authority budgets. Indeed, Hill (1997) argues that health is largely defined by the medical profession and the dominance of acute care, which is ironic when most health is determined by socio-economic factors. Ideally, formative and summative evaluation should be fed directly back into the policy-making process, but Walt (1994) questions how and which knowledge finds its way into policy. Sustainable outcomes and effects of health improvement policy may take years to identify and regular organisational change continues to interrupt this process. As Hogwood and Gunn (1984) argue, policy-making processes rely on thorough analysis early on, and politicians can frequently expect too much too soon, with a risk of insufficient resource, time and confounding factors distorting the policy process.

CONCLUSIONS

The policy process is complex and adaptive and influenced by a range of factors, most notably government, stakeholders, organisational culture and professionals, each of whom may have their own agenda, perspectives and priorities. The policy process cannot be separated from the ideology, values or interests of either those already in power, or those striving for greater power. Understanding how the policy process works and the challenges it faces in policy-making and implementation can help us reassess our own understanding of both historical and contemporary public health interventions.

Further reading

Stewart, J. (2005) 'A review of UK housing policy: ideology and public health'. *Public Health*, 119 (06): 525–34.
Mainly focused on housing and public health, but a useful summary of how ideology has informed policy since the mid-1880s.

Chapter 5

Organisation and delivery of the public health agenda

Jill Stewart, Yvonne Cornish, Stuart Lines and Ian Gray

This chapter is concerned with what we need from our public health system in terms of organisational structure, capacity and capability of the workforce across all levels, and how to access training and careers in the many areas of public health.

Learning outcomes

In this chapter you will learn how to:

- explain the public health system's organisational arrangements and operation in the context of our understanding of health determinants;

- identify the range of organisations involved in delivering public health, and why this continues to develop;

- understand the capacity and capability of the public health workforce and training requirements at different levels of public health.

WHY THE PUBLIC HEALTH AGENDA?

As Connelly and Worth (1997) observe, the history of public health in the UK is really about our history of ideas around disease and how it is caused, and therefore how we can improve health. This history includes changing patterns of disease, changing ideas about what causes disease and changes in what we can do about it. Organisations and arrangements for public health are therefore a complex response to concerns about:

- the health status of the population (issues, problems, causes – infectious disease, inequalities);
- ideas, theory and knowledge about causes – the determinants of health;
- ideas, theory and knowledge about what we should do – public health policies and strategies;
- organisational arrangements for doing it; and
- those involved – professionals, skills, knowledge – i.e. the public health workforce.

A new and more integrated approach to public health began to emerge in the 1970s and 1980s, influenced by a range of international documents including the Lalonde Report in 1974, the WHO Health for All Strategy in 1997 and the Ottawa Charter for Health Promotion in 1986 (see also Chapter 8). Health promotion began to develop a separate professional identity, mostly within the National Health Service (NHS), although there were some joint posts such as with Local Education Authorities.

The Acheson Inquiry (1998) responded to growing concern over infectious diseases, especially HIV/AIDS and hospital outbreaks of salmonella and Legionnaires' disease. His report recommended that community medicine should be renamed public health medicine, and that each Health Authority should appoint a Director of Public Health (DPH) to advise on service priorities, planning and evaluation, communicable disease control and the promotion of health and prevention of disease. The government responded by defining the role of health authorities and the roles and responsibilities of DPHs. These were to include the production of annual public health reports, health needs assessments and evaluation of health services. There was a new emphasis on information specialists and allied professionals and practitioners to support these new roles.

Public health recognises that prevention, where possible, is better than treatment and that the strategies should focus primarily on the population rather than the individual. In public health, the important issue is what happens about health improvement and health inequalities, and the success of the strategy (see Box 5.1).

Box 5.1 The scope of a modern public health system (from *Shifting the Balance of Power*, DoH, 2000)

- Health surveillance, monitoring and analysis.
- Investigating disease outbreaks, epidemics and risks to health.
- Establishing, designing and managing health promotion and disease prevention programmes.
- Enabling and empowering communities and citizens to promote health and reduce inequalities.
- Creating and sustaining cross-governmental and inter-sectoral partnerships to improve health and reduce inequalities.
- Ensuring compliance with regulations and laws to protect and promote health.
- Developing and maintaining a well-educated and trained, multi-disciplinary public health workforce.
- Research, development, evaluation and innovation.
- Quality assuring the public health function.
- Ensuring the effective performance of NHS services to meet goals in improving health, preventing disease and reducing inequalities.

THE STRUCTURE OF THE HEALTH SERVICE

Health services in England are made up of the Department of Health operating at national level via regional offices – Strategic Health Authorities (SHAs), Primary Care Trusts (PCTs), NHS Trusts (secondary and tertiary care), NHS Direct and private and voluntary hospitals and clinics. Public health has become increasingly integrated at all levels. For example, the Department of Health (DoH) oversees the Chief Medical Officer (CMO) and other national agencies such as the Food Standards Agency (see Chapter 19) and the Health Protection Agency (see Chapter 9). The NHS now comprises a mixed economy of care, with increasing numbers of contracts from outside providers.

Strategic Health Authorities' public health teams are responsible for overseeing and performance managing local health services (including PCTs), ensuring the effectiveness and organisation of clinical service networks and ensuring proper clinical governance. Regional Directors of Public Health (RDPH) oversee public health teams and have a dual role as part of the Chief Medical Officer's remit (and DoH staff), and also as a link to other government departments particularly in relation to regional regeneration programmes. PCT roles include ensuring that action is focused on improving health and reducing health inequalities, forging links with other agencies (notably local government) and ensuring that health promotion and disease prevention services are available at primary care (i.e. General Practice) level. See Figure 5.1 below.

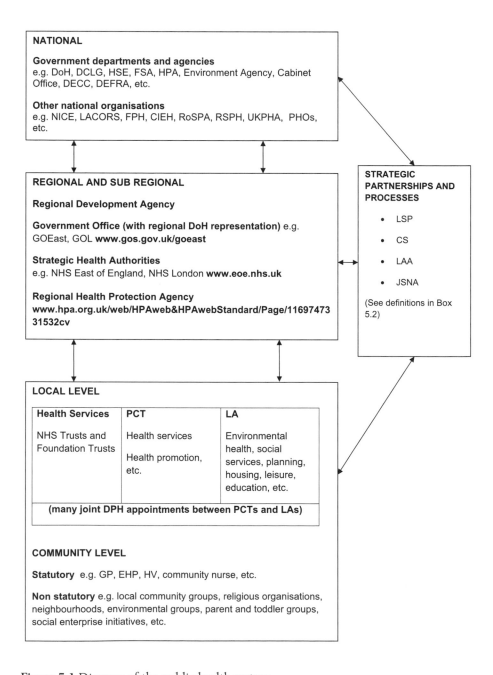

Figure 5.1 Diagram of the public health system

Other key public health agencies and organisations include Public Health Observatories (PHOs) (launched in 2000) and Cancer Intelligence Units. PHOs support public health in each region and:

- monitor health and disease trends, highlighting areas for action;
- identify gaps in health information;
- advise on methods for health and health inequality impact assessments;
- consolidate information from different sources in new ways to improve health;
- carry out projects to highlight particular health issues;
- evaluate progress by local agencies to improve health and cut inequality; and
- look ahead to give early warning of future health problems.

For further information, see the Association of Public Health Observatories website (last update 2007) at: **www.apho.org.uk**.

The Association of Public Health Observatories represents the 12 PHOs across the UK as well as the Republic of Ireland. They produce information, data and intelligence on the population's health and health care to assist practitioners, policy-makers and communities with an emphasis on turning health information into intelligence – see **www.apho.org.uk** (accessed 9 July 2009). Examples are the London Health Observatory's *Health Inequalities Health Intervention Tool* (**www.lho.org.uk/HEALTH_ INEQUALITIES/Health_Inequalities_Tool.aspx**) (accessed 9 July 2009), which supports PCTs in planning and commissioning, and the development of models for estimating disease prevalence, such as the PBS Phase 3 Diabetes Population Prevalence Model (**www.yhpho.org.uk/ PBS_diabetes.aspx**) (accessed 9 July 2009).

LOCAL AUTHORITIES AND PUBLIC HEALTH

Most DPH posts are now joint appointments. The advantage of joint appointments is that the DPH is a high-level post within both organisations, leading strategic direction. This is important as, while the NHS falls under the remit of the Department of Health, much of the public health work of local government falls under the auspices of the Department for Communities and Local Government (DCLG).

Local authorities have many roles to play in public health, and the local authority workforce comprises a range of professionals and practitioners who are involved in health improvement, protection and promotion.

Those involved include planners, housing officers, sport and leisure workers, teachers and lecturers, social workers and environmental health practitioners, many of whom already work in successful health improvement partnerships, including Local Strategic Partnerships (LSPs) and Community Strategies and, more recently, Local Area Agreements (LAAs) have provided further impetus for partnership working (see Box 5.2). An example is provided by the joint working between Newham PCT and the London Borough of Newham, in partnership with the British Heart Foundation, around a targeted community-based approach to tackling high mortality rates from cardiovascular disease (CVD) in certain wards in Newham (see also the example in Chapter 18, Box 18.1).

Box 5.2 Partnership-based strategies for public health

Local Strategic Partnerships

The LSP is a non-statutory body that brings together the different parts of the public, private, voluntary and community sectors, working at a local level. The aim is that the LSP should operate at a strategic level while remaining close enough to local people to allow them to be involved in decisions that affect their communities.

The local council is the lead player in the LSP, which will include key statutory bodies such as the police and the PCT, and representatives of the voluntary and third sector and business and private sectors. The LSP ensures that the different organisations work together to deliver services more effectively. There are many different models for the organisational structures of LSPs, but it is usual to have a single LSP for a unitary, metropolitan council or London borough and some counties have a single LSP that covers the areas of several district authorities.

Joint Strategic Needs Assessment

In 2007, the Local Government and Public Involvement in Health Act set out the requirement for PCTs and local authorities to produce a Joint Strategic Needs Assessment (JSNA) to establish the current and future health and wellbeing needs of their population, leading to improved outcomes and reductions in health inequalities.

The Department of Health describes the production of the JSNA as a 'partnership duty' that involves a range of statutory and non-statutory partners, informing commissioning and the development of appropriate, sustainable and effective services, and that will inform both LAAs and the *Sustainable Communities Strategy* (Department of Communities and Local Government, 2005).

Local Area Agreements

An important requirement for each LSP is to produce a LAA. The LAA sets out the priorities agreed between central government and a local area (the local authority and LSP) and other key partners at the local level. This is usually in the form of a negotiation with officers from regional government offices representing central government. The aim of the LAA is to simplify the provision of central funding as well as to help join up public services more effectively and allow greater flexibility for local solutions to local circumstances. The reasoning behind the LAA includes to:

- recognise that 'one size does not fit all' and local services should reflect what local people want;
- give more flexibility to local authorities and other public sector organisations in the ways they deliver services for local people;
- make local authorities and other public services more accountable to local people;
- reduce red tape and improve value for money; and,
- enable local people to get more involved in decisions about local service.

(Information provided by Rachel Flowers, Consultant in Public Health.)

LACORS

The Local Authority Coordinators of Regulatory Services (LACORS) is responsible for overseeing local authority regulatory services delivered by local authorities across the UK. It covers areas such as food safety, private sector housing, environmental protection of air, land, water and noise, and health and safety at work – in fact many areas under the remit of EHPs. LACORS promotes quality regulation, policy development and advice, guidance and good practice. For further information, visit www.lacors.gov.uk/lacors/static.aspx?N=0&Ne=0+2000+3000+4000+ 5000+6000+7000+8000+9000+10000+11000&groupid=1 (accessed 9 July 2009).

The academic community

The academic community also has an important role to play in public health. The University of Greenwich, for example, has several Schools contributing to health research and professional practice, including delivering undergraduate and postgraduate courses. Academics from the Schools of Health and Social Care and Architecture and Construction have worked closely in joint publishing on health and housing across tenures. The wider approach to public health is also exemplified by the university's outreach work and it is working with and through third sector organisations to improve community capacity and health determinants to lessen inequalities in health in the Thames Gateway region. This requires collaborative and flexible working across sectors and organisations and has included strengthening community organisations and sharing skills and expertise, including developing enterprise awareness. An example of an issue which is belatedly being recognised in public health is child neglect and the university is also involved in contributing to this area.

NICE

Various organisations have been involved in developing responses to and providing evidence for addressing some of the 'gaps' in public health information and lifestyle behaviours identified in *Choosing Health* (2004). Perhaps most notably the National Institute for Health and Clinical Excellence (NICE) (which absorbed the now defunct Health Development Agency's work) has been pivotal in producing public health programme and intervention guidance to improve health for professionals and practitioners in the NHS and local government (for further information, visit **www.nice.org.uk/aboutnice/whatwedo/ aboutpublichealthguidance/about_public_health_guidance.jsp**) (accessed 9 July 2009).

Others involved in public health

There is a range of other organisations and professional bodies involved in public health and some are identified in Figure 5.1.

COORDINATING THE WORKFORCE: CAPACITY AND CAPABILITY

The Chief Medical Officer (DoH, 2001a) in 'Strengthening Public Health' called for a wider understanding of health, better and more coordinated public health function, partnership working, community development and public involvement, a more capable and increased public health workforce and increased health protection. Wanless (2004) added to this in *Securing Good Health for the Whole Population*, questioning the cost-effectiveness of action and calling for more rigorous and long-term implementation of sustainable solutions often lacking due to a poor public health information and evidence base. Many of these areas continue to develop as policy emphasises the need for increased information, advice and support to enable healthier decisions based on informed choices for individuals, communities and across public and private sectors (for example, *Choosing Health*, DoH, 2004).

During recent years there has been a major renewal of interest and action in public health and it has come to occupy centre stage in the political agendas of each of the governments and administrations of the UK, as evidenced by their major policy publications such as, in England, *Choosing Health: Making Healthy Choices Easier* (DoH, 2004), in Wales, *Health Challenge Wales* (Welsh Assembly Government (2006 and 2007) and *Designed for Life* (Welsh Assembly Government, 2005), in Scotland, *Improving Health in Scotland: The Challenge* (Scottish Executive, 2003) and in Northern Ireland, *Investing for Health* (Northern Ireland Executive, 2002).

Fundamental to the delivery of these national strategies is the development of a 'wider public health workforce'. This concept was initially described as a 'wider public health community' by Kenneth Calman, as Chief Medical Officer (England) (Calman, 1998) and he also identified the environmental health officer (EHO) as being the only officer within the local authority who falls within the definition of a public health practitioner (see also Chapter 18 on environmental health practice).

A useful summary of the range of initiatives that are being undertaken in order to deliver the 'wider public health workforce' is set out in the June 2006 edition of the Faculty of Public Health Newsletter at **www.fphm. com** (accessed 9 July 2009) (Faculty of Public Health, 2006). In her editorial to this publication Mala Rao, Head of Public Health Workforce and Capacity, Department of Health (England) stated:

It is now accepted wisdom that improving public health requires strengthening both capacity and capability at the levels of the wider workforce, public health practitioners, and public health specialists. It also needs to take account of all three domains of public health – health improvement, health protection and health and social care quality – as well as the fact that it means building the workforce engaged in 'service' public health, the academic community, and the public health information and intelligence workforce.

Added impetus has also been given to the need for this work with the publication of the report of Derek Wanless (Wanless, 2004) who stated: 'Adequate workforce capacity will need to be created with appropriately broad skill mixes. Because more of the activity will be concerned with monitoring, interpreting data, identifying risk, educating people and motivating them to change behaviour, the required mix of skills will change.' This report focused on prevention and the wider determinants of health in England and on the cost-effectiveness of action that can be taken to improve the health of the whole population and to reduce health inequalities.

Standard-setting bodies in public health

There are a number of standard-setting bodies in relation to public health. These include the Faculty of Public Health, which sets standards for consultants and some public health specialists. Occupational standards for other public health practitioners come under the remit of the Skills for Health Council, which are now discussed.

National occupation standards for the practice of public health

If the wider public health workforce is to be truly integrated then it is important to identify and codify the common knowledge and skill areas, as well as those specific to defined areas of practice. A project to produce national occupational standards was led by Skills for Health, the UK-wide Sector Skills Council for Health, and commissioned and overseen by the four UK Health Departments and a Core Stakeholders Group that included representatives of regulatory bodies and professional bodies (including the Chartered Institute of Environmental Health [CIEH]).

The foreword to the guide to the national occupational standards document (Skills for Health, 2004) states:

These national occupational standards describe good practice in the practice of public health. The standards have been developed as a means of improving the capacity and capability of the public health workforce. The standards make the links between what needs to happen to improve people's health and what individuals need to do to contribute to this effort effectively. These standards have been designed to be used across service, organisational and individual levels across all sectors – to develop services, plan workforces, guide practice and the management of people, and form the basis of education, training and qualifications.

The standards were developed on a multi-agency and multi-disciplinary basis and were approved as UK-wide national occupational standards by all of the important education regulatory authorities. They are therefore proving to be an appropriate benchmark for all who contribute, or wish to contribute, to improving the health of the public, wherever they work and whatever their work role.

UK (Voluntary) Public Health Register

The creation and adoption of standards is important, but so too are measures to ensure that they are being observed. The UK Public Health Register (UKPHR) was established to promote public confidence in specialist public health practice in the UK through independent regulation. It provides public protection by ensuring that only competent public health professionals are registered and that high standards of practice are maintained.

The UKPHR created a standards framework to ensure that multi-disciplinary specialists in public health are appropriately qualified and competent. The register is truly multi-disciplinary and includes people from backgrounds including public health sciences, environmental health, social science, medicine, nursing, health promotion, pharmacy, psychology and dentistry. Whatever their professional background, and wherever they may work, all such specialists have to demonstrate a common core of knowledge, skills and experience, and work (or have the ability and potential to work) at a strategic or senior management level. Details of the standards and routes to registration are obtainable from the UKPHR website (**www.publichealthregister.org.uk**) (accessed 9 July 2009). The UKPHR is currently developing a practitioner route to registration that will come into effect during 2009.

QUALIFYING IN PUBLIC HEALTH

Directors of Public Health and Consultants in Public Health have traditionally been doctors who have opted to undertake extensive training in public health, either by a higher degree in public health or membership by examination of the Faculty of Public Health. However, since 2000, post-publication of *Saving Lives: Our Healthier Nation*, non-medical public health practitioners have been able to access many public health training programmes. There are also other levels for practitioners to enter the public health profession and positively contribute to health improvement and this second tier includes environmental health practitioners, housing officers, nurses, GPs, community development workers and others. The third tier includes those whose work impacts on public health, including health visitors and social workers (Lines, cited in Stewart, Bushell and Habgood, 2005).

General requirements

The training route for entrance into public health for doctors requires full General Medical Council (GMC) registration and completion of an F2 programme or the equivalent competencies. Those from other backgrounds require either a good first degree (minimum 2:1) in a subject relevant to public health, a higher degree (i.e. Masters or PhD), or a health professional qualification, for example, nursing. Relevant degrees could include any of the health sciences, such as clinical psychology and pharmacology, or other subject areas where the relevance can be shown, such as environmental science. At least three years' post-degree work experience in an area relevant to public health is also necessary.

Most trainees from a medical background will enter public health specialist training directly on completion of Foundation programmes. Some of these may have spent four months in a public health Foundation Year 2 slot but this is not a prerequisite. Entrants from disciplines other than medicine enter after a minimum of three years' postgraduate/post registration experience in service work in a health-related field. Doctors may also apply to enter after a variable period in another specialist training programme.

Application for public health training is currently made through the Medical Training Application System (MTAS). Invitations are published in the medical press in December/January each year. Applicants are able to apply for posts in two geographical areas (see also Public Health Training Curriculum 2007 at **www.pmetb.org.uk/index.php?id=640**) (accessed 9 July 2009).

Overview of public health training

Registration with the Faculty of Public Health/National Training Numbers

The Faculty of Public Health is the standard-setting body for professionals in public health. All trainees register and enrol with the Faculty. Enrolment, for which there is a fee, and this is a prerequisite of eligibility to sit the Membership exams (MFPH). MFPH is a requirement for the Certificate of Completion of Training (CCT). Trainees will also be allocated a deanery training number, which is a unique identifier during training.

The basic training structure

Speciality training as a Specialist Trainee (StR) in public health takes five years' whole time equivalent and proportionately longer for trainees working less than full time. The current curriculum is based on an understanding of what a consultant in public health needs to know and needs to be able to do. The curriculum builds basic skills on to a knowledge platform and consolidates those skills in increasingly complex work and diverse environments.

Training is delivered across three phases. The first phase concentrates on the acquisition of knowledge relevant to public health practice and gives an opportunity for development of basic skills. The second phase allows development of a wider set of skills in increasingly complex service work and exposure to health protection work. The final phase of training allows consolidation of competencies and the development of specialist skills in an area of interest or possible future career options. Each phase of training has a set of expected learning outcomes to be achieved and phases one and two have examination milestones as well.

Satisfactory completion of training leads to a CCT and registration on either the GMC specialist register or the UKVRPHS. Specialist registration is mandatory to practice as a consultant in public health in the UK. StRs may begin to apply for consultant level posts within six months of their CCT but cannot take up post until completion of training.

Academic courses

The curriculum for public health requires a sound knowledge foundation that is delivered in phase one of training and assessed through the Part A MFPH. Most trainees will gain this academic foundation through a Masters course in public health.

Placements

A series of training placements will be undertaken during the training programme. The initial placement is generally with a PCT. It is a requirement of training that all StRs are exposed to a variety of organisations and learning environments. Trainees are encouraged to experience a variety of training placements to widen their understanding of public health practice such as health protection and academic public health.

Examinations and assessment

The MFPH examination consists of a two-part exam. Part A MFPH is a knowledge-based exam. Part B MFPH is an Observed Structured Public Health Examination (OSPHE) and is normally taken six to nine months after passing Part A and must be passed with two years left of training. It is designed as a 'show how' assessment of trainees' ability to apply relevant knowledge, skills and attitudes to the practice of public health.

Workplace assessment

Trainees are required to show evidence of achievement of learning outcomes for each phase of training through a training portfolio, the ARCP (Annual Review of Competence Progression) formerly the RITA (Record of In-Training Assessment). It is a requirement under the *Gold Guide* (this governs the delivery of speciality training, see **www. mmc.nhs.uk/default.aspx?page=281**) that all StRs have an annual assessment of progress. This process is conducted under the direction of the postgraduate dean through the programme director. The process is designed to ensure satisfactory progress through training in accordance with curricula requirements and milestones.

The portfolio route

Until 31 May 2006, an option was open for an individual who had not undergone formal training to be recognised as a 'Generalist Public Health Specialist', based on retrospective assessment of a portfolio of work. Completion of this 'portfolio route' made participants eligible for the UK Voluntary Register of Public Health Specialists.

A new portfolio route superseded this on 1 June 2006, also for individuals who have not undergone formal training but who wish to appear on the Voluntary Register as 'Defined Specialists', working in one particular field of public health. Individuals who wish to become general public health specialists at consultant level are now all expected to go through a formal training scheme, as described above.

Public health skills and careers – bringing it all together

UK-wide Public Health Skills and Careers Framework

To help us all find our way through the extensive panorama that is the wider public health workforce, a public health career framework has been developed for use across the UK (Skills for Health and PHRU, 2008). This brings together public health competences, underpinning knowledge, training and qualification routes, registration requirements and a database of job descriptions across nine career levels as follows:

Level 1: Initial Entry Level Posts

Level 2: Assistants/Support Workers

Level 3: Technicians/Senior Technicians

Level 4: Assistant /Associate Practitioners

Level 5: Practitioners

Level 6: Senior/Specialist Practitioners

Level 7: Advanced Practitioners

Level 8: Consultant Practitioners

Level 9: More Senior Staff

The aim is to create a framework that can be used as a route map for careers in public health regardless of starting and intended end points and whether the intended career path is vertical or horizontal, within a single organisation or across several. All public health practitioners can make use of the public health skills and career framework (Public Health Resource Unit and NHS, 2008) in order to:

- describe and demonstrate the competences one's own profession contributes to improving population health;
- inform and facilitate closer working relationships across professional groups; and
- inform development planning for individuals, teams and professional groups.

Public Health Online Resource for Career and Skills Training – PHORCaST

To assist us further, during 2009 we will see the launch of an interactive career guidance website, PHORCaST, that will provide in one place a comprehensive e-guide to careers in public health which is a trans-disciplinary, multi-agency, multi-health system. See Figure 5.2.

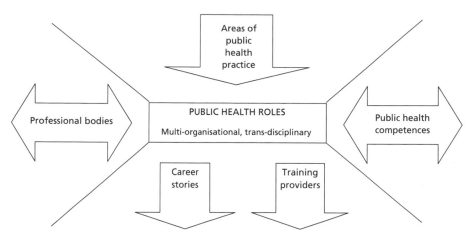

Figure 5.2 Public Health Online Resource for Career and Skills Training (PHORCaST) (illustration reproduced with kind permission of Ian Gray, a member of PHORCaST Project Board)

PHORCaST is supported by the four UK countries' Departments of Health and will contain information on the types of jobs done by people working in public health, the competences and qualifications needed for these jobs and the education and training available to achieve the required competences and qualifications.

At a time of challenging public health issues and when there is a need for greater involvement in public health as a speciality, this online resource will be an aid to recruitment and retention of a high-calibre public health workforce at all levels.

CONCLUSIONS

Roles and responsibilities in public health are wide-ranging and opportunities for those interested in a career in public health continue to develop across all levels and across a range of organisations. Training routes can largely be divided into the more academic branch of the Faculty of Public Health, or the more occupational Skills for Health. What is important is how public health practitioners are able to apply their strategies and interventions to both addressing health inequalities and improving health in the context of our contemporary understanding of what causes disease and how best to tackle it.

Useful websites

Voluntary Register for Public Health Specialists:
www.publichealthregister.org.uk

FPH training requirements: **www.fphm.org.uk/training/curriculum/
assessment/training_portfolio.asp**

Part Two: Background, Policy and Processes

Chapter 6

Environment, health and sustainability

Veronica Habgood

This chapter focuses on the links between the environment and health. It provides an overview of some of the important contemporary environmental issues relevant to the UK and contextualises the link between health, inequalities and the environment through a discussion of sustainable development. The current and nascent role of public health practitioners, working in partnership, to improve environmental quality, is explored.

Learning outcomes

In this chapter you will learn how to:

- understand and provide examples of how environmental quality influences health;

- argue that sustainable development and health are inextricably linked;

- demonstrate how public health practitioners can influence decision-making in aspects of environmental protection and can contribute towards improving environmental quality and health.

INTRODUCTION

We have established from Chapter 1 that the environment is one of the key determinants of health. It has been estimated that more than 25 per cent of disease and death, globally, can be attributed to the impact of environmental factors such as air pollution, poor water quality and climate change (WHO-UNEP, 2005). The nature of disease attributable to environmental factors, however, varies across the globe, as shown in Figure 6.1.

	Globally	**EUR-A** (WHO Sub-region including UK and most of Western Europe)
Highest ↓	Diarrhoeal disease Lower respiratory infection Cardiovascular diseases Neuropsychiatric disorders (all) Other unintentional injuries Malaria Road traffic accidents Cancers (all)	Cancers (all) Cardiovascular diseases Neuropsychiatric disorders (all) Musculoskeletal disorders (all) Asthma Road traffic accidents Other unintentional injuries Chronic obstructive pulmonary disease

Figure 6.1 Comparison between the global and EUR-A estimated burden of disease attributable to environmental factors in terms of DALYs* (adapted from Prüss-Üstün and Corvalán, 2006)

*DALYs – Disability Adjusted Life Years; a weighted measure of death, illness and disability

For the purpose of this chapter, environmental quality may be considered to encompass the quality of the atmospheric, terrestrial and aquatic environmental media but we might, additionally, consider other environmental factors such as noise, electromagnetic radiation, radon and UV radiation, although these will not be discussed in this chapter. The quality of these environmental media is shaped by natural and anthropogenic influences. We have little control over natural phenomena that affect the quality of the environment but the most significant degradation of the environment is a consequence of man's activities. Prüss-Üstün and Corvalán (2006) acknowledge that death, illness and disability could be reduced through intervention directed at reducing exposure to 'modifiable' environmental hazards, and that this can be achieved by applying technologies, policies and public health measures.

Clearly, targeting those environmental hazards that contribute most to the burden of death, illness and disability is likely to bring about most improvement in health. The discipline most closely allied to this intervention is environmental health (see Chapter 18) which focuses on the 'theory and practice of assessing and controlling factors in the environment that can potentially affect health' (WHO, 2008).

The WHO acknowledges that, for many of the determinants of health, the sphere of influence lies beyond the control of the health sector, and this is particularly the case for those determinants that relate to the environmental media (WHO, 2002). Both proactive and reactive intervention activity in respect of environmental matters tends to lie within the remit of the Environment Agencies in the UK and with local authorities (principally, environmental health but also those concerned with planning, highways and transport). There is little explicit role for those working within the health care sector. However, a core function of the Health Protection Agency (HPA) is focused on environmental threats to health, including acute and chronic exposure to chemicals and radiation. The HPA has an expectation that they will become involved in environmental issues such as contaminated land, air quality (indoor and outdoor), regulation of industrial processes and extreme weather events arising from climate change (HPA, 2008a).

SUSTAINABLE DEVELOPMENT AND HEALTH

No discussion about the environment and health would be complete without an understanding of sustainable development. A common definition is that presented in the *Brundtland Report* (UN, 1987): 'development that meets the needs of the present without compromising the ability of future generations to meet their own needs'. Achieving this will require reconciliation of the tensions between two basic aspirations of society: the need to achieve economic development to secure rising standards of living, both now and for future generations, and the need to protect and enhance the environment now and for the future. Some of the key issues facing us in achieving a sustainable future include climate change, pressure on natural resources and the environment and the inequitable distribution of wealth, leading to poverty and inequality.

International action

The Rio Earth Summit in 1992 brought together over 150 nations to discuss global action for protecting the world's environment and for promoting the eradication of poverty. The outcomes included the *Rio Declaration on Environment and Development* (an agreement on

27 principles supporting sustainable development), a *Plan of Action*, commonly known as '*Agenda 21*' to give effect to the *Declaration* and the establishment of a UN Commission on Sustainable Development.

The key principle linking health and sustainable development is the first principle, which states: 'human beings are at the centre of concerns for sustainable development. They are entitled to a healthy and productive life in harmony with nature' (UN, 1992a). *Agenda 21, the Plan of Action* (UN, 1993), recognises that health is dependent on the management of the physical, biological, spiritual, economic and social environments and acknowledges that a majority of development activities impact on the environment, which, in turn, influences health. Within *Agenda 21*, Chapter 6 is concerned specifically with protecting and promoting health and establishes five global priority actions (UN, 1993):

- meeting the primary health care need, especially in rural areas;
- controlling communicable diseases;
- protecting vulnerable groups;
- meeting the urban health challenge;
- reducing health risks from environmental pollution and hazards.

The effect of *Agenda 21*, Chapter 6 is to provide the context and incentive for global, national and local initiatives aimed at improving health for all.

The UK response

In response, the UK government has produced a series of sustainable development strategies; the most recent in 2005 (DEFRA, 2005). The Strategy proposes that the goal of sustainable development will be pursued 'in an integrated way through a sustainable, innovative and productive economy that delivers high levels of employment; a just society that promotes social inclusion, sustainable communities and personal wellbeing' (DEFRA, 2005). Arguably, the UK sustainable development strategy should be the focal point for the development of other UK policy/strategy documents, as the principles of many important policy agendas can be closely aligned with the tenets of sustainable development. Specifically, it can be argued that a majority of government policies have some impact on the determinants of health and, therefore, as proposed by Adshead *et al.* (2006), both sustainable development and public health dimensions could be incorporated into a range of policies.

Activity 6.1 Reflective exercise: UK policies and sustainable development

Consider some UK government policies with which you are familiar. To what extent do they reflect the principles of sustainable development? To what extent are these principles reflected in the policies of a health care organisation with which you are familiar?

So, how well are we doing? Progress is measured through consideration of performance across 68 indicators of success, divided into four priority areas:

- sustainable consumption and production;
- climate change and energy;
- natural resource protection and environmental enhancement;
- sustainable communities.

(DEFRA, 2008b)

Using baseline statistical data, progress can be measured on an annual basis (DEFRA, 2008a). Interestingly, many of the indicators are directly relevant to public health (see Figure 6.2).

• Employment and poverty.
 • Health inequality:
 – infant mortality;
 – life expectancy.
 • Health life expectancy.
 • Mortality rates:
 – circulatory disease;
 – cancers;
 – suicide.
 • Smoking:
 – in adults;
 – in 'routine' and 'manual'
    socio-economic groups.
	• Childhood obesity.
	 • Diet.
	 • Air quality and health.
	 • Housing conditions:
	 – social sector homes;
	 – vulnerable households in private sector
	    homes.
	 • Households living in fuel poverty:
	 – pensioners;
	 – households with children;
	 – long-term sick and disabled.
	 • Wellbeing.

Figure 6.2 Key Indicators: sustainable development and health (adapted from DEFRA, 2008b)

Environmental justice

It has been suggested that it is incumbent upon us to ensure a healthy environment for future generations but also to ensure that 'development does not create environmental problems or distribute environmental resources in ways which damage other people's health' (ESRC, 2001: 3). Environmental justice relates to the concerns that those who live in deprived areas experience a disproportionate environmental burden where, potentially, they may be subject to greater exposure to environmental pollutants and experience an environmental quality less conducive to, for example, walking, cycling and outdoor recreational activities. This can widen existing health and social inequalities in the population. The concept of environmental justice can also relate to the extent to which individuals and communities have access to information about environmental matters sufficient to enable them to participate in decision-making which may influence local environmental quality.

There is evidence that, in the UK, deprived areas are more likely to be in close proximity to the most polluting industries (Walker, et al., 2005) and experience poorer environmental quality (Pye, et al., 2006; Fairburn, et al., 2009). The evidence is less certain, however, about the adverse impacts on health as a consequence of these environmental inequalities (Fairburn, et al., 2009).

Bulkeley and Walker (2005) assert that environmental justice can be seen as a means of bringing together the sustainable development and social justice agendas. With a focus on health and social inequalities influenced by environmental quality, the concept of environmental justice further underpins the role for public health practitioners in sustainable development.

Linking sustainable development and public health

The convergence of public health and sustainable development is already beginning to become established. The UK public health strategy, *Choosing Health: Making Healthier Choices Easier* (DoH, 2004) has, as its main goals, two of the key priorities established by the UN Commission on Sustainable Development: improving health and reducing health inequalities. More recently, the UKPHA has published *Climates and Change: The Urgent Need to Connect Health and Sustainable Development* (UKPHA, 2008). The UKPHA (2008: 16) sets out the principles on which it believes the integration of health and sustainable development should be established: 'holistic, evidence-based and analytic, inclusive and equitable, clear and understandable, efficient and effective'.

Adshead *et al.* (2006) note, however, that making the link between sustainable development and public health practice will require effort and a focused emphasis on working in partnership with others.

Box 6.1 Case study: Nottingham Health and Environment Partnership

The Nottingham Health and Environment Partnership was launched in 2007. It is a multi-sector partnership that works strategically to contribute towards sustainable development through:

- achieving the best possible health, wellbeing and health services;
- tackling health inequalities; and
- addressing environmental causes of ill health

for all people living in the Greater Nottingham area.

The Partnership comprises:

- Nottingham City PCT, Nottinghamshire Teaching PCT;
- six local authorities: Nottinghamshire County, Nottingham City, Ashfield, Broxtowe, Gedling and Rushcliffe;
- Hospital and Ambulance Trusts in Greater Nottingham;
- Health in your Environment Voluntary Sector Forum;
- Local Strategic Partnerships;
- Private sector organisations;
- Nottingham Trent University.

The Partnership supports service development such as increasing energy efficiency in homes and organisations, promoting walking and cycling instead of car use and the consumption of healthy food from sustainable sources and, in respect of the Nottingham Local Area Agreement, is the lead for the priority theme of reducing Nottingham's impact on the environment in relation to climate change.

Specific achievements include:

- the Food Initiatives Group, which encourages organisations and individuals to consume healthy, safe, affordable food from sustainable sources, including locally produced food and organic food;
- the Healthy Housing Referral Service, which tackles fuel poverty by providing information and advice to people who need help keeping their homes warm in winter at a price they can afford;
- the Ridewise Cycling Training Service, which provides training to people wishing to cycle safely with confidence to national standards;
- the development of the Local Agenda 21 Health Strategy.

Source: East Midlands Regional Assembly: Nottingham Health and Environment Partnership.

CLIMATE CHANGE

As already noted, climate change is identified as one of the important priorities in the UK sustainable development strategy (DEFRA, 2005). It is recognised that climate change is likely to be the most significant environmental problem over the next century (DoH/HPA, 2008). Research indicates that the average global temperature is 15°C, an increase of 0.76°C in the period 1850–99 and 2001–05 (IPCC, 2007). The period 1995–2006 included 11 of the 12 warmest years since 1850 and sea levels have risen, caused by thermal expansion, at an increasing rate over the period 1993–2003 (IPCC, 2007). The emission of anthropogenic greenhouse gases is considered to be the cause of these changes (IPCC, 2007).

These greenhouse gases include carbon dioxide, methane, nitrous oxide, fluorinated compounds plus other synthetic chemicals. The predominant greenhouse gas is carbon dioxide, released during combustion, which in the UK accounts for 77 per cent of greenhouse gas emissions (DEFRA, 2006a).

It is widely recognised that climate change will have an impact on health and the likely change in the distribution of vector-borne disease is of interest globally because of the large populations at risk, particularly in developing countries (UNEPL/GRID-Arendal, 2008). In the UK, ongoing research commissioned by the DoH/HPA is attempting to predict the likely impacts on health in the UK as a consequence of the environmental impact of climate change. Some of these impacts of relevance to public health practitioners are summarised in Figure 6.3.

Impacts on the atmospheric environment.	Overall, interventions to reduce emissions to atmosphere will lower ambient concentrations of priority air pollutants, reducing adverse impacts on health; however, a predicted rise in ozone concentrations will result in increased hospital admissions and deaths from respiratory disease.
Impacts on the aquatic environment.	• More bacteria (for example, Giardia and Cryptosporidium) in surface waters used for the abstraction of drinking water following heavy rains, placing a greater emphasis on the need for advanced water treatments. • A greater likelihood of algal blooms, resulting in unsuitability for use of water for drinking and recreational purposes. • A decrease in the efficiency of some water treatments that render water suitable for potable and food preparation purposes. • A greater number of people at risk of flooding with potential impacts on mental health and the development of disease associated with chemical and sewage contamination of flood waters.
Food-related impacts.	• A rise in the number of food-borne diseases (for example, Salmonellosis and campylobacter infections) associated with ambient temperature increases.
Disease.	• Skin cancers expected to increase as a consequence of behavioural changes (more outdoor activity; lighter clothing = more sun exposure) • Potential for changes in the distribution and abundance of arthropod vectors of disease.

Figure 6.3 Predicted health impacts of climate change in the UK (adapted from DoH/ HPA, 2008)

Tackling climate change

Tackling climate change is one of the key priorities for sustainable development and the UN *Framework Convention on Climate Change* (UN, 1992b) to stabilise greenhouse gas emissions was agreed during the Rio

Earth Summit in 1992. The *Kyoto Protocol* (UN, 1998) sets targets and timetables for reducing greenhouse gas emissions from 2000. In the UK, the *Climate Change Strategy* (DEFRA, 2006a) sets targets for reducing carbon dioxide emissions (which account for 70 per cent of greenhouse gases) with recently revised targets of reductions to 26 per cent below 1990 levels by 2020 and an 80 per cent reduction in greenhouse gas emissions by 2050 (Climate Change Act, 2008). Estimates suggest that the UK has easily met its commitments under the *Kyoto protocol* but is likely to fall short of the UN targets for 2010 (DEFRA, 2008c).

A range of strategies focuses on six sectors: transport, business, the energy supply industry, domestic, agriculture and government. *The Strategy* acknowledges that the role of individuals is important in reducing greenhouse gas emissions, embracing one of the enduring tenets of sustainable development to 'think globally; act locally'. In recognition of the need for the public to have information and advice about climate change and how sustainable choices and living can be achieved, the Tomorrow's Climate; Today's Challenge initiative was introduced. This has resulted in some highly visual publicity drawing attention to the issue of climate change and how individuals can make a difference. Evidence suggests, however, that although recognition of climate change among laymen has risen in recent years, there is a reliance on national institutions to instigate action rather than individuals taking the initiative to modify their habits and lifestyles (Anable, *et al.*, 2006).

The role of public health practitioners

Recently, the role of public health practitioners in tackling climate change has received greater attention with the publication of guidance from the Department of Health (DoH, 2008) where there is a clear statement that 'climate change should be at the core of the public health agenda'. Both the UKPHA and Faculty of Public Health are also raising the profile of public health and proposing approaches for action. The DoH guidance suggests a range of measures to address climate change and promote sustainable development (DoH, 2008a). These include:

* partnership and collaborative working across a range of organisations on climate change initiatives and policy development;
* supporting the development of action planning through a consideration of the health impacts of climate change on vulnerable groups;
* engaging with communities to foster understanding of the health impacts of climate change and encourage lifestyle and behavioural changes to promote sustainable living;

- ensuring that strategic planning and organisational decision-making and activity routinely consider climate change.

The UKPHA (2008: 28), however, suggests that 'the community of health professionals has yet to embrace climate change as a priority'. Perhaps by way of encouragement to public health practitioners, the UKPHA (2008) proposes action that includes the need to ensure that sustainable development and health-related matters are embedded within health professional curricula and CPD activities.

From a practical health promotion perspective, public health practitioners can, for example:

- encourage individuals to take advantage of energy-saving measures such as, for example: insulation of lofts and cavity walls, using energy-saving light bulbs, promoting the subsidies available to low-income households. These measures can reduce energy bills, improve the comfort of the home and help to tackle fuel poverty and will contribute towards a reduction in carbon dioxide emissions. Over five million households have benefited to date (DEFRA, 2008c);
- support and promote initiatives that encourage walking, cycling and the use of public transport, rather than using a private vehicle;
- initiate and promote the consumption of locally-produced food;
- encourage individuals to carry out an estimation of their personal or household carbon footprint. The 'ACT ON CO_2' online calculator (DECC, 2009) will determine the carbon use arising from the home, appliance use and transport and generate an action plan.

AIR QUALITY

Poor air quality and too much traffic have been identified by Londoners as the factors they consider most likely to impact on health (McCarthy and Ferguson, 1999). Since the 1960s, the trend towards ownership of private motor vehicles (7 732 thousand vehicles licensed in 1965, cf. 26 878 in 2007 [DfT, 2008]) has significantly changed the nature of air pollution. Today, the UK recognises ten priority air pollutants (see Figure 6.4). Of these, all except sulphur dioxide, lead and ammonia are related to the use of petrol and diesel-powered vehicles.

- Oxides of nitrogen (NO_x);
- Particulate matter (PM_{10} and $PM_{2.5}$);
- Sulphur dioxide;
- Carbon monoxide;
- Ozone;
- Lead;
- Benzene;
- 1,3-butadiene;
- Polycyclic aromatic hydrocarbons (PAHs);
- Ammonia.

Figure 6.4 UK priority pollutants (source: DEFRA, 2007)

These priority pollutants have been identified as presenting a risk to human health, based on current scientific and medical research. Indeed, it has been estimated that poor air quality in the UK will reduce the life expectancy of every person by an average of seven to eight months (DEFRA, 2007). Poor air quality impacts on the most vulnerable: children, the aged, those with pre-existing respiratory and heart disease and the socio-economically deprived (WHO, 2004). In England, the most deprived wards with the lowest incomes have the highest levels of PM_{10} and NO_x pollution and associated mortality (Environment Agency, 2005).

The primary route of exposure for air pollutants is inhalation and pollutants are in a physical form that enables them to be inhaled deep into the lung issue, where pathological changes may occur. Health impacts are, therefore, largely related to the respiratory and cardiovascular systems giving rise to, for example, impaired lung function, exacerbation of pre-existing respiratory conditions and the promotion of cancers.

In the UK, the *Air Quality Strategy* (DEFRA, 2007) is focused on reducing the risk to health and the environment from air pollution and identifies a range of new and ongoing policy options to improve air quality, both in the immediate and longer term, with the aim of reducing the impact on average life expectancy by five months by 2010 (DEFRA, 2007). The leading governmental players are DEFRA, DH and DfT but local authorities (planning, highways and environmental health functions, in particular) and the Environment Agencies give practical effect to many initiatives focusing on both industrial and transport-related sources of air pollutants.

Controlling emissions from industry

Emissions from industry have been falling in the last ten years as a consequence of more stringent European-influenced legislation. Large combustion plant (including power-generation and waste incineration plant), waste installations and the most polluting industries are regulated through an environmental permitting system overseen by the Environment Agencies. Local authorities are responsible for less complex industrial processes. Permits enable the Environment Agencies and local authorities to control emissions to the environment (air, water or land) to ensure that health and the environment are protected and that there is ongoing improvement in environmental quality over time. Applications for permits are subject to consultation with (among others) the local community, local authorities and the Primary Care Trust (PCT) (or Local Health Board (LHB) in Wales). Permits will not be issued if the health of the local people will be adversely affected by emissions (Environment Agency, 2005). The HPA Chemical Hazards and Poisons Division has provided guidance to PCTs and LHBs to enable them to fully participate in their role as public consultees and, while the guidance notes that 'the statutory consultee role should be seen as a real opportunity to address environment and health issues', the process should not be resource-intensive (HPA, 2008a). Indeed, HPA guidance suggests that PCTs and LHBs are unlikely to offer comments where the emissions are primarily atmospheric. Because of the potential technical complexity of many applications for environmental permits, it is reported that many PCTs have discharged their responsibility to the HPA (HPA, 2008a).

Transport and air quality

Initiatives to improve health through intervention focusing on transport emissions may be a national or local responsibility. Examples of tools for action at governmental level that will help to improve air quality include:

- promoting the use of cleaner fuels;
- incentivising the use of fuel-efficient/low emission vehicles;
- exhaust emission controls;
- improvements in public transport to discourage private vehicle use.

None of these provide specific opportunities for public health practitioners to get involved.

Local authorities have been charged with responsibility for 'Local Air Quality Management'. This requires local authorities to assess and review air quality within their boundaries to establish whether or not the air quality objectives for seven of the priority pollutants listed in Figure 6.4 have been or are likely to be exceeded. Where air quality objectives have not been met, local authorities must declare an Air Quality Management Area and draw up an action plan. Over 200 local authorities have declared an Air Quality Management Area, mostly for the exceeding of the road transport-related pollutants NO_x and PM_{10} (DEFRA, 2007). Development of an action plan requires local authorities to engage with a wide range of stakeholders, including PCTs.

Tools for action at a local level include:

- traffic management schemes, including low emission zones;
- promotion of green travel plans for local businesses;
- congestion charging schemes;
- provision of access to information about ambient air quality;
- consideration of air quality integral to the planning process;
- park and ride schemes, walking and cycling initiatives.

Air quality partnerships have been established by some local authorities, working closely with PCTs, community groups and other agencies. The following case study is an example of one well-established air quality partnership.

Box 6.2 Case study: Sussex-air Air Quality Partnership

The Sussex-air Air Quality Partnership was formed in 1995 with the guiding principle: 'To promote and encourage the improvement of air quality throughout Sussex, to protect public health, quality of life and the environment'. Specifically, the aims are:

- to maximise the opportunities for improving air quality throughout Sussex;
- to engage in and respond to the development of local, regional, UK and EU air quality-related legislation and strategies;
- to provide a framework for dealing with Sussex air quality issues in partnership with regional stakeholders;
- to ensure air quality is fully considered by public authorities when carrying out their functions and duties;

- to encourage air quality to be considered by residents, businesses and organisations when making decisions about their behaviour;
- to promote the importance of air quality as a determinant of public health and wellbeing;
- to integrate air quality more widely into sustainability and climate change policies.

The Partnership comprises:

- five PCTs – Brighton and Hove City, East Sussex Downs, Hastings and Rother, Weald and West Sussex;
- 14 local authorities – East Sussex County, West Sussex County, Adur, Arun, Brighton and Hove City, Chichester, Crawley, Eastbourne, Hastings, Horsham, Lewes, Rother, Wealden, Worthing;
- the HPA;
- the Environment Agency;
- Brighton and Sussex Universities and King's College Environment Research Group.

One specific initiative is the airALERT service. This service is for asthma sufferers identified through the PCTs and asthma clinics in Sussex. Where there is a forecast of 'moderate' or 'high' air pollution for the following day, a voice or text message is sent to a home or mobile telephone, the aim being to provide useful health-related information that could contribute towards personal wellbeing. The service was evaluated in 2006 and provided evidence of significant health management improvements for patients and service providers in primary and secondary care. Specific aspects of airALERT were:

1. raised awareness of pollution episodes;
2. health behaviour modification – service users were able to make informed choices and behavioural changes that included preventative medication, choosing activities to lessen exposure and choosing where they went;
3. enabling health empowerment – service users had access to information and the power to make decisions that impacted on their health and wellbeing.

Source: Sussex-air Air Quality Partnership

Activity 6.2 Reflective exercise: Air Quality Management Areas

More than 200 local authorities have declared an Air Quality Management Area (AQMA). In respect of the local authority where you live (or an adjoining one), access the AQMA Action Plan and/or relevant web pages.

- How much evidence is there of input from public health practitioners?
- What initiatives/plans have direct health benefits, in addition to air quality improvement (for example, cycling schemes, walking, buses)?
- Can you think of any other initiatives/schemes that will have a benefit both to health and air quality?

OTHER ENVIRONMENTAL ISSUES

Land contamination

The contamination of land may present a risk to health either directly or indirectly: ground and surface waters may become polluted; growth of food crops may be inhibited or contaminants may be taken up and stored prior to consumption; gases, vapours and particulates may be inhaled; there may be an increased risk of fire or explosion; physical injury may arise. Land may become contaminated through the controlled disposal of solid and liquid wastes (landfill), through the uncontrolled tipping of wastes or through land use (for example, industry, mining, railways, petrol filling stations). There are thousands of contaminated land sites throughout the UK (Environment Agency, 2008) and the government has made a commitment to redevelop those sites, including their use for housing (for example, the O_2 Arena and the new Greenwich Millennium Village are constructed on the former site of the largest gasworks in Europe).

Research focusing on the health impacts of landfill sites has suggested some risk to health. For example, Elliot *et al.* (2001) noted that the rate of congenital anomalies and low birth-weight babies was slightly more than expected near to landfills. The outcome of a health impact assessment on a landfill site conducted by North Sheffield PCT concluded that there was some evidence of a causal link between proximity to the landfill site and self-reported nasal irritation but, significantly, factors such as smoking, unemployment and poor housing probably contributed far more to ill health than living close to the landfill site (North Sheffield PCT, 2005).

The approach to managing the health risks associated with the terrestrial environment is primarily the function of the Environment Agencies and local authorities, with local authorities taking the lead for most contaminated land sites. The regulation of waste management sites is undertaken by the Environment Agencies through the environmental permitting regime described above and public health practitioners can, therefore, influence the regulation of such sites. Mohan *et al.* (2006), however, call upon public health practitioners to become more involved and, in particular, suggest that public health practitioners should ensure that:

• health impact assessments are carried out on waste management strategies and installations;
• adverse impacts from the location of waste management installations do not fall disproportionately on the poor;
• the voice of the local community can be articulated through the facilitation of meetings with waste installation operators.

The concern, presented by Mohan *et al.* (2006) is that, without public health input, the wider debate around sustainable development and waste management will continue to have a technical and economic focus.

Water quality

In the UK, we tend to take potable water quality and effective waste water treatment for granted, and tend not to consider that the quality of the aquatic environment is constantly under threat from our use of water for both utility purposes and as a receptacle for our waste. Common, controllable contaminants of water in the UK include nitrates and pesticides, the contamination arising principally as a consequence of agricultural practices. In older properties, lead pipework in regions with naturally plumbosolvent waters may give rise to elevated concentrations of lead in tap water.

Intervention activity to protect public health lies largely with the agencies concerned with environmental matters: specifically, the Environment Agencies, sewerage undertakers and Drinking Water Inspectorate. These agencies employ a range of legal and policy tools to both proactively protect health and respond to incidents that threaten health. Discharges to sewers and rivers are regulated, ensuring that water quality is maintained and water for drinking and food preparation purposes is required to comply with a set of parametric values based on the WHO drinking water guidelines (WHO, 2006). While there is no direct role for public health practitioners, the HPA Chemical Hazards and Poisons Division will provide specialist advice to these agencies and to health professionals about the health risks of chemicals in water. Furthermore, the HPA's Health Protection Units provide a local response to, for example, the investigation and management of incidents such as an outbreak of cryptosporidosis.

CONCLUSION

Improving and protecting environmental quality is an essential element in securing and promoting health and wellbeing. Industrialisation and the pressure for economic growth have resulted in environmental degradation and climate change and the consequent threats to health and wellbeing. Sustainable development provides a context for action at the global, national and local level to deal with environmental issues and improve public health.

While much of this action has rested with policy-makers and regulators, this chapter has shown that public health practitioners, working in partnership, can, and should, play an increasingly prominent role in decision-making on aspects of environmental protection and can actively participate in initiatives to improve environmental quality and public health. Perhaps, more significantly, we are beginning to see, within the UK, greater convergence of the health, environment and sustainable development agendas and the emergence of public health practitioners willing to embrace this holistic perspective.

Further reading and useful websites

Landon, M. (2006) *Environment, Health and Sustainable Development (Understanding Public Health)*. Buckinghamshire: OUP. Very useful text linking environment and health.

Nottingham Health and Environment Partnership: **www.emra. gov.uk/what-we-do/regional-communities-policy/success-stories/ nottinghamshire/nottingham-health-and-environment-partnership** (accessed 6 March 2009)
Helen Ross
Nottingham City PCT
1 Standard Court
Park Row
Nottingham
NG1 6GN
helen.ross@nottinghamcity-pct.nhs.uk

Sussex-air: Air Quality Partnership: **www.sussex-air.net/index.html** (accessed 6 May 2009)
Project Development Officer
Planning and Environmental Health
Lewes District Council
Southover House
Southover Road
Lewes
BN7 1AB
website@sussex-air.net

Chapter 7

Meeting the challenges of poverty, inequality and social exclusion

Anneyce Knight

This chapter discusses the context of health, inequality and social exclusion, and focuses on poverty and social exclusion in the twenty-first century, outlining the causes and the costs to individuals and society. It assesses and evaluates poverty and social exclusion. It presents three case studies concerned with geography, occupation and older people and asks what might be done to meet the challenges of poverty, inequality and social exclusion in each instance.

Learning outcomes

In this chapter you will learn how to:

- understand the relationship between poverty, inequality and social exclusion;

- consider a range of evidence available to the public health practitioner relating to poverty, inequality and social exclusion;

- meet the challenges presented in three case studies and evaluate possible options and outcomes.

THE CONTEXT OF POVERTY, INEQUALITY AND SOCIAL EXCLUSION

Despite numerous historical policy documents and interventions – some of which are addressed in Chapters 2 and 3 – poverty and social exclusion have remained challenging areas for the government. For the New Labour Government of 1997, addressing these challenges was central to their political agenda, together with tackling the 'new' issue of social exclusion with a range of publications informing policy and a programme of social and welfare reforms has emerged to tackle poverty, inequality and social exclusion.

Defining poverty and social exclusion

Regardless of whether poverty is defined in absolute or relative terms, it is the impact of poverty on the day-to-day lives of individuals that must be acknowledged and not underestimated. As one person stated in a study exploring the experience of poverty, 'I feel less than others . . .' (Green, 2007: 12).

The European Commission provides a comprehensive definition that reflects the realities of living in relative poverty:

> People are said to be living in poverty if their income and resources are so inadequate as to preclude them from having a standard of living considered to be acceptable in the society in which they live. Because of their poverty they may experience multiple disadvantage through unemployment, low income, poor housing, inadequate health care and barriers to lifelong learning, culture, sports and recreation. They are often excluded and marginalised from participating in activities (economic, social and cultural) that are the norm for other people and their access to fundamental rights may be restricted. (European Commission, 2004: 8)

As 'social exclusion' is defined as 'what can happen when people or areas suffer from a combination of linked problems such as unemployment, poor skills, poor housing, high-crime environments, bad health and family breakdown' (ODPM, 2004a: 2), it can be seen that poverty and social exclusion are interwoven and cannot be explored in isolation, with health inequalities forming an integral part of the equation. It is important to note that living in poverty is not a predictor of social exclusion.

Causes and costs of poverty and social exclusion

There are many factors that currently predispose to social exclusion and poverty. Low income is a key reason that particularly affects women, young people, older males, people with long-term health conditions, the disabled and people from ethnic minorities (ODPM, 2004b). Lack of educational attainment is a further issue leading to reduced earning capacity and limited employment options. Other causative factors include:

- demographic trends – an ageing population;
- mental health issues;
- teenage pregnancy;
- drug and alcohol misuse;
- homelessness;
- access to affordable transport;
- possession of a criminal record;
- lone parenthood.

(ODPM, 2004b)

The personal costs of poverty and social exclusion include reduced life choices and loss of control over personal environment, poorer health and reduced social participation. In addition, there are wider social costs. For example, a joint report published by The Prince's Trust and The Royal Bank of Scotland Group (2007) highlighted that youth unemployment, at that time, was 1.2 million and cost the UK economy £10 million a day in lost productivity and £20 million a week in Jobseeker's Allowance. The financial cost to the UK economy, and the desire to maintain and improve the UK's global status, are incentives for the challenges of poverty, inequality and social exclusion to be met.

Reducing child poverty

In 1999, the government identified the challenge to halve child poverty by 2010 and eradicate it by 2020. This target has become a central focus for policy-making because of the impact childhood has on an individual's adult life and life choices. It is also acknowledged that a cycle of deprivation exists (HM Treasury, et al., 2008). To achieve the target there has been cross-governmental working between departments to develop integrated approaches. The result of this has been to decrease the number of children living in absolute poverty by half from 3.4 million to 1.6 million, and have 600 000 children no longer living in relative poverty (HM Treasury, et al. 2008). Nevertheless, despite interventions such as Tax Credits and the ongoing implementation of the *Every Child Matters* reforms, 2.8 million children continue to live in poverty in the UK (HM

Treasury, *et al.* 2008). The End Child Poverty campaign suggests the rate may be as high as 3.9 million (End Child Poverty, 2009) and Palmer *et al.* (2006) suggest progress has been limited since 2003.

ASSESSING AND EVALUATING POVERTY AND SOCIAL EXCLUSION

A variety of government departments and individual organisations use a range of tools to assess, measure and evaluate deprivation, providing a wealth of empirical data that contributes to building a contemporary picture of poverty and social exclusion in the UK. These include the Department for Communities and Local Government, the Joseph Rowntree Foundation, and the Social Exclusion Unit.

Department for Communities and Local Government

The Department for Communities and Local Government is now responsible for the publication of the *Indices of Deprivation*. The methodology for these *Indices* was devised in 2002 and updated in 2004 and now includes seven domains: income; employment; health deprivation and disability; education, skills and training; barriers to housing and services; crime and the living environment. The collation of the data under these domains provides a detailed measurement of deprivation for every 'Super Output Area' and every local authority. A Super Output Area is a unit of geography, developed by National Statistics, used to analyse statistics in a more detailed way and, currently, there are 32 482 lower layers in England and Wales. Slight modifications were made to some indicators for the 2007 Indices.

Activity 7.1 Reflective exercise: English Indices of Deprivation

Visit the two websites below and select and compare data between The English Indices of Deprivation (2007) and The English Indices of Deprivation revised (2004) and reflect on the strengths and weaknesses of this data.

The English Indices of Deprivation (2007) can be found at: **www. communities.gov.uk/documents/communities/pdf/733520. pdf** (accessed 9 July 2009)

The English Indices of Deprivation Revised (2004) can be found at: **www.communities.gov.uk/documents/communities/ pdf/131209.pdf** (accessed 9 July 2009)

Joseph Rowntree Trust (JRT)

At a similar time to the development of the *Indices of Deprivation*, the JRT published the first national study on poverty and social exclusion in the UK in 2000. In this detailed report they used income, the lack of necessities and subjective measurements to explore poverty and social exclusion at the end of the twentieth century (Gordon, *et al.*, 2000 cited in Stewart, *et al.*, 2005). Individual perceptions of which items were regarded as necessary were identified. The report, as well as providing benchmarks, supplied measurable evidence that poverty had increased from the 1980s and that the reality for many adults and children was that they did not have necessities such as adequate housing, essential clothing and access to social activities – the reality of day-to-day lives.

In its tenth annual report, *Monitoring Poverty and Social Exclusion*, generated by the New Policy Institute for the JRT in 2008, data was collected and collated into themes such as debt, education, economic circumstances across the lifespan and, again, represents the reality of poverty and social exclusion (Palmer, *et al.*, 2006). This report provides an overview and evaluation of ten years of New Labour's approach to poverty and social exclusion. Areas are highlighted that have improved (for example, the number of 16-year-olds getting 5 A–C grades at GCSE), areas that have worsened (for example, the number of 16–19 year olds not in work and households in fuel poverty) or areas that have remained static (for example, children in workless households and children permanently excluded from school) (Palmer, *et al.*, 2006). This document also provides a key benchmarking tool as the analysis took place before the UK was officially declared to be in recession and subsequent publications will reflect the real impact of the 'Credit Crunch'.

Social Exclusion Unit

The Social Exclusion Unit (SEU) was set up in 1997 to ensure cross-government working to provide 'Joined-up solutions to joined-up problems' for socially excluded groups (ODPM, 2004a: 2). Experts were chosen from different government departments, with secondments from external organisations as appropriate, to report on projects identified by the Prime Minister via the Deputy Prime Minister. The SEU was required to produce recommendations to prevent social exclusion and to ensure access to services for all. Reports published have included: *Reducing Reoffending by Ex-Prisoners* (2002), *Transport and Social Exclusion: Making the Connection* (2003), and *Mental Health and Social*

Exclusion (2004). In addition, the SEU has also been required to publish an annual report, *Opportunities for All*, documenting the government's strategies and evaluating their effectiveness in relation to poverty and social exclusion.

Breaking the Cycle (ODPM, 2004c) summarised the progress that had been made in the first seven years of the SEU. Within this report, government approaches were outlined for the prevention of social exclusion and progress made in social exclusion was explored. Strategies for breaking the cycle of deprivation, the reintegration of socially excluded individuals and the minimum standard for the provision of services were focused on. One of the key areas identified, where progress had been made, was in relation to child poverty, which has been discussed earlier in this chapter. The increase, throughout all key stages, in educational attainment for children was also cited, as was the reduction in rough sleepers. The report highlighted the need to continue to tackle the cycle of deprivation and focus on key causes of social exclusion, namely: health inequalities, homelessness, high crime areas including focusing on the economic drivers of social exclusion, especially unemployment.

The recently published *UK National Report on Strategies for Social Protection and Social Inclusion 2008–10* (HM Government, 2008a) sets out, for the European Commission, the UK's agenda to continue to tackle child poverty, improve access to quality services such as transport and address inequalities. It also provides a national strategy for pensions and a national plan for health and long-term care. Although the SEU is being closed and its work in the future will be undertaken within the Cabinet Office by a smaller workforce, both this and Government reports suggest that key challenges still have to be tackled if poverty, inequality and social exclusion are to be eradicated in the UK. The three case studies below illustrate some of these challenges.

MEETING THE CHALLENGES OF POVERTY, INEQUALITY AND SOCIAL EXCLUSION: GEOGRAPHY AND HEALTH; OCCUPATION AND HEALTH; AGE AND HEALTH

Geography (place) and health – the Kent coast

Place and health, or the geography of health, is increasingly seen as important in debates around health inequality. Thus, it is an issue that needs directly addressing within the public health agenda, particularly as geographical location is a wider determinant of health (Dahlgren and Whitehead, 1991).

The role of the Kent coast has played an important part in seafaring history both to the UK and the local economy; Chatham and Sheerness developed as dockyard towns and Margate and Ramsgate as seaside resorts (Kent County Council, 2008). The Office of the Deputy Prime Minister (ODPM) (2006) in its *Coastal Towns Evidence* identified that traditional seaside towns have faced challenges since 1950 and coastal economies have particular difficulties, summarised as follows:

- competition for land use zones;
- social isolation – rural and peripheral;
- low wages, low-skill economy, seasonal employment (also informal economy);
- high dependency on single industry;
- out-migration of young people, poor educational standards, in-migrants trapped into low wage with a seasonal economy;
- higher than average residents over 65 years;
- poor transport infrastructure;
- combination of factors leading to low aspiration and intergenerational poverty and dependence.

The population of the Kent coastal region therefore faces the many challenges of poverty, health inequalities and social exclusion as a result of its changing role. The social and economic changes have directly resulted from the loss of tourism, modernisation of the Navy and loss of coastal industries specific to the region, such as the Sally Line at Ramsgate. Indeed, Steven Fothergill (cited in ODPM, 2006) has noted that seaside resorts are the least understood of Britain's problem areas and have not been able to attract resources such as those available to inner city or rural areas.

A French-British project, part-funded by the EU under Interreg IIIA, compared the health of people in Nord Pas-de-Calais and Kent and Medway in south-east England – Comparison of Santé/Public Health (COSPH) (Palmer, *et al.* 2007). The project focused on health, health-related behaviours, health inequalities, social cohesion, use of services and users' views. The project was a collaborative partnership between universities and health-related organisations within the Euro-region. Comparing data has proved challenging because of the different ways that data is collected within the respective countries, as the countries use different indicators and collate different census material. The Howe Townsend Index was used to analyse data across the two geographical regions (Palmer, *et al.* 2007).

Using 14 socio-economically and geographically representative focus groups, the lay perceptions of health determinants, status and opportunities for health were identified in the Kent and Medway region. The overall results revealed that the public have indeed traditionally viewed the English coast as health-giving, '. . . where people used to go to get better' (Focus Group 2) but, more recently, they recognised that there has been an alteration in status (Meerabeau and Stewart, 2007).

The coastal areas were seen as run-down 'dumping' grounds for inner city problem families causing rising levels of benefit claimants. For example:

> And also, a lot of . . . particularly in the Thanet area I think, isn't it the case that . . . well the London area ships down their teenagers and things like that, who very often are depressed as well and they probably live rough after a while. It's got a lot to do with it . . . (Focus Group 12)

> It's not good living within sea air! It's because of the bed and breakfast classes, because it's a migrant population. Well, in Ramsgate, it always struck me that a lot of the mothers who came into school were slightly depressed, they were down . . . (Focus Group 12)

This alteration was seen to have changed the entire nature of the resorts in a downward spiral, creating a new socially-excluded community of low income households living in bed and breakfast accommodation, presenting major new challenges for regional policy makers (Meerabeau and Stewart, 2007).

Acknowledgement

EU Interreg IIIA for partial funding, COSPH project colleagues and supporters, and the PCTs and health authorities who commissioned the surveys in England.

> ## Activity 7.2 Reflective exercise: action to address multiple deprivation at the coast
>
> Reflect on the quotations above and consider what measures can be taken regionally to tackle the issues raised.
>
> Further information relating to inequalities and public health information in Kent can be found on:
>
> **www.kentphil.nhs.uk**
>
> Specific information relating to Kent coastal towns can be found under Dover LA and Eastern and Coastal NHS Health Profile.

Occupation – gender and health issues for sex workers

On 16 January 2008, at a meeting in the Houses of Parliament, the impending Criminal Justice and Immigration Bill was debated. Within this Bill it was proposed that there would be an offence relating to persistent soliciting and the compulsory rehabilitation of sex workers. Those present at the meeting considered that this had the potential to drive prostitution further underground and, as a result of this, compound safety issues relating directly to sex workers' health and wellbeing. There was overwhelming support for the decriminalisation of prostitution in the UK. (All Women Count, 2008.)

Later in the year, on 3 August 2008, two long-standing members of Hampshire Women's Institute, Shirley Landels and Jean Johnson, travelled the world to discover the facts about sex working in the documentary *The WI Ladies' Guide to Brothels*. Not only did they explore issues around safe practice, but they also promoted the decriminalisation of prostitution. The documentary implicitly highlighted other issues behind sex working such as poverty and drug dependency; Shirley Landels has spoken of this in a subsequent personal interview. The proposed legislation, the documentary and ongoing campaigning have raised the issue of sex workers within the public arena.

The Home Office, in its consultation document on prostitution in 2004, identified several risk factors that may explain why children and adults become sex workers. Among those factors were homelessness, debt, drug use, experience of violence or abuse, truancy and poor educational attainment. Underlying these are the key themes of poverty and social exclusion.

The government has put in place, since 1997, measures and guidance to address many of the above risk factors (for example, *Working Together to Safeguard Children* (2006), *Young Runaways* (2001), The Homelessness Act (2002), JobCentre Plus, Connexions and SureStart Children's Centres) as part of its wider agenda to tackle health inequalities and social exclusion. In the current 'Credit Crunch' factors such as debt, unemployment and homelessness will probably increase with the possible consequence of driving more into sex working out of economic necessity.

The Home Office cited that the number of sex workers in the UK in 2004 may have been in the region of 80 000. The English Collective of Prostitutes (2004) suggests that this was underestimated as it only included those who were on the streets and excluded those engaged in prostitution off-street or involved in a casual or a part-time way. The available information about ethnicity is limited but, according to Home Office-funded research, the ethnicity data that was available during one study reflected the sex workers' geographical areas (Hester and Westmarland, 2004).

Although both genders can be sex workers, without a doubt the majority are female. It is estimated that 70 per cent of prostitutes are mothers and, of these, many are lone parents (English Collective of Prostitutes, 2004). It is well documented that children of lone parents are at risk of child poverty as their parent/carer is more likely to be in part-time or low-paid or low-status work (TUC, 2008). Thus the link between prostitution and child poverty cannot be ignored.

As a result of their occupation, sex workers have been socially excluded from mainstream services. At the Royal College of Nursing's annual conference in 2005 access to health care for sex workers was identified as a priority, as it was felt that they were being excluded from health services (Ryan, 2005). Andrea Sypropoulos identified that sex workers had been 'stigmatised, marginalised and denied access to healthcare' and seen by some as undeserving of care (Ryan, 2005). The result of this stigmatisation and marginalisation was a lack of uptake of health care provision such as general health care, dentistry and social services by sex workers (Ryan, 2005). Furthermore, Jeal and Salisbury (2004) identified in their health needs assessment of street-based prostitution that the health and social inequalities 'experienced by this group are much worse than any group highlighted in the Tackling Health Inequalities Review (2002)' (Jeal and Salisbury, 2004: 147). Shirley Landels and Jean Johnson promoted decriminalisation of prostitution as a way to improve access to health screening and services that would contribute to reducing health inequalities for this group.

John McDonnell (2007), the MP for Hayes and Harlington, in his response to the Criminal Justice and Immigration Bill, stated in parliament that there was a need for 'early intervention, multi-agency working, training professionals, outreach workers, one-to-one support, fast-tracking into drugs programmes . . . , fast-tracking into emergency accommodation, advice and assistance and specialised support for victims of domestic violence'. Education of staff within commissioning and provider services and integrated services would seem to have a role to meet the needs of this marginalised sector of society.

Acknowledgement

With thanks to the English Collective of Prostitutes.

Activity 7.3 Reflective exercise: sex workers and health

Consider John McDonnell's statement and then reflect on whether these address the issues of poverty, inequality and social exclusion he cites:

- the Swedish Government's model where the individual paying for sex is criminalised and outreach programmes have been set up, which has led to a reduction in the number of on-street sex workers (Home Office, 2004 and COI, 2006).
- the New Zealand model where prostitution has been decriminalised and brothels are obliged to adhere to government legislation such as, for example, employment and health laws (Home Office, 2004, and *The WI Ladies' Guide to Brothels*).

Older people and inclusion

Life expectancy in the UK and Europe as a whole is increasing. The increase is due in part to the decline in fertility rates, an increased life expectancy of at least ten years in the last 50 years and the post-World War II increase in births – the baby boomers (Walker, 2005). The population of pensionable age, that is to say women over the age of 60 and men over the age of 65, is estimated to have been 11.4 million in 2006 and is anticipated to be 12.2. million by 2011 and 13.9 million by 2026 (Age Concern, 2007). This demographic change brings challenges for policy-makers as there will be an imbalance between those who are in work, as opposed to those in education or retired, and the increasing dependency needs of an ageing population.

Many older people in the UK face poverty. Walker (2005) states that the UK has a higher amount of older people who live on low incomes compared with Italy, the Netherlands and Sweden. Currently, the basic pension for 2008/09 for a single person is £90.70 per week based on full National Insurance contributions (Age Concern, 2008a). Rates vary depending on eligibility based on contributions and marital/civil partnership status. This state pension is currently paid to women aged 60 and over and men aged 65 and over but, between 2010 and 2020, both will receive their pension at 65. For anyone born after 5 April 1959, the age at which the pension will be paid in the future will increase gradually to 68 for both men and women between 2024 and 2046 (Age Concern, 2008a). This has potentially significant implications for levels of poverty for older people in the future.

This issue of poverty for older people in the future is further compounded by the fact that, although two-thirds of people between 50 and retirement age were in paid employment in 2002, over half were involved in caring either for grandchildren or elderly relatives (Mooney, *et al.*, 2002). As dependency increases, the demands of this caring role may mean that individuals retire early without having a full occupational pension or may be restricted in their career progression because of their caring roles, thus reducing the financial provision they may be able to make for their retirement. This is particularly the case for women (Mooney, *et al.*, 2002 and Walker and Walker, 2005). In addition, balancing work and caring needs can increase personal stress and lead to poorer health in older age (Mooney *et al.*, 2002).

Older people also face issues of social exclusion such as, for example, access to transport, particularly when no longer able to drive and especially in rural areas where public transport can be limited. Discrimination in the form of ageism is also a cause of concern and can be both organisational and/or individual such as, for example, being unable to access specialist health care or losing a job because of age (Age Concern, 2008b). The Employment Equality (Age) Regulations Act 2006 seeks to tackle age discrimination by providing protection for people of all ages whether in employment, training or adult education. Furthermore, the *National*

Service Framework for Older People (DoH, 2001a) sought to standardise health provision for older people within its eight standards, including a standard specifically aimed at rooting out age discrimination.

The government sought to address the needs of an ageing society in its strategy *Opportunity Age: Meeting the Challenges of Ageing in the 21st Century* (DWP, 2005). This strategy focused on:

- work and income, to enable people over 50 to manage their careers;
- health and personal commitments;
- active ageing;
- service provision in order for individuals to maintain their independence and control over their lives;
- development of the pensioner service to tackle poverty.

This strategy is currently under review (HM Government, 2008b).

The UK is a multicultural society with a rich ethnic diversity, which is also reflected within the older population. The census of 2001 noted the following ethnic groups were represented in those over 65 (see Table 7.1)

Percentage	Ethnic origin
11%	Black-Caribbean
2%	Black-African
7%	Indian
4%	Pakistani
3%	Bangladeshi
5%	Chinese
68%	White

Table 7.1 UK ethnic make-up in the older population (source: Age Concern, 2007)

For older people from black and minority ethnic (BME) groups, poverty in retirement is an issue resulting from lower than average incomes during their working life, in particular for Pakistanis (Walker and Walker, 2005). Ageism and discrimination based on ethnicity can also be further compounding factors that can promote social exclusion and health inequalities for older people from ethnic minorities. The *National Service Framework for Older People* (DoH, 2001a) and the Race Relations

(Amendment) Act 2000 have sought to address this. The challenge to all organisations and their employees is to meet all older people's needs in an individual and culturally competent way that respects diversity.

Activity 7.4 Reflective exercise: inclusive services for older people

Reflect on how your service provision meets the needs of older people from BME groups and what changes can be made to meet the challenges they face.

CONCLUSION

It can be seen that the government, since 1997, has sought to address the issues of poverty, inequality and social exclusion but many challenges remain, such as, for example, those identified within the case studies. The government has yet to reach its target for eradicating child poverty, a challenge seemingly further compounded by the current recession in the UK. The wealth of evidence assessing, measuring and evaluating poverty, inequality and social exclusion provides public health practitioners with comprehensive data that can be utilised to develop innovative and evidence-based practice to meet local and individual needs, delivered within a culturally competent framework. Cross-organisational working, both at national and local levels, continues to be necessary to meet the challenges of poverty, inequality and social exclusion.

Further reading

Byrne, D. (2005) (reprinted 2008) *Social Exclusion*. Maidenhead: Open University Press
This book provides a detailed exploration of social exclusion.

Curtis, S. (2004) *Health and Inequality; Geographical Perspectives*. London: Sage
One of the key writers on place and health, a recommended read.

Gattrell, A.C. and Elliot, S.J. (2009) *Geographies of Health: an introduction* (2nd Ed.). Oxford: Wiley Blackwell
Key writers on place and health, a recommended read of a very contemporary text.

Smith, G.D., Dorling, D. and Shaw, M. (2004 reprinted) *Poverty, Inequality and Health in Britain 1800–2000: a reader*. Bristol: The Policy Press
A book of extracts from key texts relating to poverty, inequality and social exclusion providing a contextual background to these areas.

This chapter is dedicated to Shirley Landels who inspired so many.

Chapter 8

Health promotion: a multi-causal approach

Suri Thomas and Ben Bruneau

This chapter presents a multi-causal approach to health promotion. It first takes a sociological approach, using the Beattie Model as an analytical tool, and then provides a psychological approach using the Theory of Planned Behaviour. It particularly focuses on examples of obesity and smoking and on the way in which these approaches can help to improve health. This chapter does not seek to address social marketing.

Learning outcomes

In this chapter you will learn how to:

- define health promotion in the context of the public health agenda and what it seeks to sustainably achieve;

- apply the constructs of the Beattie Model and those of the Theory of Planned Behaviour across a range of health promotion strategies and interventions with particular reference to obesity and smoking;

- use the Beattie Model with the Theory of Planned Behaviour to help improve health and prevent illness.

INTRODUCTION

Health promotion activities seek to sustainably address health inequalities at the level at which they are determined and to improve health, particularly through partnerships between statutory and non-statutory health agencies and the community.

As our understanding and application of public health has developed so, of course, have health promotion activities. A century and a half ago the 'sanitary movement' saw that environmental factors were central to health, followed by the 'personal hygiene movement' in the early twentieth century. The emphases of the second phase were education and individual responsibility, which were viewed by the critics as a 'victim blaming' philosophy. The responsibility of being healthy was firmly located in the individuals and their lifestyles, thereby reducing the need to address the effects of capital production (Turshen, 1989). The prevailing Conservative ideologies at the time (1979 to 1997) subscribed to these values and were consolidated in *The Health of the Nation* document (DoH, 1992).

The subsequent White Paper *Saving Lives: Our Healthier Nation* (DoH, 1999a) used a more communitarian approach to health improvements. Operating in this way provides the opportunity for trusting relationships to develop between health and social care professionals, clients and their families, enabling the potential for positive public health outcomes for both individuals and at community level. The Beattie Model of health promotion offers a structural and analytical framework to help practitioners maximise their actions by understanding, questioning and positively adapting their role within public health.

This chapter applies Graham and Kelly's (2004) concept of a causal chain of socio-economic factors at the macro level and psychological factors at the individual level to the health issues of obesity and smoking. This application uses the Model of Health Promotion (Beattie, 1991) and the Theory of Planned Behaviour (Ajzen, 1991), which best exemplify the interrelationships between sociological and psychological constructs vis-à-vis the two health issues.

THE CONTEXT AND PHILOSOPHY OF HEALTH PROMOTION

The purpose of the public health initiative is to prevent ill health and protect health through organised interventions, directed at the public or at the community level. Health promotion provides the means to organise and achieve the goals of these interventions. The government's perspective is that a joint approach to health promotion through regeneration and community empowerment can more comprehensively and sustainably address health determinants and thereby help reduce health inequality. This relies on organisational and community-based partnerships, heralding new community-based responsibilities and participation, with government, communities and individuals mutually responsible for improving health (DoH, 1998a and 1999a).

In order to be effective, new partnership strategies must incorporate sustainable health promotion strategies that are viable and sustainable and there needs to be local involvement, participation, partnership working and sound accountability mechanisms, even when the programme(s) is completed and the state 'exits'.

THE BEATTIE MODEL OF HEALTH PROMOTION

Health promotion represents mediation between people and their milieu. In other words, the role and actions of health promotion involve looking at the total environment, which enhances health. Therefore, health promotion activities not only include improving food, income, housing and skills but also creating supportive environments resulting in personal and community empowerment (Dines and Cribb, 1993). These are achieved through education, legislation and community-based social actions. The WHO 1986a and 1986b documents express these as their core values underpinning health promotion. A closer look at the WHO health promotion definition shows the amalgamation of old and new public health views '. . . synthesising personal choice and social responsibility in health to create a healthier future' (WHO, 1984: 2). It sets the scene for a dynamic relationship between individuals and their wider social world thereby asking each one to act 'local' and think 'global'.

Health promotion is very much a 'hands on' activity. It is in the business of prevention, the active management of disease and the creation of healthy environments, adding years to life and life to years – an ideal to which health and social care professionals can subscribe. Primary care 'is the first level of contact for individuals' of the health system and therefore is identified as the core location for health promotion. Key professionals in health and social care are in an excellent position to enable people to take control of their lives, reduce health deficits, achieve equity in health and help to build social capital. Communities with a high level of social capital are better able to overcome acute and chronic illness because there is a feeling of wellbeing from increased community activity (Baum and Saunders, 1995). (See also Chapter 14.)

Understanding and applying the Beattie Model of Health Promotion

Beattie (1991) offers an analytical model that enables us to critically evaluate the different approaches used by successive governments. The Beattie Model has four quadrants and each quadrant conveys the means by which professionals may promote health. Importantly, each quadrant is infused with its own philosophies, beliefs and values and outcome measurements in relation to health promotion. The approaches can be directed at an individual or at population level. The manner of delivery can be authoritarian and therefore top-down or negotiated and bottom-up. The top-down approaches are labelled as health persuasion techniques for health (HPT) and legislation for health (LAH), the bottom-up approaches are named personal counselling for health (PCH) and community development for health (CDH). The aims of the top-down approaches are to redirect unhealthy behaviours; the bottom-up approach aims to increase individual and community empowerment.

The Beattie Model is represented in Figure 8.1, which demonstrates the way in which it can be used as an analytical tool to explore and contextualise health promotion under various headings or themes.

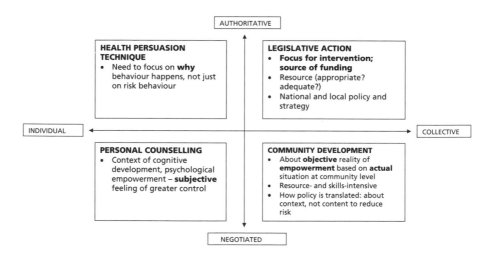

Figure 8.1 The Beattie Model of Health Promotion, (adapted from Beattie (1982) cited in Beattie A (1991) 'Knowledge and control in health promotion: a test case for social policy and social theory' in J. Gabe, M. Calnan and M. Bury (Eds) (1994) *The Sociology of the Health Service*. London: Routledge

Health persuasion

The health persuasion technique is a popular approach both with professionals and politicians. It seemingly addresses health risk factors, it is cheap and easy to deliver. Health professionals have done their bit and politicians have acknowledged medical knowledge and even manufacturers of unhealthy products are pleased. After all, evidence suggests that only limited change may be expected from such an approach. At no time are the social and economic determinants of health questioned. Therefore, this is often seen as a 'victim blaming' approach. It disables and increases the feeling of powerlessness in individuals; the total opposite to empowerment and taking control of one's life.

Yet, a focused and consolidated use of this method can increase awareness and 'set the agenda' for changes in legislation. The use of mobile telephones while driving was highly publicised prior to new legislation, demonstrating HPT in use. There has been a 15 per cent increase in the incidence of HIV and AIDS in UK, supporting the thesis that knowledge does not always translate into attitude and behaviour change (Rutter and Quine, 2002).

Legislation for health

Legislation for health is benevolent in approach and it aims to redirect behaviour at the macro level. Historically this is a proven method – the Race Relations Act and the Clean Air Act are examples. However, Acts of Parliament use utilitarian principles and are therefore unlikely to meet everyone's needs equally. Legislation acts on the local and immediate environment and does not really question the actions of producers of harmful products. Selling cigarettes to children is forbidden, which is helpful, but it does not confront cigarette manufacturers. The interests of commerce and industry, those with least stake in the local environment, are not challenged. The failure to challenge producers does demonstrate the limits of such an approach.

Personal counselling for health

The personal counselling for health starts at where the user is. Through a process of active listening and reflection it aims to empower the individual to become more capable of making genuine choices. A biographical and value clarification approach is employed and works on the understanding that individual(s) have the capacity to make genuine choices. Examples are as follows: self-monitoring, goal setting, problem-solving and self-reward.

The glaring weakness is that the client may return to an unchanged environment to practise new skills. It could pose difficulties initially, at least until skills are transferred to address the new problems. If budgeting is the new expertise then sufficient income is required to practise this skill. Essentially an empowered individual would be able to participate more fully in community development.

Community development for health

The community development for health approach provides people in similar situations of need with opportunities to work together to seek changes in their environment. It does require an enabler to maintain focus and coordinate services. An example is when parents living in an inner city area want to control pollution levels during playtime. They could request a reduction of traffic during playtime. This of course requires negotiation, collaboration by the community and statutory and non-statutory services. Mabhala and Lesiamo (2009) allude to the importance of 'health literacy' skills. They maintain that much health information in the form of literature or professional advice may not be understood and that people may lack competence to take advantage of health information. In such circumstances, with an enabler, CDH can improve literacy skills in given communities to improve health literacy. This could ameliorate social disadvantages like low self-esteem as identified by Marmot and Wilkinson (2006).

CDH can be hijacked if the enabler's goal is to deliver predetermined objectives. It then effectively becomes a route to reach 'hard to get' groups of people. An example will be a needle exchange service where an individual is helped through a caring group process but which does not involve community participation.

Activity 8.1 Reflective exercise: understanding and applying the Beattie Model

Health Persuasion Technique (HPT)
- What are the advantages of this approach?
- What are the disadvantages of this approach?
- Would you like to receive this form of health promotion?
- What is the aim of this approach?
- How would you measure success?

Legislation for Health (LAH)
- What are the advantages of this approach?
- What are the disadvantages of this approach?
- Would you like to receive this form of health promotion?
- What is the aim of this approach?
- How would you measure success?

Personal Counselling for Health (PCH)
- What are the advantages of this approach?
- What are the disadvantages of this approach?
- Would you like to receive this form of health promotion?
- What is the aim of this approach?
- How would you measure success?
- What are the advantages of this approach?

Community Health Development (CDH)
- Would you like to receive this form of health promotion?
- What is the aim of this approach?
- How would you measure success?
- What are the advantages of this approach?
- What are the disadvantages of this approach?

Activity 8.2 Reflective exercise: applying theory to practice

Consider the different health promotion approaches that have been used on you. For example:

- school-based health education such as, for example, the school nurse and sex education;
- information from a GP nurse, such as for example, weight reduction or smoking cessation advice;
- targeted health information in the media such as, for example, drink-driving at Christmas and fireworks safety on Guy Fawkes night.

How effective was it at changing behaviour? How do you know? What evidence supports your views?

OBESITY: THE HEALTH PROMOTION CHALLENGES

It is estimated by the Department of Health in the *Foresight – Tackling Inequalities in Health Future Choice Project* (2007) that, in future, 60 per cent of men and 50 per cent of women will be clinically obese and the related health cost could amount to £45.5 billion per year. To remedy this epidemic requires a holistic approach.

Using the Beattie Model Health Persuasion Technique quadrant, for example, the government is backing a £375 million campaign called Change4Life which commenced in January 2009. The focus is on 'shock tactics', showing fat oozing or clogged up arteries. This may increase awareness of the problem but is unlikely on its own to result in behaviour change. This view is supported by a spokesman for the National Obesity Forum who said that 'posters or leaflets will not persuade the poorest, hard-to-reach groups most likely to have weight problems' (Rose, 2008: 25).

In terms of obesity management and the HPT approach, Davies (2008) supports the use of a screening tool called MUST. The tool is used to measure weight loss and weight gain and, based on the results, to refer patients to appropriate local resources. While the power still remains with the professional, the tool does provide an objective measure to approach a delicate but seemingly obvious problem. Another method is the use of drug therapy. Kanumilli (2006) has put forward the use of statins as a relatively effective pharmacological intervention. Murray *et al.* (2007) in their West Scotland Coronary Prevention study of 6 595 men with an average age of 55, support this view. The research found that the cholesterol-lowering drugs statins had the ability to provide ten years of protection against heart disease after patients stop taking the drug. Sengupta (2009) points out the need for a multi-dimensional package of activities for interventions in order to be successful.

Similarly, 'junk food' advertising before the 9 p.m. watershed is another example of the power of vested interests in the food industry. To combat obesity the National Health Service (NHS) National Service Framework for Coronary Heart Disease and Mental Health policy has been established (DoH, 2000c). However, Pearson (2005: 87) states that 'this has not led to effective strategies for tacking obesity'.

Hogston and Simpson (2002) state that eating is pleasurable and therefore changing eating behaviour can be difficult. Food is the centrepiece at weddings and funerals and many other festive occasions. It acts as a mood stabiliser at times of happiness and sadness. The PCH approach, through a process of active listening, seeks to engage with the individual and their relationship to food. The result may be the requirement for menu planning, shopping and cooking. The problem now has shifted from obesity to life skills attainment. Low self-esteem has been attributed to the development of mental problems in some cases, particularly as Western societies value 'thinness' as a desired body image. Sarafino (2002) makes a clear link between low self-esteem and negative attitude which then poses a problem for behaviour change.

The obesity epidemic represents a major challenge to health promotion professionals. A health promotion model like the Beattie Model acknowledges this complex area. In order to make any impact at all it requires the synthesis between personal responsibility and a supportive environment. For example, HPT takes into account risk factors and engages with the client/patient to take action in health management. PCH, on the other hand, considers the individual relationship to food including psychological factors through a reflective process. LAH utilises policies like the National Framework for Health, which puts obesity on the health agenda. Finally, CDH uses a group approach for people in similar situations to find collective solutions.

SMOKING: THE HEALTH PROMOTION CHALLENGES

It is also useful to consider how the Beattie Model can be applied to smoking, another major lifestyle factor currently being addressed in public health. Recent years have seen the government introduce a smoking ban in public places across the UK. The Beattie Model shown in Figure 8.2 below demonstrates the range of techniques required to help people to quit smoking, encouraged and supported by a range of legal and community measures and then to retain their smoking cessation.

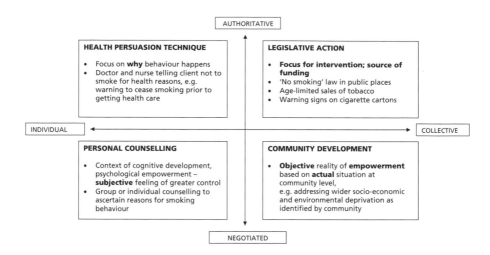

Figure 8.2 The Beattie Model of Health Promotion using smoking as a theme, adapted from Beattie (1982) cited in Beattie, A. (1991) 'Knowledge and control in health promotion: a test case for social policy and social theory' in J. Gabe, M. Calnan and M. Bury (eds) (1994) *The Sociology of the Health Service*. London: Routledge

Activity 8.3 Reflective exercise: health promotion and smoking

Read the example of how the Beattie Model can be applied to food and health and think about this in the context of smoking prevention initiatives. Also think about the following questions:

- HPT – Should doctors ask patients to stop smoking before providing treatment? (Refer also to Chapter 15 on ethics.)
- LAH – Can you find evidence to support the view that the smoking ban has reduced smoking morbidity and mortality?
- PCH – How effective are smoking cessation clinics? Evidence?
- CDH – Find out what communities would need to improve their living and working environments so that they do not require chemical comforters such as cigarettes and/or alcohol to reduce their stress.

THE CONTRIBUTION OF A PSYCHOLOGICAL APPROACH

The change of behaviour posited by the Beattie Model of Health Promotion requires that attention be paid to the individual's personal qualities in the prevention of disease and the restoration of health. This is considered in the left lower quadrant of the model and suggests the link with psychological factors. The health behaviour model, the Theory of Planned Behaviour, (TPB) (Azjen, 1991) and the five constructs that it represents can subsequently satisfy the consideration needed for a comprehensive health promotion strategy. In this strategy, what the individual wants to do, or is seen as capable of doing, depends on three kinds of considerations or three sets of beliefs (Ajzen, 1991; Gollwitzer, 1999):

- beliefs about the possible results of a behaviour, and the evaluations of these results (behavioural beliefs);
- beliefs about what people in the individual's community expect and the individual's motivation to comply with these expectations (normative beliefs); and
- beliefs on what factors in the community can assist or impede the occurrence of the behaviour and the perceived strength of these factors (control beliefs).

Individually, behavioural beliefs can lead to a positive or negative attitude toward a behaviour; normative beliefs can produce social pressure (or subjective norm); control beliefs can provide a perceived behavioural control. In combination, however, these beliefs lead to an individual's intention to perform a behaviour (that is, the intention to act in a certain way). The stronger these beliefs are, the stronger is the intention, and the higher the degree of actual control, the higher the likelihood that the intention will translate into the behaviour.

TPB can predict a wide range of health-related behaviours (Armitage and Conner, 2001; Godin and Kok, 1996), including smoking (Godin, et al., 1996; McMillan and Conner, 2003; Moan and Rise, 2005), eating a low-fat diet (Conner, et al., 2000) and exercising (Sheeran and Abraham, 2003). TPB, therefore, provides a useful conceptual framework for understanding and predicting how individuals can and will act to give up smoking and, for example, through exercise, to reduce their weight to combat obesity. In the exercise situation, for instance, the theory becomes valuable in predicting and understanding the motivational influences that are not wholly under a person's control (Horodynski, *et al.*, 2007). There is also ample evidence to support the theory's capabilities to predict physical activity intention and behaviour (Ajzen and Driver, 1992; Armitage and Conner, 2001; Rhodes and Courneya, 2003). It explains the informational and motivational influences on physical activity intentions and behaviour (Hagger, *et al.*, 2002; Symons Downs and Hausenblas, 2005). Thus, it can provide guidance on how and where to target strategies for changing behaviour. This prediction can best be derived from the information given by an obese person using the self-report inventory indicated in Box 8.1, after receiving an explanation that exercise can help in the reduction of weight.

Box 8.1: Self-report inventory in changing behaviour: an example

Attention to obesity: exercise to deal with overweight problem
Please answer the following questions by placing a tick (✓) in the appropriate space.

The desired behaviour
In the course of the past month, how often have you tried to exercise for at least 30 minutes?

___ Every day   ___ Almost every day   ___Most days

___ On about half the days ___ A number of times, but less than half

___ A few times   ___ Never

Please estimate how often you have exercised for at least 30 minutes in the past month.
Check the interval on the following scale that best represents your estimate.

Never: ___: ___: ___: ___: ___: ___: ___: ___: ___: ___: Every day

Attitude toward exercise
For me to exercise for at least 30 minutes each day in the following month is:

harmful: ___: ___: ___: ___: ___: ___: ___: beneficial

pleasant: ___: ___: ___: ___: ___: ___: ___: unpleasant

---

good: ___: ___: ___: ___: ___: ___: ___: bad

worthless: ___: ___: ___: ___: ___: ___: ___: valuable

enjoyable: ___: ___: ___: ___: ___: ___: ___: unenjoyable

Subjective norm
Most people who are important to me think that:

I should:___: ___: ___: ___: ___: ___: ___:I should not

exercise at least 30 minutes each day in the forthcoming month.

It is expected of me that I exercise for at least 30 minutes each day in the forthcoming month.

Extremely likely: ___: ___: ___: ___: ___: ___: ___: extremely unlikely

The people in my life whose opinions I value would:

approve: ___: ___: ___: ___: ___: ___: ___: disapprove

of my exercising for at least 30 minutes each day in the forthcoming month.

Most people like me exercise for at least 30 minutes each day.

Extremely likely: ___: ___: ___: : ___: ___: extremely unlikely

Perceived behavioural control
For me to exercise for at least 30 minutes each day in the forthcoming month would be:

Impossible: ___: ___: ___: ___: ___: ___: ___: possible

If I wanted to I could exercise for at least 30 minutes each day in the forthcoming month.

Definitely true: ___: ___: ___: ___: ___: ___: ___: definitely false

How much control do you believe you have over exercising for at least 30 minutes each day in the following month?

No control ___: ___: ___: ___: ___: ___: ___: complete control

It is mostly up to me whether or not I exercise for at least 30 minutes each day in the forthcoming month.

Strongly agree: ___: ___: ___: ___: ___: ___: ___: strongly disagree

From this questionnaire it would be possible, therefore, to predict an individual's intention to exercise. That intention, which will lead to the performance of the behaviour, is sequenced in Figure 8.3. Similar principles can be applied when a health promotion strategy is aimed at encouraging individuals to give up smoking.

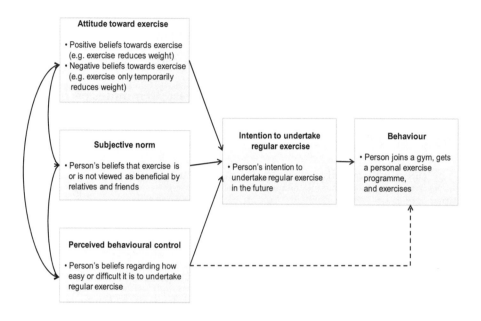

Figure 8.3 Application of the Theory of Planned Behaviour (adapted from Ajzen, 1991)

CONCLUSION

Health promotion is a fundamental part of tackling health inequalities and improving health and there is a range of theories and approaches. This chapter has focused on the Beattie Model as a sociological approach and how it can be supported as part of a holistic approach by a psychological approach in the form of the Theory of Planned Behaviour. A health promotion strategy that considers the principles of the Beattie Model is likely to be at its most effective when it is used in combination with another model that emphasises the individual's role and contribution in enacting a desired behaviour. Here the examples of obesity and smoking have been considered as current high-profile issues in public health, but other topics such as sexually transmitted disease, breastfeeding or accident prevention, to name but a few, could equally be considered within these models.

Chapter 9

Health protection

Yvonne Cornish

This chapter provides an introduction to public health practice in relation to health protection, with a particular focus on the ways in which public health organisations, and the people within them, work together to protect the population from the spread of infectious (communicable) diseases. Health protection is a specialist area within public health practice, and those who undertake this work require specialist training – which usually includes gaining 'hands on' experience of working in a local health protection unit (see below). However, all public health practitioners, whatever their area of work, can benefit from developing a greater awareness and understanding of the public health roles and responsibilities in relation to health protection.

Learning outcomes

In this chapter you will learn how to:

- appreciate the importance of communicable disease control and other aspects of health protection;

- understand the principle modes of transmission of communicable diseases;

- describe some of the measures used to control the spread of communicable diseases within populations;

- relate communicable disease control to the wider context of health protection;

- describe the structure, roles and responsibility of the Health Protection Agency.

HEALTH PROTECTION: AN INTRODUCTION

The term 'health protection' encompasses the prevention and control of infectious diseases and other environmental threats to health. While infectious diseases represent the main biological threat to health, there are a number of other hazards present in the physical environment that regularly impact on the health of individuals and communities, including, for example, chemical and radiological incidents (DoH, 2002a). There are therefore a number of threads to this work, including:

- preventing and controlling the spread of infectious diseases in the community and in institutions such as hospitals and care homes;
- responding to environmental hazards, for example, by assessing the health effects of exposure to hazardous chemicals in air, water, soil and waste;
- looking at the public health risks of radiation from natural and man-made sources;
- developing responses to the deliberate or accidental release of biological, chemical or radiological agents.

Within the UK, the policy and organisational arrangements to support health protection have their roots in nineteenth-century public health practice, and have at times seemed fragmented (Grey, *et al.*, 2007). Until quite recently, responsibility for health protection was split between the Department of Health, the NHS and local government, with support for communicable disease control provided by the Communicable Diseases Surveillance Centre (CDSC) and the Public Health Laboratory Service (PHLS). However, at the beginning of the twenty-first century, a major review of the arrangements for communicable disease control and other aspects of health protection recommended a more integrated approach (DoH, 2002a). In order to implement these recommendations, the government established the Health Protection Agency (HPA) in 2003. The new organisation brings together the Centre for Infections (previously CDSC and PHLS), the Centre for Radiation, Chemical and Environmental Hazards and the Centre for Emergency Preparedness. More information on the structure, roles and responsibilities of the Health Protection Agency is provided later in this chapter. The next section will look at the issues around communicable disease control in a little more detail.

COMMUNICABLE DISEASE CONTROL

What do we mean by 'communicable' diseases?

Communicable diseases – also described as infectious, or contagious diseases – are caused by micro-organisms that can be transmitted from person to person, either directly or indirectly. Most communicable diseases found in the UK are caused by either bacteria or viruses, and many have humans as their only host – although there are a number of exceptions (Donaldson and Donaldson, 2003). Pathogenic (i.e. disease-causing) micro-organisms can be transmitted in a variety of ways, and understanding the mode of transmission is important for public health practitioners who often need to develop or implement measures to control the spread of infection (Gillam, *et al.*, 2007). The development of our understanding of the source and mode of transmission provides insight into the complex relationship between pathogenic micro-organisms and populations, the measures taken to control their spread, and the ways in which these have changed (and will continue to change) over time.

Communicable diseases in context

Controlling the spread of communicable diseases has been important to society throughout recorded history. Rosen (1993) argues that the first clear-cut accounts of communicable disease appear in the literature of classical Greece, and that the infectious nature of many diseases was recognised long before the ways in which they were passed from person to person were understood. The Romans are known to have experienced periodic epidemics of infectious diseases, including at least one epidemic of bubonic plague, and historical evidence suggests that, from the Middle Ages onward, epidemics of infectious diseases such as leprosy, plague, smallpox and cholera repeatedly swept through Western Europe (Rosen, 1993). These repeated epidemics appear to have held back population growth in pre-industrial Europe (Gray, 2001).

Furthermore, this pattern of infectious diseases was not historically static. While leprosy seems to have been prevalent throughout Europe and the Mediterranean for centuries, plague arrived suddenly in Europe in 1348, and disappeared just as suddenly in 1666 (Gray, 2001: 110). The death toll from these epidemics was considerable: for example, in 1348, plague reduced the population of Venice by half, and the 'Great Plague' of 1655 is estimated to have killed over 80 000 people in London alone, producing more deaths in London that year than in any single year before (Porter, 2003). In Victorian England, infectious diseases such as smallpox, typhus, typhoid, dysentery, diphtheria and scarlet fever were continually present in urban communities, occasionally reaching epidemic proportions and taking a heavy toll on human life (Rosen, 1993: 251). For example, an epidemic of smallpox during the late 1830s killed 42 000 people (DoH, 2002a). Other infectious diseases reached the UK during periods of pandemic. Examples of these include a number of cholera epidemics that swept through Europe during the mid-nineteenth century (Rosen, 1993) and, in the early twentieth century, the Great Flu Pandemic of 1918, which is estimated to have claimed the lives of 228 000 Britons (Honigsbaum, 2009).

Approaches to the control of these epidemics varied historically and geographically, and were informed by competing theories about the mode of transmission (Lupton, 1995). Contagion theory led to the isolation of the sick (for example, in leper colonies and plague houses outside city boundaries), restriction on movement of people and goods, and the introduction of quarantine. Miasmic theory, on the other hand, resulted in the adoption of sanitary reforms (such as the introduction of clean water supplies and the development of sewage systems) and underpinned the Victorian public health movement in the UK. It was not until towards the end of the nineteenth century that 'germ theory' – the idea that contagious diseases were caused by specific micro-organisms, which could be transmitted in a number of different ways – began to inform public health interventions aimed at controlling the spread of infectious diseases. From this point in time, increasing emphasis was placed on individual (rather than population) interventions, such as improving personal hygiene (Armstrong, 1993).

Activity 9.1 Reflective exercise

In response to what you have read so far, make a list of infectious diseases that have caused epidemics historically. Are there any others you can think of? If so, add these to your list, then try to answer the following questions.

- How many of these diseases do you think still pose a threat to population health in the twenty-first century?
- If you think that some of the diseases on your list are no longer a threat, what factors have influenced this change?
- Are there any 'old' diseases that are still a major threat to public health? If so, why do you think this is?

Controlling communicable diseases in the twenty-first century – basic principles

To achieve effective control of infectious diseases, it is important to understand the ways in which they spread through populations. This involves not only identifying the 'source' of the infection (i.e. the pathogen causing the disease) but also the 'mode of transmission' and the 'susceptibility of the recipient'. As we saw above, the source of an infectious disease in the UK is usually viral or bacterial. Fungal infections (such as *candida*, which causes thrush and athletes foot) can also be transmitted from person to person, but do not usually cause serious illness, except in people whose immune system is already impaired. Other pathogenic organisms occasionally causing communicable diseases in the UK include protozoa (for example, *cryptosporidia*) and prions (abnormal protein particles thought to be responsible for BSE and vCJD). Some pathogens are transmitted directly, by close physical contact (including sexual contact). Others may be spread indirectly, for example: via infected food or a contaminated water supply; via an insect vector (such as fleas, ticks or mosquitoes); or through sharing inanimate objects. Some pathogens are also capable of airborne transmission (Donaldson and Donaldson, 2003). Box 9.1 contains some brief descriptions of main modes of transmission, together with examples of communicable diseases usually spread via each route. (However, please note that some pathogens can be transmitted by more than one route.)

Box 9.1 Main modes of transmission of communicable diseases

- **Airborne**: Many viral and bacterial respiratory infections are spread by airborne droplets, or aerosols, which are then inhaled. Pathogens transmitted in this way include the viruses responsible for the common cold and influenza, as well as bacteria causing infections such as Legionnaires' disease and TB. Infections such as measles, mumps, rubella and whooping cough are also usually transmitted by airborne droplets; though rubella can also be transmitted from a pregnant women to her unborn child across the placenta.
- **Food-borne**: A wide variety of human and animal pathogens can enter food at a number of stages in its production and preparation and cause gastro-intestinal infections. Common examples include salmonella and campylobacter, both of which

---

are frequent causes of food poisoning. Other examples of food-borne pathogens implicated in recent outbreaks of severe food poisoning include *E. coli* 0157.

- **Contaminated water**: Water-borne infections such as cholera and dysentery are now infrequent in the developed world, where there is access to clean water and safe disposal of treated sewage. However, the protozoan organism *cryptosporidium* has caused a number of outbreaks of diarrhoeal disease in the UK in recent years when domestic water supplies have become contaminated. The bacterium responsible for Legionnaires' disease is sometimes categorised as water-borne, as it is found in environments such as showers, whirlpool spas and air conditioning systems, though it is usually transmitted to humans by aerosols (see above).

- **Sexually transmitted diseases**: Many infectious diseases can be transmitted directly, by sexual contact. These include HIV/AIDS, gonorrhoea, syphilis and chlamydia. Sexually transmitted infections (STIs) are of particular importance to public health, because of the challenge they present in terms of surveillance and control, as well as their potential impact on the health of the population.

- **Blood-borne**: Blood-borne viruses (BBVs) such as HIV/AIDS and hepatitis B and C pose a potential risk to health care workers, especially those who experience needle-stick injuries or come into contact with contaminated blood. Other groups at risk of contracting blood-borne viruses include injecting drug users who share needles.

- **Vertical transmission**: Pregnant mothers can pass a number of infections to their unborn babies, across the placental barrier. HIV, congenital syphilis and rubella can all be transmitted in this way.

- **Other**: There are a number of other ways in which infectious diseases can be transmitted. These include animal bites (for example, rabies), insect bites (malaria) and via fomites (objects harbouring an infectious agent).

(Adapted from Donaldson and Donaldson, 2003 and Gillam, 2007)

Communicable disease epidemiologists usually work with a theory of disease causation referred to as the 'epidemiological triangle,' which sees diseases as the product of an interaction between an agent, a host and the environment (Locker, 1997: 20). This takes account of the major limitation of germ theory – i.e. that not everyone exposed to a pathogen will necessarily become ill. Whether or not a person develops an infectious disease after contact with any given pathogen will depend on whether or not they are a 'susceptible recipient'. This is influenced by a number of factors, including their age, general health, nutritional status, previous exposure, whether or not they have been immunised and so on (Donaldson and Donaldson, 2003).

Public health interventions to prevent and control communicable diseases are frequently targeted at the mode of transmission – for example, typhoid and cholera can be prevented by the safe disposal of sewage and the provision of uncontaminated drinking water (Donaldson and Donaldson, 2003: 369) and many of the organisms causing food poisoning can be controlled by good food hygiene, not only within the home, but also across all stages of the production process. Host susceptibility to a number of infectious diseases can be reduced by effective vaccination programmes – for example, diphtheria, tetanus and whooping cough; measles, mumps and rubella; and poliomyelitis. Communicable disease control experts frequently argue that, together with sanitation, vaccines are the most effective means of disease prevention currently available (Noah, 2006).

Communicable diseases: the current situation

Many of the epidemics that affected Victorian Britain were gradually brought under control by a combination of a general rise in living standards (particularly in terms of improved housing conditions and better nutrition) and sanitary reform (the introduction of clean water and safe disposal of sewage). During the twentieth century, the introduction of vaccines and antibiotics also played a significant part. Nevertheless, at the beginning of the twenty-first century, infectious diseases continue to pose a major threat to the health of populations, especially in low-income countries, where children are often the group worst affected. Estimates suggest that 41 per cent of the global burden of disease, and 25 per cent of deaths worldwide, are caused by infectious diseases. Three diseases, HIV/AIDS, Malaria and TB, are together responsible for more than 13 million deaths worldwide every year (DoH, 2002a).

However, the threat to health from infectious diseases is by no means confined to low-income countries. Although the decline in deaths from infectious diseases which occurred in developed countries throughout the late nineteenth and early twentieth century has been dramatic, the hope that all infectious diseases could eventually be eradicated by a combination of immunisation and antibiotic therapy has so far proved unfounded. The development of an effective vaccine for some diseases (most notably, HIV/AIDS) still seems to be some years away, and antimicrobial resistance is becoming an increasing area of concern. Resistant strains already exist in many common pathogens, including those causing TB and malaria, and multi-resistant *Staphyloccus aureus* (MRSA) is a frequent cause of hospital-acquired infections.

Since the 1970s, a number of new infectious diseases have been identified (for example, HIV/AIDS, Legionnaires' disease and SARS) and some diseases previously thought to be under control, such as TB, have 're-emerged' as a serious threat to public health (Coker, *et al.*, 2005). Within the UK, there have been a number of high-profile community and hospital-acquired outbreaks of infectious diseases over recent years, leading policy-makers to acknowledge the need to strengthen arrangements for communicable disease surveillance and control (DoH, 2002a). There has also been a growing recognition of the role of globalisation in influencing both the impact of infectious diseases and the public health response to them (Weinberg, 2005). Examples of some high-profile outbreaks of infectious diseases which have influenced public health policy in England are given in Box 9.2.

Box 9.2 Some examples of high-profile disease outbreaks

- **Legionnaires' disease:** There have been a number of outbreaks of this severe form of pneumonia since its first appearance in the 1970s. The name is derived from the first recorded outbreak, which occurred in the US in 1976, among a group of elderly people attending an American Legion convention. There were over 200 cases, which included 34 fatalities. The first cases of this new disease were diagnosed in the UK in 1977, and a series of outbreaks followed throughout the 1980s, usually associated with water-cooled air conditioning systems and cooling towers. A major outbreak in Stafford during 1985 affected 68 people, of whom 23 died (DoH, 2002a). This led to a Government Committee of Inquiry, which went on to influence changes in the way that public health services were organised in England through the 1990s.
- **BSE/nvCJD:** A new disease in cattle, Bovine Spongiform Encephalopathy (BSE) was first diagnosed in England in 1986. By the end of 2001, over 179 000 cows in Great Britain had

---

developed BSE (DoH, 2002a). At the height of the epidemic, in 1993, nearly 1 000 cases of BSE were being reported in British cattle every week. In 1995, a new form of Creutzfeld-Jacob disease (vCJD), also a spongiform encephalopathy, was detected in humans and further research provided evidence that the agent causing both diseases was the same. A Government advisory committee subsequently concluded that the most likely explanation for the emergence of vCJD was that it had been transmitted to people who had eaten meat from infected cattle (Donaldson and Donaldson, 2003: 381).

- **Salmonella**: There was a severe outbreak of salmonella food poisoning in 1984, in the Stanley Royd Hospital, Wakefield. It affected over half the patients in the hospital, and led to 19 deaths. This outbreak attracted a considerable amount of adverse publicity at the time, which included allegations of mismanagement at the hospital and criticisms of the way in which the outbreak was handled. A Committee of Inquiry was set up to investigate further. This found that food-handling procedures were not being followed, and that this failure had contributed to the outbreak of disease.

- **Severe Acute Respiratory Syndrome (SARS)**: In February 2003, the outbreak of a severe acute respiratory infection, initially involving 300 cases and leading to five deaths, occurred in Southern China. This new human virus spread rapidly to Hong Kong and then to Singapore. Further cases were soon reported in other parts of South East Asia, and then in Canada. The WHO issued a global health alert, and declared SARS a worldwide health threat. As no vaccination or treatment was available, intensive public health measures (disease surveillance, case management, contact tracing, advice to the public on travel to South East Asia, etc.) were required to bring the outbreak under control (Noah, 2006).

- **_E. coli_ 0157**: Most _E. coli_ bacteria found in humans are harmless, but some strains produce toxins that can cause serious illness and sometimes death. In 1996 an outbreak of Vero-toxin producing _E. coli_ 0157 occurred in Preston, associated with consumption of commercially-produced beefburgers. Another outbreak, in Lanarkshire Scotland during 1996, caused serious illness in 496 people and resulted in 17 deaths. Following this outbreak, the government appointed Professor Hugh Pennington to lead an expert group to advise on the implications for food safety and lessons learned. Despite the work undertaken by Professor

Pennington and his colleagues, outbreaks of *E. coli* 0157 continue to occur. In 2005, an outbreak in South Wales, linked to a local meat supplier, affected 44 schools, and resulted in the death of a five-year old child. More than 150 people were taken ill and 31 were admitted to hospital (DoH, 2001c; FSA, 2009).

OTHER ASPECTS OF HEALTH PROTECTION

Infectious diseases are only one of the threats to population health arising from the external environment (DoH, 2002a). Other examples of risks to health included under the remit of health protection include risks from chemical and radiation incidents. The rationale for this is twofold. Firstly, at the outset of an incident, it may not be immediately clear whether the cause is an infectious disease, or exposure to a non-infectious environmental hazard. Also, many of the systems for investigating and managing infections are broadly similar to those required for managing other environmental risks and hazards. Examples of some non-infectious incidents involving potential risk to population health, and causing widespread public concern, are highlighted in Box 9.3.

Box 9.3 Examples of health protection incidents involving chemical hazards

- **The Lowermore incident**: In July 1998, a lorry driver delivering a consignment of aluminium sulphate to a water treatment works near Camelford, in North Cornwall, mistakenly dumped 20 tonnes of this chemical into the wrong tank, contaminating the drinking water supply. Local residents experienced a number of unpleasant symptoms following this incident and demanded further investigation. This incident led to a series of detailed inquiries and to litigation. While major changes have been made to prevent such incidents occurring in future, there are still people who feel that all their concerns have not been met, and research into the potential longer-term effects of this incident continues (adapted from DoH, 2002a: 122–123).

- **Buncefield oil depot fire**: in December 2005, an oil depot containing diesel oil, kerosene and aviation fuel exploded in Hemel Hempstead. The resulting fire took four days to bring under control, and caused a plume of dense black smoke over the area. Despite initial concerns about the potential health impact of this and air quality monitoring at the time of the incident, further investigations since have concluded that the risk to health was low. Public anxiety reduced during the weeks following the investigation. A recent report by the HPA has concluded that a number of lessons have been learnt from this incident that will enable them to respond better to future incidents (HPA, 2006a).

CURRENT ARRANGEMENTS FOR HEALTH PROTECTION

The Health Protection Agency (HPA) was established in 2003, in response to recommendations set out in *Getting Ahead of the Curve: A Strategy for Combating Infectious Diseases* (DoH, 2002a). This strategy established a number of priorities for action in relation to the present and future threat from infectious diseases, and proposed the setting up of a new national agency to act as a source of expertise in health protection (DoH, 2002a). The HPA brought together a number of functions previously provided by local communicable disease consultants in the NHS and national structures such as the Public Health Laboratory Service, the Centre for Applied Microbiology and Research and the National Focus for Chemical Incidents. Since its establishment, it has continued to grow. The National Radiological Protection Board and the National Institute for Biological Standards and Control are now also part of the HPA. The current structure is based around the Centre for Infections at Collingdale, the Centre for Emergency Preparedness and Response at Porton, and the Centre for Radiation, Chemical and Environmental Hazards at Chilton. However, it has a large network of staff based regionally and locally throughout England (different arrangements are in place in Scotland and Wales), mostly in local health protection units (see below). Other organisations involved in health protection at a national level include the Department of Health, the Department for Environmental and Rural Affairs, the Food Standards Agency, the Health and Safety Executive, the Environment Agency and the Drinking Water Inspectorate. The HPA works with these organisations as appropriate, depending on the nature of the risk involved.

Local Health Protection Units

There are currently 26 local Health Protection Units (HPUs) in England. These units are part of the HPA, but work very closely with the NHS and local government to provide an integrated health protection service. HPUs are staffed by a range of professionals, including consultants in communicable disease control (CCDCs), nurses with expertise in infection control and other public health specialists. They are supported in this work by regional and national structures and specialist expertise (see above).

Current functions of the HPA include primary prevention, surveillance, investigation and control of any hazard to health arising from infectious diseases, chemical and poisons, or radiation incidents. To achieve this it:

- monitors and investigates occurrences of infections, locally and nationally;
- provides specialist and reference laboratory services;
- investigates outbreaks of disease and coordinates the response to major epidemics or other infectious disease emergencies;
- provides authoritative information and advice to government, professionals and the public;
- manufactures vaccines and studies safety and effectiveness;
- undertakes research and development.

An example of how multiple agencies worked together in addressing a chemical incident is presented in Box 9.4 below.

Box 9.4 Case study: multi-agency support to chemical incident management

A significant level of multi-agency working and coordination is required to provide effective advice and support to front-line health protection practitioners and emergency services dealing with accidental exposures to chemical substances.

Early in February 2009, a local fire and rescue service dealt with an unusual incident involving a 23-acre facility, some 100 feet underground and in a former mine, used for storage of ex-military equipment. Fire had been detected in a five-acre chamber, initially thought to have been caused by a fork lift truck igniting. Response was severely hampered by thick smoke and the complexity of the underground site layout, and a decision was made to withdraw and consider how to contain the blaze. All outlets from the underground areas were sealed to prevent emissions and reduce available oxygen.

The site operator was able to provide a vital snapshot of potential hazards such as the extent of asbestos cement linings throughout and also an inventory of the stored equipment. Hazard identification and risk assessment focused initially on potential exposure to white asbestos fibres, detached and airborne, as a result of fire damage. However, previous research by the HPA has shown that the risk of exposure in this type of incident is very low. In the interim, advice from the Mines Rescue Service led to the introduction of controlled quantities of liquid nitrogen into the sealed space to reduce temperature and available combustion air.

Consideration of potential releases of toxins and other harmful substances from heat-damaged, stored electrical equipment included:

- transformers (polychlorinated biphenyls);
- switch gear (mercury);
- control panels and motherboards (lead, copper and other metaliferous solders); and
- equipment casings and insulation (unsaturated hydrocarbons such as styrene).

The task for multi-agency responders was how best to advise on protecting nearby residents from exposure when the fire and its combustion products were eventually vented to surface level.

The public health response was led by the Director of Public Health from the NHS Primary Care Trust (PCT) supported by the Environment Agency and HPA specialists, including:

- medical health protection consultants and nurses from the local HPU (support and specialist advice to PCT);
- environmental health scientists and risk assessment experts from the Chemical Hazards and Poisons Division (health effects and properties of hazardous emissions and design of monitoring and sampling);

- Environment Agency inspectors (environmental effects monitoring); and
- communications managers from HPA Regional Office, fire, police, Primary Care Trust and county council emergency planning service (risk communication and promulgation of public health advice).

Further support was enlisted from:

- Met Office atmospheric modelling teams (providing constant weather and wind predictions and specialised dispersion modelling capacity);
- asbestos and air quality sampling teams tasked by Environment Agency, county council emergency planning and the Primary Care Trust.

When the fire was eventually extinguished, the underground spaces were ventilated to atmosphere, under controlled conditions determined by the multi-agency coordination group. The comprehensive range of skills and expertise brought together to support the incident ensured that this final phase of the incident was safely completed with adequate protection for public health.

(This case study is reproduced with the kind permission of Mike Studden of the Health Protection Agency's Environmental Health and Risk Assessment Unit, Stonehouse, Gloucestershire.)

CONCLUSION

The potential threats to health from infectious diseases and non-infectious environmental hazards such as chemicals, poisons and radiation are varied and complex. This chapter has introduced you to some of these hazards, and begun to explore many of the ways in which public health practitioners across a number of organisations are working together to reduce and/or contain these hazards. It has focused particularly on the issue of communicable disease control, explaining why infectious diseases continue to be a public health issue in the twenty-first century, and introduced you to some of the principles underpinning communicable disease control, as well as the agencies involved in health protection more generally. However, health protection is a large field of work and it has only been possible to scratch the surface in an introduction such as this. For those who wish to find out more, a great deal of information on all aspects of health protection, including communicable disease control, is available on the Health Protection Agency website. Some suggestions for further reading are also given below.

Further reading

Hawker, J., Begg, N., Blair, I., Reintjes, R. and Weinberg, J. (2005) *Communicable Disease Control Handbook* (2nd Ed). Oxford: Wiley-Blackwell
This book has been written for those working in the field of communicable disease control. It is comprehensive, clearly laid out and written in a style that makes it accessible for students as well as experts.

Useful website

The Health Protection Agency: **www.hpa.org.uk** (accessed 15 July 2009)

Chapter 10

Health needs assessment

Jill Stewart, Yvonne Cornish and Swatee Patel

This chapter explores a range of health needs assessment (HNA) approaches and their increasing importance in the fair and equitable distribution of limited resources to meet health needs at a local level. It provides an overview of where to source data and examples of how HNA can be used in practice.

Learning outcomes

In this chapter you will learn how to:

- define and discuss health needs assessment;

- discuss the concepts of health and need;

- understand how health and need can be measured, giving examples;

- provide a range of examples of HNAs and their suitability to a given application in helping ensure sufficient allocation of resources.

WHAT IS A HEALTH NEEDS ASSESSMENT?

The purpose of health needs assessment (HNA) is to identify the health assets and needs of a given population to inform decisions about service delivery to improve health and reduce health inequalities. The HNA role for Primary Care Trusts (PCTs), local authorities (LAs) and other health agencies is: to determine and justify service priorities and targets; to strengthen links with GP practices and public health programmes; to inform strategic partnership activities; and to identify staff and training needs. HNAs provide the opportunity to build alliances with other agencies and the community, to focus activity and to meet government objectives to provide services to those in greatest need.

HNAs are becoming increasingly important to the inclusion agenda in addressing inequality by concentrating on where needs are greatest and delivering resources accordingly. They may challenge existing conceptions about resource delivery and profile health and needs more accurately so that resources are targeted to where they will have most impact. HNAs help to address health inequalities by recognising health determinants; to concentrate resources on areas or communities of greatest need; to challenge existing conceptions about resource delivery; and to map health and need, analyse overlaps and relationships and develop local integrated solutions that recognise and take into account environmental health determinants. They increasingly play an advocacy role for marginal communities.

PCTs and LAs are now required to produce a Joint Strategic Needs Assessment (JSNA) of the health and wellbeing of their local community (see also Chapters 5 and 18). This involves stakeholders, engaging with communities and linking to other strategies. It helps inform local commissioning, based on locally-led decisions. The objectives are to enhance service outcomes and improve accountability. An overriding emphasis is on partnership work focusing on local health and wellbeing issues so that they are better understood and addressed (DoH, 2007).

HEALTH

Health is a dynamic and holistic concept. It has physical and emotional dimensions and social, sexual, spiritual, environmental and societal contexts. It can be difficult to reach a shared meaning of health and it is a contested topic, with different people assigning different meanings. Negative definitions of health are concerned with an absence of disease and epidemiologists tend to work with the simple dichotomy of disease being present or absent according to normality or abnormality, with diagnosis based on symptoms, signs or test results. For this reason, epidemiologists need definitions that are clearly stated, easy to use and understand and easy to measure.

The most commonly referred to positive definition of health is that of the World Health Organisation (WHO) (1946): 'A state of complete physical, mental and social wellbeing and not merely the absence of disease or infirmity'. Positive definitions also refer to the ability of an individual or group to realise aspiration and cope with their environment. It can therefore be seen as a resource – even foundation – for living, concerned with social, personal and physical capabilities and empowerment and enables people to cope with stress, maintain relationships and have peace of mind (Seedhouse, 2001; Ewles and Simnet, 1999; Naidoo and Wills, 2000).

Lay concepts of health take a wider understanding of health and take account of people's own experience of illness and disease. Blaxter (1995), for example, demonstrated that lay perceptions of health include factors such as being 'not ill', a reserve of energy, behaviour, physical fitness, social relations and psychosocial wellbeing.

Sociologists of health, illness and medicine distinguish between illness and disease. They see illness as describing people's experience of symptoms such as pain, discomfort or feeling generally unwell. They use disease to describe a pathological state and a deviation from the biological norm, whether the patient perceives this as illness or not.

Each definition has strengths and weakness in relation to finding consensus for a health needs assessment and the definitions are contested. Health means different things to different people in different roles. Meanings change over time and across different cultures. This has clear implications for how epidemiologist and health researchers measure health and disease; how public health practitioners undertake health needs and impact assessments; and how health promotion specialists work to improve individual and community health; and there are also implications for service planning and use.

NEED

Need is a 'gap' somewhere in the provision of, and access to, health and health care. It has already been established that health inequalities exist, which suggest a differential in need: some individuals and communities are in greater need than others. Need, however, takes on different contexts according to who is assessing it. An individual or community may or may not see that they have needs and the government or health care provider may or may not identify that community's need in a similar way, because of their own objectives and ideologies. Need is a dynamic concept about what a current heath status is and what it should – or perhaps could – be.

Maslow (1954, cited in Naidoo and Wills, 2000) suggests that all human needs are health needs. Maslow categorises need into a hierarchy starting with basic physiological needs (hunger, thirst) at the bottom, rising to safety (feeling secure and out of danger), belongingness and love (concerned with relationships, belonging), esteem (achievement, gaining approval and recognition) to self-actualisation (fulfilling one's potential) at the top of the hierarchy.

Doyal and Gough (1991) focus on 'fundamental rights' and develop Maslow's perspective that in order for human beings to be able to participate fully in society, their needs must be met. They argue that fundamental rights – which focus largely around access to public health issues – include adequate nutritional food and clean water, adequate protective housing, non-hazardous physical and working environments, appropriate health care, security in childhood, significant primary relationships, security, education, safe birth control and safe child rearing.

However, Bradshaw (1994, cited in Popay and Williams, 1994) provides a different perspective and looks at need from the perspective of those who are determining it. Bradshaw places need into four categories as normative needs, felt needs, expressed needs and comparative needs, which helps provide a basis for the perspective of the person or organisation identifying need:

- **Normative needs** are defined in a professional's judgment about how a person deviates from an established or predefined standard. Normative needs are judged in relation to what intervention is able to be provided, by the provider;
- **Felt needs (or service needs)** are about what people want, or about how a person feels, and therefore have a subjective dimension, which can be limited by the perception or cultural background of the person;
- **Expressed needs** exist when felt needs are requested. Service provision may not reflect felt need, but may be all that is available, and may be accepted due to lack of alternate provision opportunity. Clearly, people and communities (as well as service providers) are differentially empowered in their needs and, indeed, in accessing appropriate interventions; and
- **Comparative needs** relate to people or communities sharing similarities, where needs relate differential access to similar people or communities, and this is a matter of equity and similar provision for similar need and may be based on resource availability.

It is important to assess need so that the health of a given community can be improved, health potential can be maximised, variations and inequalities in health can be reduced and that resources are delivered equitably. A joint understanding and agreement on what constitutes need is therefore key in community empowerment, in being able to challenge existing medical provision and being able to seek alternative complementary therapy interventions to tackle ill health and to help promote wellbeing.

Other ways of looking at need

A great deal of work was carried out in the early 1990s to help understand 'need'. One example was the Department of Health's Project discussion paper (NHS Management Executive, 1991), which identified three approaches:

- epidemiological;
- comparative assessment; and
- corporate.

Epidemiological needs assessment

Epidemiological assessment has probably been the most influential model in public health. It is disease-based, looks at incidence and prevalence, the ability to treat and the cost-effectiveness of this. Stevens (1991) took an epidemiological approach to HNA, defining 'need' as the ability to benefit from health care interventions, and this approach is still very influential in the NHS, both in developing new services and reconfiguring existing services. This led to a series of epidemiological reviews for the Department of Health based on the paradigm of need, demand and supply (Stevens and Raftery, 1997).

Need is defined as a dynamic, rational concept that people can benefit from. Demand is what people ask for, and is changeable. It can be influenced by social and educational background, media and medical professionals. Supply, on the other hand, is what is actually provided, which is also subject to change and is influenced by the public, political and professional factors, economics, technology and so on. There is a range of information sources to help establish (medical) need. Utilisation rates measure supply, which may or may not be needed, and may or may not be supplied. Waiting lists measure demand, which again may or may not be needed, and may or may not be supplied.

Comparative needs assessment

Comparative needs assessment compares health performance across and between local communities, disease groups, client groups, services providers and so on, and is important in the debate around equity and health inequality. Sources of information can be local, including data on the local population, local service provision and local health status as compared with national or other similar local (or even international) settings.

Corporate needs assessment

Corporate needs assessment combines the views of professionals, local communities or groups, other interested parties and policy-makers. Eliciting views and ensuring that they and professional views are properly weighted requires skill.

Box 10.1: Epidemiological and corporate HNA: tackling teenage pregnancy in Brent

Teenage pregnancy has become an important government priority due to the UK's high rate of teenage conception and has been closely associated with a cycle of deprivation across generations.

Brent – an area with some of England's most deprived wards and around half its population belonging to an ethnic minority – saw teenage pregnancy rates increase between 1998 and 2003, and this was found to correlate closely to socio-economic and environmental disadvantage. Pillaye (2004) undertook an epidemiological and corporate approach to HNA, analysing conception rates, sexually transmitted infections and qualitative service mapping. A literature review identified effective interventions.

The epidemiological needs assessment used data from the Office for National Statistics (ONS), abortion data, sexually transmitted disease (STI) data, family planning services, community family clinics and Geographical Information System (GIS) from the local authority. The corporate needs assessment relied on a participative inquiry workshop to glean knowledge and generate ideas from stakeholders, experts, community and voluntary groups. Teenagers' and stakeholders' views were obtained via focus groups and participatory workshops.

The findings were that services were erratic and uncoordinated with less offered in the more deprived wards where need is highest. Brent teenagers had varying levels of understanding about contraception and felt that services offered were inaccessible due to timing or location, and that teenagers were concerned they might meet someone they knew, breaching their confidentiality. Results were used to plan local service improvements. Brent teenagers needed more information on sexual health at an earlier age through targeted, youth-focused services with reference to community risk factors. It is clear that teenage sexual behaviour and pregnancy rates are multi-faceted and that appropriate and timely messages in a trusting, friendly and confidential environment are paramount to help break the cycle of deprivation by improving prevention and access services and to provide support for teenage parents.

Source: adapted from Pillaye (2004), with permission.

Need – demand – supply

One current problem in 'need' is that it is still frequently seen from a medical model and perspective that is generally about the absence of disease, rather than the promotion of socio-economic status, wellbeing, self-esteem, etc. In this respect, need often relates to existing, reactive medical data where gaps in provision are normally represented by data in the form of statistics. The data is normally negative, and emphasises what is needed in provision, not what communities may feel they need – or may even know exists – as part of a bottom-up approach with potential clients at the centre of needs assessment. Using qualitative data can help focus on positive health-related issues as a subjective reality, relating to emotional and social wellbeing, where complementary therapies may prove very appropriate as interventions.

To reduce health inequality, it is therefore necessary to assess the current health of a community through a health needs assessment before jointly deciding appropriate strategic interventions arising from joint agreement on definitions of health and need from all perspectives.

MEASURING HEALTH AND DISEASE FOR HNA

There are many sources available for qualitative and quantitative data. Quantitative data tends to focus on what is missing (negative) and emphasises what is needed. Conversely qualitative data can focus on positive health-related issues, including social capital (see Chapter 14), and can help provide baseline evidence and data to map progress in reducing health inequalities.

Epidemiology is the study of disease and risk factors in populations, providing a key method for population health surveillance. Epidemiology informs service planning and delivery and can be used to assess the health needs of local populations and communities and to underpin service monitoring and evaluation.

The International Classification of Disease (ICD) is produced by the WHO and is periodically revised. It is used by many countries as the principal means of classifying and coding mortality and morbidity. In the UK, there has been a legal requirement to register deaths since the early nineteenth century, which is organised by the Office for National Statistics (ONS) through local Registrars. Deaths are certified by doctors and statistics returned weekly to the ONS. The quality of this data is extensive and accurate. It is often used as a proxy for disease (morbidity).

Descriptive epidemiology describes the occurrence of disease in terms of person, place and time.

- **person** – characteristics of people who are affected by disease, in terms of age, sex, social class, etc;
- **place** – where people are geographically (local, regional, national and international) when they get diseases and how incidence and prevalence vary;
- **time** – when people get diseases and how it changes over time.

An example of person, place and time of disease is illustrated in Patel, Jarvelin and Little (2008), where a complete review of worldwide variations of asthmatic symptoms in children is reported in all studies published over a 16-year period between 1990 and 2005. This review reports the ages of children, the place and time of the study, and reports that the rate of increase in asthmatic symptoms was significantly higher in Australia than the UK.

Disease can be measured by mortality (deaths) or morbidity (incidence or prevalence).

Mortality

Mortality data is good for comparing causes of death across and between different populations and is an important part of epidemiological and comparative needs assessment. It can be used by epidemiologists to describe the health status of a population and to investigate causal links and risk factors. The rate of mortality is a unit of measurement as a numerator (number of deaths), denominator (population at risk) and time (period under consideration). Crude death rates are usually expressed as deaths per 1 000, or 10 000 for rarer conditions.

It is more usual to use standardised mortality rates. These take into account the age or sex structure of the population and allow experience to be compared, such as data from a local study being compared with data for a whole country or another similar area.

Morbidity

Measuring disease, or morbidity, is less straightforward as there is no single, routine source of information, or any overall comprehensive picture. Data is normally incomplete due to undercounting and it may not be fully valid or fully extensive. Morbidity is expressed by incidence and prevalence. Incidence is the number of new cases of a specific disease or condition in a given person. Prevalence is the number of people with a particular disease/condition at a given time (point prevalence) during a given period (period prevalence). Although incidence and prevalence do not equate with need, they are both important in describing the population burden of disease. Incidence is the number of new cases with disease in a specified period (for example, one year). Prevalence is the total number of cases, existing cases plus new cases, as a proportion of the total population, at a given point in time (point prevalence) or during a given period (period prevalence, for example, one year).

Sources of health information in the UK

Sources of health information include disease data sets. The Cancer Intelligence Unit maintains records of individual cancer notification and provides aggregate data by age, sex, type, site, stage and so on. Disease registers are largely under the auspices of primary care and are being increasingly established in areas such as asthma, CHD, diabetes and so on. Infectious disease data is collected by the Health Protection Agency (see Chapter 9) for notifiable diseases including anthrax, cholera, mumps, rabies and others.

There are other more qualitative ways of collecting data at national and local levels on health and lifestyle. These include the Health Survey for England and, at a more local level, Healthquest (for the South East of England). The General Household Survey includes information on acute and chronic conditions, the use of health services and smoking and drinking habits.

Wellbeing and quality of life are of increasing importance in public health and information sources include the General Health Questionnaire, EuroQol or EQ5D and SF36. There are other tools in use or being developed, including level of social deprivation (SES, IMD) and concepts such as social capital.

Routine sources of data can only provide limited descriptions of disease. For more detail on the possible links between disease and possible risk factors, special surveys may be required. There are three main types of epidemiological surveys: prevalence surveys (cross-sectional), longitudinal survey (cohort studies), and case-control studies (usually used for rare diseases such as childhood leukemia). It is important to identify the possible risk factors of disease, to aid prevention of disease and hence reduce the burden of health needs.

Undertaking an epidemiological survey costs time and money and there should be a clear aim for the study. What disease and risk factors are being measured? What is a case definition in terms of disease? What is the population of interest? It is essential to calculate the correct sample size for the survey and this is done on the basis of a balance between the need for precision (the more precise the estimates of incidence and prevalence required, the larger the sample size) and available resources in terms of time and money. The next step is to decide on how individuals are to be selected for the survey. The most common sampling methods are simple random sampling, systematic sampling, stratified sampling, cluster sampling and so on. The questionnaire used should be reliable, valid and repeatable. Finally, a high response rate is essential for results to be generalisable to the population.

ASSESSING COMMUNITY HEALTH NEEDS

There has been a recent revival in community HNA arising from a combination of factors including public sector management, the modernisation agenda, delivery of care services, urban policy initiatives and a return to the concept of 'community'. The purpose of a community needs assessment is to assist local statutory and non-statutory agencies in exploring the need for a new or enhanced service. It has become of increasing importance in bidding for funds, such as Single Regeneration Budget or Lottery funding. For community workers, it is an initial stage in community development.

Community needs assessment is a wide-ranging concept. It differs due to the definition of community, the type of needs being assessed, who does the assessment and the methods used for the collection and analysis of data. The community may be classified as being a geographical community, an institutional community or a community of interest (Percy-Smith, 1996). A geographical community is locality-based and may comprise neighbourhoods, electoral ward, Primary Care Trust (PCT) population, or housing estate. It may include the resident population only, or all those who live and work there. An institution-based community may include a service provider, school, hospital or nursing home and may be an assessment of those who live there or an assessment of those who use its services. A community of interest is independent of locality and may be dispersed. It is based on shared interest, values and identity and may, for example, comprise older people, young mothers or an ethnic community.

Methods of HNA depend on its purpose: for example, whether it is for advocacy or an agency requirement. It is subject to resources and, as such, depends on resources available, including money, time, those involved, expertise required and equipment required. Data sources may be primary, secondary, qualitative and/or quantitative. The approach may be participative or non-participative.

Participatory health needs assessment

A participatory needs assessment is both an approach and a set of methods that involves the community at all stages of the process, so that both the task and process are equally important (see, for example, Wainwright, 1994 and Box 10.2; Rowley and Bhuhi, 1999).

Participatory health needs assessment is used to identify a range of needs, including health needs, social needs, environmental needs or a combination of these, and it can help to assist communities in identifying their own needs. It is linked to community development and aims to help communities mobilise their own resources. Participatory needs assessment aims to bring about change in local communities through developing consultation, advocacy and relationships (partnerships) with local groups. A range of methods may include collection and collation of secondary data and usually includes standard social science research methods such as interviews and focus groups. Other methods may include rapid participatory appraisal and citizens' juries and panels.

Box 10.2: Participative HNA

The Waterfront Health Action Project (WHAP) at Greenwich and Bexley

Wainwright (1994) provided a (then) new focus for HNA, moving away from a 'professionals know best' and 'market is the best provider' perspective, towards a new form of participative needs assessment focusing around communities themselves. This provided a context of a HNA in terms of people's wants, and what others perceive them to need.

The Waterfront Health Action Project (WHAP) at Greenwich and Bexley was among the first in seeking a new approach to community needs assessment. It sought to develop skills and resources to identify community health needs based on rational inquiry, analysis and democracy. A main objective was to create an independent and critical body of knowledge with scientific validity, but also representing the needs of the population from their perspective.

The process involved professionals radically altering their own perspective, but using their skills of analysing statistical data and drawing rational conclusions. This enables professionals to look at problems through 'new eyes' and develop new strategies to address social and economic relations, not just to reconfigure existing agencies to fit perceived need.

Actioning WHAP's objectives took several months of outreach work and South East Thames Regional Health Authority grant aid for a community development worker who, in turn, contacted local community groups and individuals. This outreach work enabled subjective health concerns to be identified and other trained lay volunteers to become involved in the project.

The second part of the project involved a community health survey and a new partnership between professionals and volunteers. This led to a questionnaire that trained local volunteers could administer and that local residents understood, but that was also of sufficient scientific rigour. It covered health status, social and economic

---

position, lifestyle beliefs regarding causes of ill health, attitudes toward existing services and views of local heath actions. Analysis was statistical and also focused on the structure of power relations. The emphasis on group work with appropriate training meant that data was presented and discussed in a group forum and further information arising was able to be incorporated.

The final report included an account of current health status and an analysis of socio-economic and environmental influences on health. The report also included priorities for local health action, a critique of existing health service provision, and a report of local residents' views on community health action. Wainwright argues that such systematic and detailed assessment of health needs may be an early stage in overcoming some of the entrenched barriers people face in health, and it is about turning knowledge into practical activities. Source: adapted from Wainwright (1994), with permission.

Rapid participatory appraisal

Rapid participatory appraisal has been developed from ethnographical approaches used in anthropology. Key features may include interviews with key informants, focus groups and observation within the community. It is usually undertaken by key people working within commissioning and provider agencies.

There are advantages and disadvantages to rapid participatory assessments. They are usually small scale, carried out in a short time, and often used in deprived areas. They require time and commitment and those involved may unintentionally influence the findings. 'Key informants' may be self-selected and may not fully represent their community. In addition, some communities have been subjected to numerous attempts at social research and disheartened with few perceived changes as a result.

Participatory approaches to HNA are fundamentally about: identifying perceived needs of local communities; exploring how these impact on people's lives; developing creative solutions to the problems identified; and building capacity within the community to bring about changes that improve health and wellbeing (Ong and Humphries, cited in Popay and Williams, 1994).

CONCLUSIONS

HNA draws on a wide range of qualitative and quantitative data and measures a range of different concepts, including health, illness and disease. In carrying out a HNA it is necessary to have regard to the source and validity of the data and its robustness and to ensure that the correct approach is taken.

Further reading

Bowling, A. (2005) *Measuring Health: A Review of Quality of Life Measurement Scales* (3rd Ed). Buckinghamshire: Open University Press

Bowling, A. (2001) *Measuring Disease* (2nd Ed). Buckinghamshire: Open University Press
These are more specialist texts, aimed at researchers and written from a social science perspective.

Wright, J. (2001) 'Assessing health needs', in D. Pencheon, D. M. Guest, D. Melzer, J. A. Muir and J. A. Gray (eds) *Oxford Handbook of Public Health Practice*. Oxford: Oxford University Press
This provides a brief but comprehensive overview from a public health perspective.

Coles, L. and Porter, E. (2008) *Public Health Skills – A Practical Guide for Nurses and Public Health Practitioners*. Oxford: Blackwell Publishing
This contains three chapters on various aspects of HNA:
1. Haughey, F., 'Assessing and Identifying Health Needs: Theories and Frameworks for Practice';
2. Carlson, C., 'Health Needs Assessment: Appraising and Measuring Need';
3. Acres, J., 'Needs Assessment' – very good, though it is quite epidemiolgical/public health medical in its approach.

NICE (2005) *Health Impact Assessment, Health Equity Assessment, Health Needs Assessment Publications December 2005*. London: NHS
These are practical approaches to help PCTs, LAs and other agencies to tackle health inequalities and target resources at the greatest need – this publication draws the (then) HDA publications together and provides information on the HIA gateway. See **www.nice.org.uk/ nicemedia/pdf/HiA_HEA_HNA_recent_pubs3_dec05.pdf** (accessed 20 February 2009).

Cavanagh, S. and Chadwick, K. (2005) *Health Needs Assessment: A practical guide*. London: HDA/NICE

Hooper, J. and Longworth, P. (2002) *Health Needs Assessment Workbook*. London: HDA
These are useful documents for HNA in practice.

Chapter 11

Health impact assessment

Evelyn Gloyn

Learning outcomes

In this chapter you will learn how to:

- briefly explain the concept of health impact assessment (HIA);
- identify various approaches to HIA;
- appraise the current practical use of health impact assessment;
- recognise where health impact assessment sits within current government policy.

INTRODUCTION

Through all levels of decision-making, from local authority/Primary Care Trust level to global/international level, policies, projects, programmes and plans do not have health as a primary, or even nominal, objective, yet may have major implications for the health and wellbeing of individuals and the population. These health implications, or impacts, may be positive, neutral or negative, yet often decisions are made without an assessment of the available evidence of the impacts on health. Health impact assessment (Scott-Samuel, 1998; WHO, 1999; Cave and Curtis, 2001a; Joffe and Mindell, 2002) can add value to the decision-making process by predicting possible implications for health and by putting in place consensual improvements to mitigate, maintain or enhance levels of health, and reduce health inequalities, arising from those policies, projects, programmes or plans. It is a tool, or process, to support decision-making; it is not a decision-making tool.

The main concepts and approach to health impact assessment (HIA) were encapsulated in the Gothenburg Consensus (WHO, 1999). It is based on principles of democracy, equity, sustainable development and ethical use of evidence. The implication from this is that it should be a tool used objectively and independently of any decision-making. The approach considers evidence about expected relationships between policy and the health of a population; engagement with those affected; and provides informed understanding to enable changes to maximise positive health effects, and minimise negative health effects.

HIA can be defined as, 'a combination of procedures, methods and tools by which a policy, program or project may be judged as to its potential effects on the health of a population, and the distribution of those effects within the population' (WHO, 1999: 4). Note that the term 'project' throughout this chapter is used to denote 'policies, projects, programmes and plans'.

STEPS TO HEALTH IMPACT ASSESSMENT

HIAs generally follow a five-step sequence:

1. Screening

Is an HIA worth the time and effort? This would consider if it is plausible that the outputs or outcomes from the project will affect health. The size and quality of HIA produced should be proportionate to the policy or project being influenced.

2. Scoping

How will the HIA be conducted? This defines what the HIA will, and will not, cover, the level of resources available to conduct the HIA, potential pathways that may impact health, what kind of evidence to use, the timeframe available, how it will influence the decision-making process, how (or, for some practitioners, whether) to involve participation, a communication strategy (that explains the why, who, how, what and when), how it should be managed and how to monitor and evaluate the HIA process and its outcomes.

3. Appraisal

The what, if and when questions. This includes collection and examination of the different types of evidence from a range of disciplines and sources, each with its own limitations and concerns about research methodologies and discussions on reliability and validity. Analysis of the evidence seeks to identify and define the nature of those impacts, such as the likelihood, the magnitude, the distribution and the (positive, neutral or negative) direction of impact and, in addition, should seek out evidence on what works to change the impact. There are three types: rapid or desk-top (one to two people taking a few hours or a day); intermediate (two or more people taking days or a week); and comprehensive (a multi-disciplinary team taking weeks or months). Findings can often challenge assumptions made about health impacts.

4. Recommendations and engagement (decision-making)

'Who' and 'so what?' Projects are often implemented on the assumption that they are good for health, yet health impacts are rarely checked for or measured. Another challenge is about communication and negotiation; how to present the evidence and communicate health risk to health-literate and non-health audiences, and how to feed ideas into decision-making processes and elicit engagement from key decision-makers. Timeliness is essential; if remedial or preventative work is planned for implementation how may it reap benefits for the future?

5. Monitoring and evaluation

Does it achieve what it sets out to do? This learning is essential to improve the process of HIA, assess the accuracy of predictions made during appraisal and modify future proposals to achieve health gain. Publishing HIAs, both positive and unexpected, can add to collective learning and reflective practice. Kemm (WHO, 2007) notes that process evaluation can show if timing and content are appropriate and likely to have influenced the final decision, if the methods in the appraisal are robust and likely to produce an accurate prediction, and if participation has been effective. Outcome evaluation takes more commitment, planning, resources and time; it is an area for ongoing and future research.

Activity 11.1 Reflective exercise: objectivity and outcomes

The design and implementation of an HIA should ensure that there are no presumed outcomes; otherwise it would merely become a collection of data to support those outcomes. Which of the steps above would be essential to ensuring this does not happen?

APPROACHES TO HIA

Early approaches to HIA suggested that they could be prospective (done before implementation of the project), concurrent (conducted during implementation) or retrospective (after implementation). However Kemm (in WHO, 2007) suggests that HIA are about prediction so must be prospective; a concurrent HIA would be monitoring and a retrospective HIA an evaluation. HIA has developed out of environmental impact assessment, a legal requirement since 1988 (SI, 1988 [listed under Legislation, page 163) but limited 'to take account of concerns to *protect*

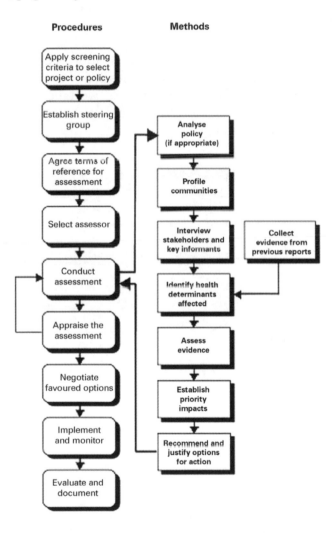

Figure 11.1 The Merseyside approach to HIA. Stages in the HIA process from the Merseyside Guidelines for Health Impact Assessment (Scott-Samuel. *et al.*, 2001). (Reproduced by kind permission of the International Health IMPACT Assessment Consortium.)

human health' (EEC, 1985), focusing on risk assessment and epidemiology and based on a biomedical model of health. Reviews and evaluations of various HIA models and frameworks have been undertaken by the London Health Commission (LHC, 1999), Mindell *et al.* (2008) and the World Health Organisation (WHO, 2007).

Since 1998 across the UK two main approaches have been used, using broader socio-economic models of health. The Merseyside approach (Scott-Samuel, 2001 2nd Ed.) was pioneered by Scott-Samuel, Birley and Arden, a team of public health professionals in Liverpool in 1998, to enable health risk to be integrated into regeneration projects. See Figure 11.1.

The Context-Mechanism-Outcome (CMO) approach was developed by Cave and Curtis (2001b), whose professional expertise is from a geographical and urban planning perspective working on regeneration projects in East London and aiming to 'ensure health gain while achieving a project's outcomes'. See Figure 11.2.

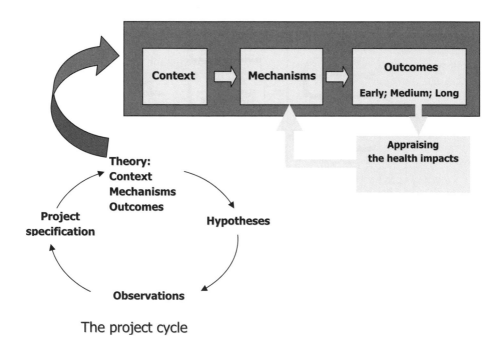

Figure 11.2 Context-Mechanism-Outcome approach to HIA. This shows the HIA process in terms of the project cycle (adapted after Cave and Curtis, 2001b).

Although both approaches follow the sequence of five steps, there is a different emphasis on each stage between the two approaches. See Table 11.1.

The CMO approach tends towards being more participatory and integrated; the Merseyside approach tends to fit with many local decision-making processes. In a global risk society (Beck, 1999) these approaches can support decision-making that in turn can lead to improved health effects and, more importantly, to redistribute those health effects within the population.

Five steps of HIA and different approaches		
HIA stage	**Merseyside**	**CMO**
Screening	Seeks to establish if a decision will be made in the foreseeable future *and* if that decision can be influenced.	Focuses on the project's outcomes, not necessarily health outcomes. It examines the context of the project and the mechanisms for the delivery of the project's planned outcomes. These include aspects of the local setting, and local knowledge and understanding of all stakeholders.
Scoping	Defines what is and is not within the HIA, its structure, content and reporting mechanisms.	Collects further information about the aims of, and stakeholders in, the project, again not necessarily looking at health outcomes.
Appraisal	Collation of health data, profiling, modelling of likely impacts, synthesis of their magnitude and direction of impact.	Identifies potential health impacts within the context and mechanisms in place. This link to the context and mechanism of project delivery may help identify possible potential pathways. Evidence to either support or challenge these pathways is then mapped onto the local profile of the area/target group. Synthesis of magnitude and direction of impacts.

Five steps of HIA and different approaches (cont'd)		
HIA stage	**Merseyside**	**CMO**
Decision-making	Dependent on stakeholders adhering to the agreed reporting mechanism; risk of personnel change with varying levels of commitment to HIA process, and risk that the report loses its level of priority within the project management hierarchy, unless significant risks are logged. Often health impacts tend to show up a long time after the project has ended, and are unlikely to be a priority to a project risk log (focused on delivery of a project within time and budget, and sometimes within a political timeframe).	Feedback into the process of planning and implementation, with suggestions for how project activities can be adjusted to maximise the potential for health gain. Process is integrated with the project and therefore may have more opportunity to engage with key stakeholders.
Monitoring and evaluation	Systems for monitoring and evaluation need to be built into the HIA process.	Systems for monitoring and evaluation need to be built into the HIA process; however, these are more likely to be built into the monitoring and evaluation of the entire project, not just the HIA.

Table 11.1 Five steps of HIA and different approaches

Current policy-making makes two main assumptions: that planning for positive health outcomes will result in better population health; and that those outcomes will be evenly distributed. To help appraise the current practical use of HIA in the UK, and as a test to these assumptions, it is worth exploring the purpose and challenges to HIA.

THE PURPOSE OF HIA

The primary purpose is to predict possible implications for health. This is achieved by using evidence to identify potential health impacts and make an assessment, based on expected relationships. The evaluation of HIAs on the London Mayoral draft strategies (LHC, 2003) further noted that the HIA process identified positive and negative impacts, and identifying both helps to maintain beneficial aspects of a strategy.

The secondary purpose is to put in place consensual improvements for health. This is achieved through engagement with those affected and a better understanding of health impacts and factors affecting them. The World Health Organisation's (2007) evaluation of the effectiveness of HIAs across Europe between 2004–07 found evidence that changes were made within decision-making processes encompassing health recommendations and, in other cases, although the decision was unchanged, the process created a stronger health consciousness. Importantly, it found no evidence that HIAs were initiated to support a preferred policy option.

Key to these purposes is effective engagement. This is facilitated through the production of HIA documentation, but the quality is dependent on the robust research skills of the complier and their abilities to present information suitable for decision-making. Such information should include the likely health impacts of implementing different options, allowing decision-makers to make better trade-offs and decisions that are better for health (Kemm, 2007).

Informed understanding goes beyond reading an executive summary. It relies on the timely use of various media and techniques to give information to, and receive information from, a wide spectrum of people; professionals, politicians, pressure groups and the public. Thus engagement considers the opinions, experiences and expectations of those affected, and confirms or challenges the assumptions about the distribution of effects within the population. If done well, it can facilitate challenge and consensus regarding people's perception of health, help people gain a better understanding of risks to health, be involved and have some element of control over the prioritisation process, in itself a healthy process (Syme, 1994; Tarlov, 1996) and, above all, reflects the move towards civic society having an influence on policy that affects its members (Arnstein, 1969; DCLG, 2006; DH, 2004). This greater openness and involvement of the public is based on a psycho social model of health. However, there are challenges regarding the way in which evidence can be presented to the lay public, and how it is assessed and prioritised. At a population level, however, engagement builds a better understanding of health issues within a community, and creates social networks; elements required for 'bridging social capital' (Putnam, 2000) that may, in turn, address health inequalities. In London (LHC, 2003) the HIA process consolidated and evaluated evidence through literature reviews and stakeholder workshops for decision-makers to consider. This process facilitated better understanding of health issues among decision-makers and better co-operation between different agencies, enabling connections to be made between transport, economic development, waste and health, which may not otherwise have been made (LHC, 2003). Readers should also refer to Chapters 4 and 14 in particular, which discuss community participation and power as well as social capital.

CHALLENGES TO HIA

Resources

HIAs are considered to be time-consuming, although this is challenged by Kemm (WHO, 2007) on the grounds that the process is made to seem overly complicated. He believes there is no need for HIA-qualified professionals to conduct the work, although the London evaluation (LHC, 2003) notes that the availability of resources, particularly the ability to commission freelance researchers to undertake rapid reviews of the evidence from research, was noted as invaluable to the process.

Availability and type of evidence

In the past there has been a lack of evidence (Mindell, *et al.*, 2001), for example, local authority interventions are often not evaluated or documented, and meta-analyses are not part of the social science library, but over the past decade this has been getting better. However, in a modern risk-based society (Beck, 1999 cited in Curtis, 2008), the nature of evidence and how it is used is questioned by Curtis (2008). Risk is based on perception and estimates of uncertainty. Curtis argues that knowledge was once based on a consensus of professional experts (the medical paradigm), but now there is a range of views about knowledge, and also dissent and conflict over the rationality and principles between the various networks of experts, whether professional or those not within a recognised profession. This then brings uncertainty in how to manage the prediction of impacts on health. Kemm (WHO, 2007) counter-argues that an HIA based on sociological reasoning draws prediction information from what those affected think is likely to happen. This takes account of their fears, perceptions and experience of living in a community that is likely to be affected (Elliott and Williams, 2004 cited in WHO, 2007). A similar theme came from the London evaluation (LHC, 2003); how should different types of evidence be managed – should evidence from research take priority over stakeholder views if they contradict each other?

Stakeholder influence

There are concerns that outcomes can be railroaded or influenced by the more powerful stakeholders, relevant stakeholders may not be engaged, the evidence used may not be the best available, and there may not be any political commitment to carry through the implementation of recommendations. These concerns are particularly significant to timescales; timeliness of engaging stakeholders and the political election agendas as determinants of health can take extensive time to properly address.

HIA IN FOCUS

HIA differs from evaluation and research. Evaluation examines the extent to which the project's objectives have been achieved; research is applied to an intervention. There are similarities between evaluation and research, including defining the theoretical framework, reviewing the evidence base, and HIA may follow similar stages and be targeted to include the same population affected by evaluation or research activities. However, HIA is a process that itself may have an interventional effect, for example in raising awareness and engaging others in the project.

HIA uses theoretical frameworks and the results of research to make predictions. Kemm (WHO, 2007) recognises that potential pathways, or 'logic paths', are key to HIA prediction. These set out what will be changed by the implementation of possible decisions and how these changes will impact on health (Joffe and Mindell, 2002). An implemented decision may be expected to change various intermediate factors (such as employment, social capital, air quality, built and natural environment) which, in turn, produce changes in specified health outcomes. A further use of the potential pathway is to enable the challenging of assumptions and reveal knowledge gaps. At the recommendation stage potential pathways help to demonstrate positive or negative impacts.

A conceptual model of potential pathways relating to housing is captured in Figure 11.3. Each potential pathway can be researched independently, proactively looking for potential paths with both positive and negative impacts on health. Taking the box on neighbourhood satisfaction, for example, investment in the neighbourhood may provide more security and a better environment. This then impacts (both positively and negatively) on personal identity, control over housing, coping mechanisms especially in the workplace, and social networks. Other research shows how these in turn impact on personal health.

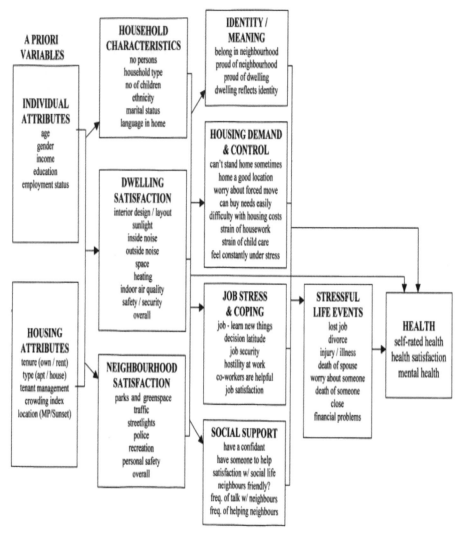

Figure 11.3 Conceptual model of housing and health pathways (see also Chapter 20), Dunn and Hayes (2000) 'Analytical model for housing and health regression analysis' reprinted from *Social Science and Medicine*, 51: 565, Copyright (2000), with permission from Elsevier.

A more recent example of a potential pathway (see Box 11.2 Case study) uses the cost-effectiveness of improving mental health in private rented properties with high burglary rates by introducing security measures such as installing 'Secured by design' windows and doors thus improving security (Nicholas *et al.*, 2005 cited in Green and Pugh, 2008); and assessing the impact of air pollution and deprivation on the health of lower-income residents (Sundquist *et al.*, 2004 cited in Green and Pugh, 2008).

Three case studies have been selected to illustrate aspects discussed above and these are presented in boxes 11.1, 11.2 and 11.3.

Box 11.1 Case study: HIA on the draft London Plan

The London Health Commission conducted an HIA on the spatial development of London in 2002. This followed the CMO approach and the process involved stakeholder and public engagement and came up with eight main recommendations:

- supporting community involvement and actively involving people in local governance;
- strengthening delivery through partnership working;
- vulnerable groups receiving mainstream attention;
- using planning conditions to benefit work opportunities;
- existing and new residents benefiting equally;
- regeneration agencies working together for evaluation and 'active learning';
- integrated impact assessment for new developments;
- maximisation existing resources.

A further impact assessment (IA) was undertaken in 2006 with a team looking at health issues arising from the alterations to the London Plan as part of a wider sustainability appraisal process. This endorsed:

good health as a key condition to enable both economic growth and sustainable development. Longer, healthier, more productive human lives deliver concrete economic benefits. Good health in this sense is the very foundation of thriving modern societies and economies, and needs to be defined in much broader terms than simply the prevention of illness. The concept of good health embraces life-long physical and mental wellbeing that is essential for people to lead meaningful, enjoyable and productive lives. (GLA, 2006, Introduction, p. iii)

Revisions to the London Plan prompted by the IA are listed as a table (GLA, 2006: 26–31) but of particular note is that there is now a greater emphasis on participation and community engagement, a recognition of the need to address issues associated with 'problem gambling' with a requirement for an action plan to mitigate its impacts, including contributions to meeting its additional health costs, and inclusion of indicators on health and health inequalities.

Source: adapted from LHC (2002) and GLA (2006)

Box 11.2 Case study: HIA on Sheffield housing policy (see also Chapter 20 on housing and health)

Sheffield First for Health and Well-being Partnership commissioned an HIA on their housing policy (Green and Pugh, 2008). This followed the Merseyside approach and listed recommendations on:

- **Access**: maintain and replenish a strong social housing sector to enhance the financial security and mental health of lower-income residents.
- **Affordability**: focus in the short term on measures to alleviate financial distress in the private housing market and maximise gains in mental health.
- **Housing quality**: cost-effective investment to improve health should focus on measures to improve security and warmth in private rented housing and in single pensioner households of all tenures.
- **Neighbourhoods**: a holistic model of successful neighbourhoods should balance environmental objectives with those for health, social cohesion and community safety.
- **Independence**: expand Sheffield's joint strategic needs assessment to include a cost-benefit analysis of housing's contribution to adding quality of life to years lived.
- **Inclusion**: provide evidence of health gain from securing a home for vulnerable and excluded people.

Source: adapted from Green and Pugh (2008)

Box 11.3 Case study: Belfast Community Health Impact Assessment

In 2004, Belfast Healthy Cities worked with two local communities to develop a Community Health Impact Assessment Project; one was a community-led HIA looking at proposals for water reform. Using elements from both the CMO and Merseyside approaches, its focus was on building capacity within the community, primarily by enhancing the skills and experience of individuals who are active within their own community, enabling them to participate more fully in future HIAs, perhaps assuming an advocacy role. The key stakeholders were selected by staff on the project and included elected representatives as well as representatives from local voluntary and community sector groups, local health and social care groups, and local housing providers. The main outcomes were a positive reception of the community profiles for each area, developed to help people understand the broader determinants of health, the ability to use the profiles to make bids for funding of local schemes, training days that brought people together from a wide range of backgrounds and experience, and the opportunity for people to extend their networks. Thus the communities were able to become involved in an appraisal of water reform from which recommendations were taken forward in the plans for water reform. The pilot project reports how the process raised health concerns but does not report on the extent to which the developers of the water reform proposal chose to implement the recommendations.

The HIA supported local decision-making by:

- raising awareness of health determinants and sustainable development;
- strengthening cross-sectoral policy implementation;
- providing a systematic framework to assess health impacts;
- promoting and integrating heath factors at local and strategic level;
- involving a range of stakeholders in planning, and encouraging awareness of participation.

Source: adapted from Belfast Healthy Cities (2004)

HEALTH IMPACT ASSESSMENT IN CURRENT UK POLICY

The UK government has shown commitment to the principle of prospective HIA with all four of the UK nations' consultative documents on public health strategy referring to the requirement for HIA of both national and local policies and projects (Secretary of State for Northern Ireland, 1997; Secretaries of State for Health, Scotland and Wales, 1998). However, over the past decade there has been an explosion in the number of impact assessments required, resulting in impact assessment fatigue. Since the issues covered in the different forms of assessment are similar they became incorporated into an integrated impact assessment (IIA). One example where IIA has been used would be the alterations to the spatial plan for London in Box 11.1 above.

Strategic environmental assessment (SEA) came into force in the UK on 20 July 2004 (SI, 2004[listed under Legislation, page 163]). The European Community Directive 2001/42/EC (European Union, 2001) requires a formal assessment for a wide range of plans and programmes (for example spatial, transport, and waste) of the likely significant effects on the environment of implementing the plan, including effects on population and human health both direct and indirect.

Specific impact tests (SITs) were introduced following a review of the Regulatory Impact Assessment guidance in 2006 by the Department for Business, Enterprise and Regulatory Reform (BERR). HIA is one of these. The driver for the review was to streamline the assessment process, focusing on the economic costs and benefits of policy-making. The new impact assessment (IA) became fully operational in 2007 and is used for proposals above £5m with sign-offs required at Options, Consultation and Final Proposal stages. The HIA screening questions are on the Department of Health's (DoH) website linked to the BERR Toolkit.

The commitments made in relation to HIA in the Health Inequalities Progress and Next Steps (DoH, 2008a) are:

- to consider how HIAs can be used more systematically and consistently;
- to improve the way these assessments are carried out by providing access to modelling tools as well as providing easy access to the evidence base and other support for these assessments;
- to develop the DoH's HIA tool, so it can be used more effectively to ensure that all policies support the government's objective of reducing health inequalities;

- to strengthen the health inequalities element of HIA through tools and support – including investment in improvement systems and support for commissioners;
- to ensure that the cross-government mandatory impact assessment, which includes HIA, is strengthened by emphasising the importance of considering health inequalities so that the impacts of cross-government policies on health inequalities are further understood and taken into account in policy-making.

The UK government has recognised that health is global (DoH, 2008b). As part of implementing the ten principles that underpin the 2008–13 strategy, the government will:

- use impact assessment to take greater account of the global health impact of and equity of foreign and domestic policies across government, as part of the new government impact assessment process;
- help reduce conflicts, to which end the DoH will support other departments in preparing global health impact assessments, which describe the global health impacts of their foreign and domestic policy.

CONCLUSION

HIA provides a way forward in a global risk world, enabling the use of evidence-based practice and public participation. It utilises the skills of environmental health practitioners (EHPs) and public health practitioners to facilitate and advocate for healthier environments (living, working and public realm), based on principles of democracy, equity, sustainable development and ethical use of evidence. However, the context in which HIA operates must guide how its processes are developed. On the one hand how it engages the decision-makers is crucial; it must appear that HIA is a cost-effective (O'Reilly *et al.*, 2006) tool to support decision-making, with emphasis on reducing the burden on decision-makers, not that health issues are more deserving of their attention. On the other hand, HIA provides a mechanism to engage people in influencing policies that affect them.

Legislation

SI 1988 No. 1199 The Town and Country Planning (Assessment of Environmental Effects) Regulations 1988
SI 2004 No1633 The Environmental Assessment of Plans and Programmes Regulations 2004

Further reading and useful websites

The HIA gateway: **http://apho.org.uk/resource/item.aspx?RID=60066**

For general interest and case studies

London HUDU: **www.healthyurbandevelopment.nhs.uk/index.html**. The website of the London healthy urban development unit, useful for regeneration or land use, special planning.

Netvibes: **www.netvibes.com/healthimpactassessment#HIA_-_England_info**. This is a type of search engine put together by HIA enthusiasts.

IMPACT: **www.liv.ac.uk/ihia/index.htm**. This is the website for the Merseyside guidelines and work in Liverpool.

Department of Health HIA pages: **www.dh.gov.uk/en/Publicationsandstatistics/Legislation/Healthassessment/index.htm www.dh.gov.uk/en/Publicationsandstatistics/Legislation/Healthassessment/index.htm**

HIA Connect: **www.hiaconnect.edu.au**. For a link to HIA in Australia.

HIA Wiki: **www.healthimpactassessment.info**. These are the wiki pages where you can contribute to developing the body of knowledge on HIA.

European Commission, Public Health Projects: **http://ec.europa.eu/health/ph_projects/2003/action1/action1_2003_20_en.htm**. This page describes the European Commission project on the evaluation of health impact assessment started in 2003.

London Health Commission: **www.londonshealth.gov.uk/hia.htm#Top** For health impact assessments in London, resources, evidence and publications.

Health Impact Assessment Support Unit Wales: **www.wales.nhs.uk/sites3/home.cfm?OrgID=522**. This is the main webpage for HIA in Wales.

Scottish Health Impact Assessment Network: **www.healthscotland.com/resources/networks/shian.aspx**. This is the main webpage for HIA in Scotland.

www.belfasthealthycities.com/health-impact-assessment.html. This is a good starting point for current practice in Northern Ireland.

(Websites all accessed 15 July 2009.)

Other commentators on health impact assessment include:

Joffe, M. (2008) 'The need for strategic impact assessment'. *European Journal of Public Health*, 18(5): 439–40

Kemm, J. (2008) 'Comments on HIA forecast: cloudy with sunny spells'. *European Journal of Public Health*, 18(5): 438–39

Thomson, H. (2008) 'HIA forecast: cloudy with sunny spells later?' *European Journal of Public Health*, 18(5): 436–38

Chapter 12

Leadership in community health development

Allan McNaught

This chapter discusses the concepts of leadership and community health development, and their relationship to public health practice, primarily in the UK. The strengths and limitations of these concepts for public health practice are explored through a review of a sample of the current literature. The discussion of these concepts and their interrelationship illustrates some of the boundary issues with political, social, organisation and management theory. The core argument of this chapter is that an understanding of 'leadership' and 'community health development' are essential for modern public health practice.

Learning outcomes

In this chapter you will learn how to:

- have a critical understanding of community development as a strategy for advancing public health;

- develop an awareness of the different definitions and notions of community in modern society, and the contrast with more traditional definitions;

- differentiate between organisational and community modes of leadership.

INTRODUCTION

It has been accepted that leadership skills are necessary for public health practitioners to be effective in their role (Faculty of Public Health, 2006;

Umble *et al.*, 2007). The community development approach is also seen as an effective strategy for public health practice in modern society. Within this, community leadership is an essential resource for galvanising and working with communities around health issues. However, community leadership is itself a complex phenomenon because of the social, political and technological developments that have resulted in more dynamic and fragmented communities than were typical in more settled and traditional societies. Because of this shift in the context and the practical evolution of communities, it could be argued that the leadership skills and abilities required by public health practitioners are very similar to those required and deployed by community leaders. More to the point, public health practitioners need to understand communities and to identify how community leadership models will enable them to work effectively with communities on health development strategies.

ON DEFINITIONS OF COMMUNITY

Traditionally, the term 'community' has been used to define or describe the people of a particular geographical area or urban neighbourhood and the network of social, psychological and economic relationships and obligations that bound them together. Belonging to such a community also acted as a constraint on the behaviour of community members. Traditional communities provided a total environment for their members, as the role of state and private organisations was more limited. Modernity led to the creation of a network of public and private organisations that invaded the community's domain and took over its welfare, social order and economic responsibility. An especially powerful force was created by the growth of capitalist work organisations that reduced the economic role of local communities and relocated work to factories, workshops and offices. While in traditional society most time was spent in the neighbourhood, in modern society the workplace is the main place for congregation and the prime social network for adults. Schooling and other educational establishments fulfil the same purpose for children and young adults. In addition, teenagers have the ability to structure their own social networks or communities because of increased social, geographical, technological, transport and commercial opportunities (Boyes-Watson, 2005; Tones, 1986).

Modernity had a direct effect on traditional notions of community. However, the term still has power, and is now used to define people who are ascribed or who claim membership of a 'community of interest', characterised by geography, gender, ethnicity, age or some other feature which they recognise, are seen to share, or which others assume they share. In the modern world we also have a variety of 'virtual communities', such as readers of particular newspapers and those brought together by internet blogs or social networking sites such as 'Facebook' (see also Chapter 14). What gives the notion of community its strengths is the self-perception and awareness of its members that they are a 'community'.

Definitions of community development

Definitions of community development are very much locked into notions of geographic neighbourhood communities. These definitions still have resonance because of the persistence of geographic concentrations of disadvantaged populations. This perception underpins area-based social action programmes, such as 'Health Action Zones', aimed at disadvantaged populations, particularly in urban neighbourhoods. The definition of community development used by the Christian Reformed World Relief Committee (CRWRC, 2004: 1) is very typical of the assumptions that underpin such initiatives: 'a long-term, indigenous, people-centered process developed from participant involvement and enthusiasm that results in transforming, measurable, individual and community change'.

The underlying assumption is that communities have a deficit of knowledge, skills, and political or economic power. The processes involve enskilling/upskilling and empowerment through participative strategies and directed resources. These strategies are clearly appropriate in both developed and undeveloped societies for populations or communities whose characteristics fit the traditional definition of community. However, even in these 'classical' settings, there remain populations and groups who are 'hard to reach' (Chiu, 2008; Carr et al., 2008).

Concepts of community development and community leadership are contested in social and political theory, which raise questions about their applicability in post-industrial, globalised society, where traditional forms of association and identification with small geographical localities and patterns of leadership are weak. There is also recognition that social inequality is a structural phenomenon, and that the organisation and mobilisation of the poor and marginalised has limited capacity to achieve significant social change (Bridgen, 2004).

While recognising these arguments and limitations, my objectives are rather utilitarian. I will look at community development and leadership as techniques and approaches to working with disadvantaged communities – however they are defined – to achieve definable change in respect of public health objectives. The social and spatial differentiation of disadvantaged communities, however, means that the operationalisation of community development techniques and the practice of leadership within this 'postmodern' context depart at many critical points from the more traditional approaches to community development.

Community health development initiatives tend to be focused on the amelioration of health inequalities, a major concern in public health in the UK. Health inequality is structural, and a reflection of social and economic disadvantage. This structural inequality manifests itself in many enduring ways. One of its most potent expressions is geographic and spatial, with poorer citizens congregating in distinct residential enclaves, as a consequence of the interaction of inequality and disadvantage on many platforms. However, the geographical reflection of inequality is simplistic, as disadvantage is individual, familial, community, social and regional. Spatial concentration does not mean homogeneity: disadvantaged communities have their own complex social structures, and the character and severity of individual disadvantage provides a severe test for conventional strategies for empowerment, engagement and upliftment (Schweigert, 2007; Kegler *et al.*, 2008).

Working with disadvantaged communities, while difficult, is easier than dealing with the more complex patterns of structural social inequality that we know exist (Curtis, 2003; Graham, 2007).

Activity 12.1 Reflective exercise: community health development

Ascertain what community health development projects exist in your area. Choose one run or funded by your own organisation and one run by a non-government organisation or by your local authority. Get hold of project documentation, and compare and contrast the following:

1. The aims and objectives of the respective projects;
2. Their definition and quantification of the target community and what they perceive as 'community development';
3. How project outcomes are specified and measured.

ON LEADERSHIP

'Leadership' is also a term that requires exploration and debate. Leadership derives essentially from group psychology. It refers to an individual who forcibly, or by consent or appointment, takes power over others in a formal or informal group. Modern society is one that is characterised by formal organisations, all with a requirement for leadership and management. It is commonly perceived that 'management' is essentially about effectiveness and efficiency in the day-to-day operations of an organisation. 'Leadership' is about something more strategic; it is about having a sense of direction, vision and the ability to interpret and judge social, environmental, political and economic forces and to facilitate the adaptation of the organisation, its workforce and processes to these forces (Kotter, 1990). Organisational leadership takes place within the context of structure, of bureaucratic organisations, in which leaders and managers have rewards, sanctions and performance management arrangements to mould behaviour.

The UK National Public Health Leadership Programme (NPHLP) recognises the importance of leadership skills and ability in advancing the public health agenda. The programme's objectives are:

- to ensure that public health considerations are included in decisions concerning health and social policy at all levels within the NHS and other relevant organisations;
- to foster better understanding of how leadership skills in people and organisations can improve health;
- to identify and support the development of self-awareness and personal leadership styles and offer additional skills;
- to promote strong multi-disciplinary and cross-sectoral working for health;
- to develop a network of peers committed to shared learning and improving population health.

This idea of leadership across networks of organisations is something that is not encompassed by the current leadership literature. In much of this literature, the leadership conundrum is about how to develop excellent organisations that are able to survive and prosper in turbulent environments (Senge, 2006; Peters and Waterman, 2004).

The underlying assumptions of the NPHLP see public health leaders as social actors in a health policy/political network characterised by organisations operating in different sectors, with a multi-disciplinary policy framework. These features and demands of public health leadership bear a strong resemblance to the challenges faced in the domain of community health development and community leadership.

Community leadership

The notion of 'community leadership' is also not straightforward in modern society. It suggests that definable communities have an identifiable leadership cadre, which has status, influence or power over others. This almost tribal concept of leadership is very apparent when we look at initiatives aimed at black and minority ethnic (BME) groups.

The power of the term, perhaps, explains its appropriation by the state. In local areas we have the overlapping jurisdiction of local government and central government agencies, as well as voluntary and community organisations. Some of these organisations aspire to exercise 'community leadership'. Central government has urged local authorities to take on the 'community leadership role', in the sense of being seen as 'bringing coherence . . . to local action in pursuit of a "shared vision"' among local stakeholders (Sullivan, 2005: 13). In pursuit of this top-down vision, local government was granted a new 'duty of community strategy', a new power of 'economic, social and environmental well-being' (Sullivan, 2005: 13).

The contribution of 'bottom-up' community leadership has long been recognised as the provision of a bridge between officialdom and communities, and as a way of motivating individuals, groups and communities to become engaged with public and community health activities. Many public health initiatives build on existing community leadership networks, or go through the process of establishing such individuals and networks to heighten the possibility of effectiveness of projects and initiatives. (See also Chapter 4).

There is, then, an inextricable link between public health, community development and community leadership. As an approach to public health practice, it can be suggested that community development has a distinctive contribution. This has been recognised by Huang and Wang (2005) who locate community development as a technique or way of working within the context of 'community health development', alongside primary health care and health promotion, as an integrated part of 'community health practice'.

This notion of community development as an active strategy and instrument for promoting public health needs to be distinguished from 'patient and public participation' strategies that, on the one hand, attempt to increase public participation in the health care governance, or those, on the other hand, that are part of a 'consumerist' initiative. Because community development stresses participation, partnership and empowerment, they sometimes overlap with these latter kinds of initiatives. However, public and patient involvement initiatives can be pursued without a community development infrastructure or philosophy.

COMMUNITY HEALTH DEVELOPMENT INITIATIVES

Within the scope of my definition of community development in health, the existing literature seems to fall into one of the following categories:

- advancing health education or health promotion;
- promoting service improvement and utilisation;
- health needs assessment.

The remainder of this section will review selected literature to illustrate the texture of initiatives in the areas identified. Within each of these categories of literature, there are examples of work and initiatives that illustrate the interaction and utilisation of public health leadership and community leadership for the purpose of community health development.

Advancing health education and health promotion

This approach is used when it is known that a particular group experiences defined health issues and where there are cultural, linguistic and behavioural barriers to health improvement. In these projects it is health workers working directly with community development methodologies or community health workers/advocates who are used to get the message across to the community. The 'Asian Mother and Baby Campaign' is a classical project of this kind. This project was designed to increase uptake of maternity services and to tackle the problem of vitamin B deficiency in Asian children. The project methodology involved the recruitment of 'Link Workers' from Asian communities.

A retrospective study was carried out comparing 1000 non-English-speaking women delivering at the Mothers' Hospital, Hackney in 1986 who had been accompanied by an advocate, with women delivering at the same hospital in 1979 and at a reference hospital, Whipps Cross. The study found significant differences between the groups in three outcomes: antenatal length of stay, induction and mode of delivery. The changes in Caesarean section were of particular note. The rates rose from 11 to 17 per cent at the reference hospital, whereas they fell from 10·8 to 8·5 per cent at the Mothers' Hospital. The authors considered it reasonable to deduce that improved communication could have influenced clinical practice, suggesting that health advocacy may offer a mechanism to address some of the adverse obstetric outcomes observed in ethnic minorities (Parsons and Day, 1992).

Promoting service improvement and utilisation

This is a variant of the first type of initiative. However, while the first was focused on information and education, this sort of project is focused on particular services, their improvement and their utilisation. Raine (2003) reported on a project designed 'to evaluate the effectiveness of peer support intervention to promote breast-feeding in a deprived area'. This initiative was developed under the umbrella of a Surestart Project that is itself designed to improve community capacity, participation and empowerment in respect of children's health and development. Among the objectives of the research were:

- to explore the development of a 'culture' of breastfeeding in a deprived area; and
- consider the potential of the project for community capacity building.

The project reported social, cultural and economic barriers to the upliftment of the area's breastfeeding rates. However, the initiative was regarded as a success as many of the volunteers went on to other formal, health-related training, and the project provided a model for other forms of community capacity building.

Millett *et al.* (1999) have reported on a project aimed at improving the quality of rheumatology, diabetes and spinal injury services in West Yorkshire through increased levels of patient participation. The methodology of this project included patient questionnaires, focus groups and increased involvement with voluntary organisations. The focus groups were deemed as particularly useful in highlighting some practical measures and systems to improve services and the patient experience. However, it is debateable if this project can be deemed to be 'community development' in the classical sense, as it does not seek to develop any identifiable community capacity other than as inputs to service improvement strategy.

In reviewing this type of strategy, Fudge *et al.* (2008) found that patient involvement tends to be in the least technical area and with least input from clinicians. They argue that user involvement may not automatically lead to improved service quality and call for better evidence for the claimed benefits of users' involvement.

Health needs assessment

Needs assessment is a persistent area for community development initiatives (for further information, see Chapter 14). Kai and Hedges (1999) recruited and trained 13 Community Project Workers to define and conduct research on psychological distress in Pakistani and Bangladeshi people in an inner city area in the UK. This work was undertaken in order to provide information and analysis for services development. The work was overseen within a local multi-disciplinary steering group, who were not able to confirm that the funding and support was or would be available. The authors recognised the value of the approach and argued that it was worth continuing.

Similar themes and problems are illustrated by Cornwall *et al.* (2003) in their report on a wellbeing assessment conducted via Participatory Action Research on a large council estate in South London. Within this project, a worker moved on to the estate, drew together a support team that built links and worked with existing social networks and organisations, and used a variety of participatory methods to develop an understanding and awareness of wellbeing issues and to identify what could be done to facilitate improvement. The work led to a detailed report, based on residents' views and experiences. It also led to the employment of a community health development worker (CHDW), who was able to work on a wider platform than the initial researcher. The CHDW began to develop a greater local constituency and also to work at a more strategic level with the health and local authority and their staff. This report made it evident that there was a gap between the findings of the report and the kind of partnerships and actions necessary to achieve improvement for residents: 'Community development work remains a long, intensive and slow process. Participatory assessments such as these are no substitute for the kinds of process of engagement that are needed to build confidence and capacity within communities' (Cornwall, *et al.*, 2003: 6).

Activity 12.2 Reflective exercise: community leadership

Review the organisation and management arrangements of the two projects that you selected for the earlier exercise above, and compare and contrast the following:

1. What leadership role is played by the sponsoring organisation?
2. Who provides day-to-day leadership of the project?
3. How do they approach the issue of community leadership?
4. If there are leadership roles in the project, how are the people recruited?

SUMMARY

Community engagement and community development strategies remain vital, but the diversification and dynamism of communities requires significant modifications in engagement strategies. This places a particular demand on leadership capacities in public health as well as in communities. Community leadership skills are more akin to political leadership, as community leaders do not have recourse to the sanctions and incentives of leaders of formal organisations. Public health leaders demand the same kind of skills when working across networks. There are differences though. Natural communities are voluntary forms of association. Professional communities and networks invariably have elements of policy, compulsion and necessity.

If we look more closely at community development in health we can see that the published literature has a number of strands. In practice, the boundaries between community developments, public and patient participation can be blurred because of the variety of methodologies that are used, and because we often do not know the background of the patient groups who contribute towards involvement events. However, we do know that such inputs do have an effect on the service providers, as evidenced by Crawford *et al.* (2002: 1) who found that 'evidence supports the notion that involving patients has contributed to changes in the provision of services across a range of different settings'. However 'an evidence base for the effects on the use of services, quality of care, satisfaction, or the health of patients does not exist'.

The effectiveness of community development also rests on the willingness of individuals to participate, to get involved in issues that do not always affect them directly. Campbell and McLean (2002) examine the impact of ethnic identity on the likelihood of people's participation in local community networks. While African-Caribbean identity played a central role in people's participation in inter-personal networks, this inter-personal solidarity did not serve to unite people at the local community level beyond particular face-to-face networks. Levels of participation in voluntary organisations and community activist networks were low.

Community development as a technique in public health is generally framed as an appropriate strategy for capturing the needs, concerns and securing the involvement of disadvantaged communities. It could be argued that it is of broader significance, given the nature of the health challenges facing Britain and other advanced societies. Orchard *et al.* (2000) have argued, in the case of Canada, that community development is necessary to promote 'a more balanced health system encouraging health promotion, illness prevention and care determined by communities – community health is shifting from a medical to a social-action approach which fosters collaboration between communities and providers'.

In exploring community development and community leadership we have to consider the situation of the community and voluntary sector. Most local community health development organisations are dependent on local authority and Primary Care Trust funding. Throughout the country, financial support to the voluntary sector has changed from grant-in-aid to service level agreements for defined services. Smaller voluntary organisations have either collapsed or operate in constrained circumstances. Local authorities have been urged by central government to take on a community leadership role. However, it would seem that the leadership of powerful local state organisations precludes local government leaders from acting with the kind of community leadership model, the essential dynamics of which 'and characteristics of leadership appear more clearly in relational patterns of thinking, acting and responding that can move in multiple directions' (Schweigert, 2007).

CONCLUSION

This chapter has argued that traditional notions of community development and community leadership are still relevant in modern public health. However, the underlying practices, assumptions and philosophy of community development need to be tailored to recognise the complexity of modern communities. Socio-demographic change has produced complex communities. Modernity, too, has resulted in the state and private organisations playing a greater role in social affairs and has contributed towards the creation of communities that are more complex than those simply defined by geographic proximity. Community, however defined, continues to be important as impersonal modern organisations and their way of working have meant that they can never get as close to the individuals as the kind of interpersonal and group relationships that are often characteristic in traditional and newer communities.

Public health leaders share the same problems and constraints as their counterparts in local government, as they too can be considered as part of the 'local state'. The notions of user and community involvement are an essential part of the leadership ideology of public sector managers. Community activists also ascribe considerable power to user and community involvement. The evidence from numerous projects and reports tends to acknowledge the difficulty of maintaining participation levels and in actually influencing services (Fudge, *et al.* 2008). On the other hand, numerous studies also report positive processes and outcomes from community health development projects and activities from the perspective of community leaders and beneficiaries.

Further reading

Adams, J., Witten, K. and Conway, K. (2009) 'Community development as health promotion: evaluating a complex locality-based project in New Zealand'. Oxford University Press and *Community Development Journal*, 44: 140–57
Much of the earlier work on health promotion and health education had a very strong community development focus, and later work is on individual behaviour, so this provides a historical perspective.

Birmingham NHS Strategic Partnership (2005) Health Project Development Toolkit for Community Groups
A useful work-through of the kind of issues and challenges faced by community organisations in influencing public health, and practitioners may learn about community organisations by reading this text.

Chapter 13

Information technology and public health (EHealth)

Anne Gill

This chapter provides an overview of the rapidly evolving role of information technology in public health and the importance of the ethical and legal issues involved. It demonstrates the importance of an effective information environment, how factors such as social disadvantage may hinder access to EHealth, and asks how EHealth might operate in the future.

Learning outcomes

In this chapter you will learn how to:

- understand the central role of information technology in the delivery of public health (EHealth);

- understand the importance of ethical and legal issues like, for example, confidentiality and freedom of information, when using information technology;

- perform an analysis of your current information environment;

- understand the characteristics of an effective information environment;

- be aware of the effects of social deprivation on the ability to access EHealth.

INTRODUCTION

Information has always played a central role in the delivery of public health but recent radical changes in the technology used to deliver information mean that both professionals and the public need to adjust to a fast-changing world. The public is being exposed to new information systems on a daily basis. This includes the internet but also new government initiatives such as 'choose and book'. This is a computer-based system that GPs use to ensure their clients have a choice of hospital to treat their condition. Other recent developments that affect nearly everyone are multi-choice telephone menus (press number 1 if you want to . . .), and the biggest change of all is the proposed access to their medical records, via computer, by all citizens. This will potentially affect everyone and could alter our approach to health information at all levels.

This emphasis on information means that all health, public health and social care professionals need to understand the importance of information systems and evaluate those available to them. In addition, all users of health-related information systems would benefit from a greater understanding of how they work. We all need to be able to influence the way information systems are introduced to make the most effective use of them. An information system is not just a question of the technology; it is essentially about how to communicate with the public and to ensure health promotion messages get to all who can benefit from them. A collective name for the above activities could be EHealth, and this term will be used in this chapter. The focus of this chapter will therefore be on the role of information technology in the delivery of public health and on the characteristics of an effective information environment.

THE ROLE OF INFORMATION TECHNOLOGY IN THE DELIVERY OF PUBLIC HEALTH (EHEALTH)

Confidentiality, ethics and the law

It is essential that all health and social care professionals understand the legal and ethical issues relating to all uses of information. Confidentiality is the key issue: there are moral issues about privacy and also legal requirements like, for example, the Data Protection Act 1998 and the Freedom of Information Act 2000. The Information Commissioner's office plays a key role in regulating information. The Information Commissioner is a government official who is responsible for the safety and confidentiality of all public information. The commissioner's office should be a frequent port of call for all involved in giving and receiving public information.

The Data Protection Act 1998

The Data Protection Act 1998 focuses on privacy and disclosure and works in two ways. Firstly, it states that anyone who processes personal information must comply with eight principles that make sure that personal information is:

- fairly and lawfully processed;
- processed for limited purposes;
- adequate, relevant and not excessive;
- accurate and up to date;
- not kept for longer than is necessary;
- processed in line with people's rights;
- secure;
- not transferred to other countries without adequate protection.

The second area covered by the Act provides individuals with important rights, including the right to find out what personal information is held on computer and most paper records (The Information Commissioner's Office, 2009a).

The Freedom of Information Act 2000

The Freedom of Information Act 2000 deals with access to official information and gives individuals or organisations the right to request information from any public authority. The Freedom of Information Act applies to all 'public authorities'. This includes:

- central and local government;
- the health service;
- schools, colleges and universities;
- the police;
- lots of other non-departmental public bodies, committees and advisory bodies.

Any individual can ask for any information at all – but some information might be withheld to protect various interests that are allowed for by the Act. If this is the case, the public authority must explain why they have withheld information (The Information Commissioner's Office, 2009b).

These two Acts are the core of the legal protection system with regard to the information that the state and private organisations hold about citizens and they apply to most of the following information sources.

Activity 13.1 Reflective exercise

- How can you ensure that your practice adheres to both ethical and legal requirements with regard to confidentiality and freedom of information?
- There are sometimes conflicting imperatives regarding privacy and disclosure. How would you reconcile these?

INFORMATION TECHNOLOGY AND PUBLIC HEALTH

That section of the public with access to the internet has a huge range of health information available to them. There are essentially two important areas with regard to this: one is the world wide web where a health query typed into a search engine will often return thousands of hits but little information on the reliability and veracity of the site; the second is the network of sites sponsored and created by the government with the intent to ensure that every citizen of the UK has access to their own personal information and also to health advice tailored to their needs.

The Spine

The Spine is part of the NHS Care Records Service (NHS CRS). A key part of the NHS CRS will be the gradual development of an electronic summary care record. Once the NHS CRS is fully implemented, having each patient's summary care record stored on The Spine will mean that wherever and whenever a patient seeks care from the NHS in England, those treating them will have secure access to summary information to assist with diagnosis and care. The intent is to provide safer, more joined-up care. However, concerns about privacy have led to the need for a voluntary opt-out, although, if this is widespread, it would compromise the effectiveness of the service (NHS Connecting for Health, 2009).

There are now indications that this development may be subjected to considerable delays. Two out of the four companies producing the system for the NHS have pulled out and the 'Care Records System' is the most at risk because the pilot projects have not gone well. While everyone appears to agree on the value of IT for the NHS, there is considerable doubt from authoritative sources such as the Committee on Public Accounts as to whether the deadlines can be met or whether the potential cost is justified (House of Commons Public Accounts Committee, 2009).

An important point to make about the summary care record is that this will not just be an information file with a static record, but will be part of a service that will provide access to a range of information that is tailored to the individual's requirements. It will essentially be a personal webpage, similar to pages created by existing providers such as Amazon and Google. This service will be known as Health Space.

Health Space

Health Space provides a personal health organiser where the individual user can record information such as weight, medications and alcohol intake. Eventually all UK citizens will be able to access their summary care record using Health Space.

Health Space also supports other systems and services, including Choose and Book and the Electronic Prescription Service (EPS). Health Space is active now and will still exist even if the summary care record has to be modified or abandoned and it will give the individuals who are able to access it personalised health advice and information.

A review of Health Space

At the moment the service is rather limited. The user can access services such as NHS Direct and Choose and Book but these can be accessed elsewhere and the personalised health advice is restricted to recording details of indicators such as weight and health history. However, there is no feedback on actions the user can take to remedy problems. When and if the summary record is added (see above section on 'The Spine'), the site will have more utility with regards to public health. The most useful service currently available is the ability to investigate local NHS services.

Choose and Book

Choose and Book is a national service that allows patients to choose their hospital or clinic and book an appointment with a specialist. Patients can choose from at least four hospitals or clinics and choose and book the date and time of their appointment. The main gatekeeper for Choose and Book is currently the general practitioner. After some difficulties Choose and Book is functioning well.

Electronic Prescription Service (EPS)

The Electronic Prescription Service replaces paper prescription forms with a safer, more convenient, electronic system that will make collecting repeat prescriptions easier for patients. This service is currently working well (NHS Connecting for Health, 2009).

UK citizens can register now for Health Space but will not be able to access their summary care record unless they are in one of the early adopter pilot areas.

There is potential for the above initiatives to give individuals greatly increased control over their health information and more control over managing their own health. Health Space will provide tailored information for each individual, enabling them to develop their own health protection programmes.

Box 13.1 Case study

In November 2007, HM Revenue and Customs lost computer discs containing the entire child benefit records, including the personal details of 25 million people, covering 7.25 million families overall. The two discs contain the names, addresses, dates of birth and bank account details of people who received child benefit. They also include National Insurance numbers. The data was essentially lost in the post. Advice to the general public to monitor their bank accounts and change passwords, particularly if they had used family names that were in their child benefit records, was necessary but did little to restore public confidence in government-held information. The Information Commissioner Richard Thomas said: 'The alarm bells must now ring in every organisation about the risks of not protecting people's personal information properly' (BBC, 2007).

Activity 13.2 Reflective exercise

Think of the individuals you know – colleagues, friends, relatives. Which individuals would be able to take advantage of the new developments outlined above and which would not? What are the differences between those who can and those who can't?

THE CHARACTERISTICS OF AN EFFECTIVE INFORMATION ENVIRONMENT

In order to create an effective information environment, the health professional needs to be able to analyse their current environment and identify any changes needed to optimise the client's access to information.

Analysis of the information environment: purpose of the information system

The starting point of analysing an information system is to ask 'what is it for and who is it for?' This question may seem obvious but is not always asked. Confusion often arises because the different people involved have very different views on what they want the system to do. The problem can be alleviated with comprehensive negotiation and communication, and by agreeing objectives. Think about these questions:

1. What are your objectives regarding an information system?
2. Who should be involved in consultations regarding these objectives?
3. Who is going to be responsible for what?

Example:
1. What are your objectives regarding an information system?

Health Care Professional
I want accurate information about my clients, preferably from a single source that is secure and accessible.

Client
I want accurate information about my health, obtainable from a single secure and accessible source. I also want clear advice on what to do with regard to potential problems.

Users of the system

It is surprising how little consideration can be given to users of the information system: who is going to have access; what levels of access will there be? With electronic patient records (EPR) the proposals include access for all professional staff and clients. However, there are ethical questions regarding confidentiality and practical problems in designing an information interface that will be accessible to all, particularly those groups who are often excluded from information technology, notably the elderly and the socially disadvantaged. (See the section on 'The effects of age and social deprivation on the ability to access EHealth' below.)

More questions

1. Who uses or will need to use the information on the system?
2. What are their information needs?
3. What language will the system need use to be understandable to all who use it?
4. What are the benefits of the system for all users, professionals and clients?

The nature of the information

Understanding the nature and qualities of the information used is essential to designing and using an information system. Health promotion and health education materials have special qualities; they must be accurate, targeted and accessible. Electronic information sources have both advantages and disadvantages in this regard. The advantages include the ability to translate in to almost any language instantly (although the quality of the translation may be questionable) the ability to set the size of print to suit the client and audio programmes that will read printed materials. Disadvantages include expense and client resistance.

Questions

1. What exactly is the information being used for – clinical, personal, educational or a mixture of all three?
2. What sorts of information are needed – for example, numeric, qualitative, identification?
3. How will the information be collected?
4. What is the quality of the information? There is an old acronym regarding information: 'GIGO', i.e. 'garbage in garbage out'. There is basically no point in creating an information system without data that is accurate, timely and reliable. The principles of evidence-based

practice are also useful here – does the information have a basis in evidence?

Information flows

Mapping information flows (see Figure 13.1) helps us to understand how information works. Take a look at your next client or at yourself and imagine them/you at the centre of a nexus of information. Ideally information should be available to all the different people involved at the push of a button; no one should have to ask for the same bit of information twice. It should always be possible to improve the information flow if we understand our own information environment. Try the following exercise to see how information works in your organisation or in your local health centre or hospital.

Questions

1. Who are the people that the information has to flow between?
2. How can information flow most effectively?
3. What is the best way to represent the information flow?

Your client arrives at your organisation. Track their quest for information or imagine yourself arriving in your local health centre or hospital.

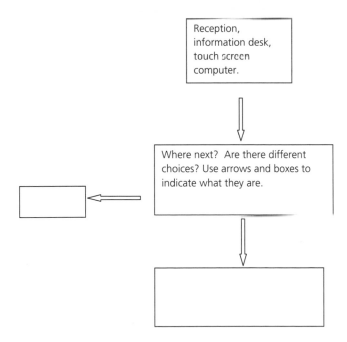

Figure 13.1 What is the starting point for information?

If your organisation or local health centre/hospital has a good information system you will be able to do this exercise as you will be aware of the choices facing your clients or yourself. If you find it very difficult to map the information flows, so will your clients. They will find it very difficult to find out what they are supposed to do or where to go. Think of yourself standing bewildered in a large outpatients department with no idea what to do next.

Create your own flow diagram based on a recent client or on you as a patient. How does the information flow around them/you? What can block the information flow and what can facilitate it?

Use of information technology: what system to use

The mistake people often make is starting at this point. They have a system and then decide what to do with it. In an ideal world no system would be purchased until all the questions in this exercise were answered but, in the real world, we have to work with what exists.

Questions

1. What information system is available – is it an IT system or is it paper-based?
2. What systems are in use?
3. Are the present systems being used well?
4. Can the systems be improved?
5. Are the systems fit for their purpose?
6. What staff/client training needs to be in place?

Evaluation

It is not a good idea to put a system in place and then figure out how you are going to evaluate it. The evaluation strategies need to be part of the preliminary planning. Internal and external review and audit can be used but, most importantly, feedback from the users of the system should be acquired.

Questions

1. What methods of evaluation will be used and how will you get the users involved?
2. What formal methods of evaluation will be used? If you are using an audit, do you have a suitable tool available?
3. How will you judge the effectiveness of the system?

If you work your way through all the above questions you will have most of the information you need to design an effective information system.

Activity 13.3 Reflective exercise

We manage information every day of our lives. Look back on your day so far. In what ways have you managed information both at work and in your home life?

PRINCIPLES OF INFORMATION MANAGEMENT

The following general principles should be borne in mind with respect to information management.

- Be aware of the information sources available to you, such as, for example, clients, relatives, the local hospital trusts, the local authority, the world wide web. How are you utilising these sources? Clients and relatives often complain that they are not listened to; the lack of 'joined-up care' is cited as a cause of both complaint and of mistakes. Whom do you talk to and who talks to you?
- Be aware of the quality and meaning of the information you use. The quality of your decisions depends on the quality of the information and your ability to analyse it. Skills of evidence analysis and critical thinking are useful here. Most good information sources have indications of reliability and validity, but some lack these qualities.
- Know how and where to obtain the information you need. Public health practitioners need these skills above all others.
- Know how to apply the information you use and how to communicate information to others (Scott and Gill, 2008).

Activity 13.4 Reflective exercise

List your information sources, then categorise them according to reliability and usefulness in particular situations. This could be the beginning of a very useful personalised public health database.

THE EFFECTS OF AGE AND SOCIAL DEPRIVATION ON THE ABILITY TO ACCESS EHEALTH

There is research regarding access to health information that indicates that those at greatest risk of not being able to access and use these services are the elderly and the socially disadvantaged. There is still a significant proportion of the public that does not have internet access or basic computer skills. The latest figures indicate that 65 per cent of UK households now have an internet connection (Ofcom, 2007), with a significant minority of 35 per cent that do not. Only 20 per cent of the elderly have an internet connection and the data suggests that the main driver of internet usage is income.

The digitally disadvantaged

The elderly and social class DE are the most likely to lack resources such as the internet. A profile of these individuals indicates multiple disadvantages including lack of transport, low home ownership, meagre educational qualifications, and a high proportion of individuals who are widowed, single or divorced. It is evident that digital exclusion cannot be solved in isolation from other policy areas. A projection for internet use in 2025, which must be treated with caution of course, is that internet use overall will increase but the proportionate difference between the young and old will remain, with 10 per cent of the 15–24 group excluded and 45 per cent of 75+ (Department for Communities and Local Government, 2008).

It is evident that both time and resources need to be targeted at the excluded groups. This is not an insuperable barrier. Health and social care professionals will have an increasing role in enabling access to electronically produced information. This will not be different in kind to their current role but will include different skills and abilities.

Box 13.2 Case study

The following case studies imagine the digital world of public health in 2025:

- It is 2025. Marge is a Public Health Information Officer working in the East End of London. Her electric van is fitted with a mobile internet connection and she is a familiar figure at the local supermarkets where locals can come in and ask questions or use the touch screen on the side of the van.

- Eric is a community care practitioner who works in Glasgow. His beat is the local Extra Care Housing Project, a thriving estate that is specially designed for the frail elderly. He takes his large print touch screen on all his visits, backing up his advice with printouts and audio recordings depending on the abilities of his clients.
- Jennifer, a health education specialist who works in the Highlands and Islands, never leaves her office. She communicates with the local schools, elderly care centres and nurseries using the screens installed in all public organisations. She can tailor her presentations for her audience and talk to groups and individuals as if she were present in the room. The addition of 3D technology and sensori-vision, which includes smells and tactile sensations, has greatly expanded her repertoire.
- Irena is responsible for designing rehabilitation programmes for stroke victims. Each client has a terminal in their home where they can talk to Irena on a regular basis. She can design individual programmes for them using physiological data obtained from a touch-sensitive monitor in the client's home. All the client has to do is place their hand upon the monitor for Irena to receive an up-to-date analysis of their progress.

CONCLUSION

GPs are already guiding their patients through Choose and Book and will be the key gatekeepers for information access as they always have been. However, health care professionals at all levels will also be involved and it is possible to envisage a time when the laptop is as essential an item in the health and public health practitioner's kit as the notebook and pen is now. The important issue for both professionals and clients is not technical proficiency but the ability to use the information provided. The responsibility of the professional will be to create an effective information environment that is accessible to all. Public health practitioners will have an important role to play. Current activities, including writing lively and informative leaflets and making good quality videos, are of course important, but these materials are of little use if they do not get to the public they are intended for. It is also important to realise that the socially deprived are often cut off from all sources of information and not just the online world.

In order to create an effective information environment, the most important factors are the needs and capabilities of the client group and the capabilities and resources of the health and social care professionals. Professionals may have to reframe both their working methods and their relationship with the client. The 'active information client', who will use all the information sources available, may need guidance as to the reliability and validity of the sources they are accessing, particularly the unregulated information available on the world wide web. The 'passive information client', on the other hand, is unlikely to access EHealth sources without active assistance and help from the professionals. A professional with a large group of the elderly and socially disadvantaged could spend a high proportion of their time as navigator through the information network, but it could be said that this is time well spent.

Useful websites

The Information Commissioner's Office: **www.ico.gov.uk**
(accessed 15 July 2009)
This site contains useful information on the Data Protection Act 1998 and the Freedom of Information Act 2000 for both the public and professionals.

Health Space: **www.healthspace.nhs.uk/visitor/default.aspx**
(accessed 15 July 2009).
Health Space is a free, secure online personal health organiser. It can help you to manage your health, store important health information securely, or find out about NHS services near you. Anyone living in England aged 16 or over, with a valid email address, can register for a Health Space account.

Chapter 14

Social capital, social enterprise and community development

Charles Oham, Jill Stewart and Yvonne Cornish

This chapter provides a brief overview of social capital before exploring the concept of social enterprises (businesses) and considering their eminence and strategic importance in delivering health outcomes. The chapter carries out an analysis of social enterprise frameworks, and the opportunities and challenges presented within the context of public health. The term 'social enterprise' will be interchangeably used with 'social business' to broaden the scope.

Learning outcomes

By the end of this chapter you should be able to:

- define social capital and appreciate its potential role in health improvement;

- critically evaluate the concept of social enterprise and its importance as a business model in driving through social change by analysing the concept and differentiating it from other forms of business;

- discuss the implementation and use of a business analytical tool (PESTLE) to evaluate the external business environment in which social enterprises operate;

- make critical judgements of the opportunities available for social businesses to exploit and their role in public health value creation by assessing the merits of this business model.

SOCIAL CAPITAL

Social capital can be broadly defined as the networks and levels of values, trust and reciprocity between communities held together through shared norms and values. It includes citizenship, neighbourliness, social networks and civic participation and is concerned with what is happening outside the remit of governmental organisations (Swann and Morgan, 2002). It has become important in the public health agenda (Baum, 1999 and 2000), and areas higher in social capital are generally associated with better heath. The Office for National Statistics (ONS, 2003) reports that areas with high levels of social capital are associated with:

- lower crime rates;
- better health and improved longevity;
- higher educational attainment;
- greater income equality;
- improved child health and lower rates of child abuse; less corrupt and more effective government; and enhanced economic development.

The concept of social capital has had a 'meteoric rise' in public health rhetoric in recent years (Lynch, *et al.*, 2000). Participation is seen as an important health promotion strategy (cited in Campbell and McLean, 2002) and participation by grassroots communities can make strategy more democratic and services more accessible, particularly by previously excluded groups. If local people participate in health promotions, behaviour change is more likely to be sustainable and there is growing recognition that participation yields positive effects on health through enhanced community networks. The government is keen to enhance social capital as part of strengthening marginalised communities to help reduce health inequalities, as a stage in the development of the social model of health, and to help buffer against some of the worst effects of deprivation (Cattrell and Herring, 2002).

Social capital can be bonding, bridging and linking. Bonding social capital is concerned with connections between people such as family members, close friends and ethnic groups. Bridging social capital is about more distant connections, and works across groups or work associations. Linking social capital is concerned with still more distant connections between people in organisations (see, for example, Putnam, 2000; Swann and Morgan, 2002).

There are (very valid) arguments about how government sees the role for social capital now and in the future, and ideological arguments about the role of the state and its ability to withdraw if social capital is seen to be sufficient in an area. Conversely, others see the government as key in nurturing social capital, particularly in more deprived areas where it is depleted.

Measuring social capital is not straightforward, but can include indicators like social relations, formal and informal social networks, levels of trust, civic engagement, reciprocity, membership of clubs, etc. and levels of social contact. Most studies to date have been secondary data analysis of existing data sources, with much being carried out in the USA.

A social approach to addressing health inequality and health improvement is now paramount. Social capital can help buffer against the worst effects of deprivation (Swann and Morgan, 2002). Building on social capital locally requires culturally sensitive and appropriate strategies and takes time, facilities, motivation and empowerment.

Activity 14.1 Reflective exercise: measuring social capital

Think about factors involved in social capital such as belonging to clubs, community groups, neighbourliness, trust and reciprocity.
- How might you assess whether an area is depleted or high in social capital?
- What would you set out to 'measure': how and why?
- In an area or setting you are familiar with, do you think that social capital is inclusive or exclusive?

SOCIAL ENTERPRISES

Social enterprises and entrepreneurs are an emerging business model gaining widespread acceptance and support on a global scale. Many terms have been used to describe social businesses and these include social enterprise, charitable trading businesses, community businesses and not-for-profit companies. Social businesses have been around for several hundreds of years and examples were reported in the Bible where Christians were selling their possessions and giving the proceeds to those who had need, signifying some kind of social action through trading activity. Within the doctrines of other religions, social action and businesses play an integral part in the propagation of community and human development. Social businesses are about equity and corporate benefit.

Social enterprises are actively involved in assisting the UK's public health agenda and 'social enterprises' began to gain prominence in the 1990s and early 2000. It would be unrealistic to incarcerate the concept of social enterprises in a set of structures, systems and procedures, as they exist in innovative and creative forms. There seems to be a sense of convergence between practitioners and academia on building the capacity of social entrepreneurs to foster efficiency and sustainability and capture social impact.

One position all stakeholders must avoid is having a 'one size fits all' outlook, which conceptualises rigidly the *modus operandi* of what makes a business a social enterprise. This attempt could be detrimental to enterprise incubation and development. It is essential that practitioners and academics embrace the culture of knowledge transfer for innovative and applicable models for managing social enterprises within the community. Most social entrepreneurs require accessibility to scarce resources and this can be achieved by the formulation and implementation of value adding frameworks for the participants in this economy. Mawson (2008), one of Britain's prolific social entrepreneurs, states that social entrepreneurs worth their salt do not follow convention; their views of the world begin with people, passion, experience and story – not policy, statistics and theory. It is important that social entrepreneurial activity is not stifled by policies and programmes that do not build capacity.

Defining social enterprises

There are five key characteristics that can be used to describe the philosophy that exists within the social enterprise community:

- people orientation;
- community ownership;
- social response;
- enterprise; and
- innovation.

Social enterprise exists to benefit people; whether it has environmental, health or community objectives, the bottom line is enhancing the quality of human life. An orientation towards people is the foundation block that social enterprises build on. A social enterprise starts and continues with people. The social response angle illustrates a proactive disposition to align with the moral values of society and tackle a local, national or global challenge. While some disciplines may analyse, social enterprises tend to deliver on social responsibility (Gil, 1973 cited in Lavalat and Pratt, 2006).

The enterprise dimension is a distinguishing feature of social enterprises in comparison with other forms of non-profit endeavour. It demonstrates a non-dependent strategic intent to break away from a total reliance on long-term funding and grant aid models that may restrict their objectives owing to funding and investment variables. The innovation element of a social enterprise typifies a relentless resolve on the part of the organisation to design novel services (or products/processes) that satisfy pressing needs.

Therefore, several definitions exist on what social enterprises are. There seems to be an unclear consensus on the definitions, but there is a common thread that links them.

The Office of the Third Sector/DTI (2005) defines a social enterprise as:

> A business with primarily social objectives, whose surpluses are principally reinvested for that purpose; in the business or in the community, rather than being driven by the need to maximise profit for shareholders and owners.

An American definition:

> A social enterprise is any business venture created for a social purpose – mitigating/reducing a social problem or a market failure and to generate social value while operating with the financial discipline, innovation and determination of a private sector business. (Kim, 2003)

Social enterprises can also be defined as stakeholder-managed, non-profit sharing business ventures, whose resources are committed to social causes at a local, national or global level.

However restrictive or difficult these definitions may be, they assist us in starting the process of understanding the core values of social businesses. Social enterprises, apart from tackling social challenges and reinvesting surpluses, contribute a weightier dimension to society: they give the marginalised access to engineer or reengineer their future, imparting a sense of ownership to the volunteers and staff as they participate in the creation of social capital. The social enterprise model attempts to redress the imbalance of profit maximisation and social responsibility that is prevalent in corporate practice.

Social enterprises in public health

Many organisations are involved in social entrepreneurial activity, from churches, mosques and community groups to charities and businesses. Some have a formal structure while others are informal. Notable social enterprises on our high streets in Britain are Barnardo's, Oxfam, the Red Cross, Cancer Research and the British Heart Foundation. However, the legitimacy of these organisations as social businesses may be argued. Some recent ones include the *Big Issue* Magazine, Hackney Community Transport (CT PLUS), Fairtrade and Divine Chocolate. They play a key role in public health either through prevention, health promotion, treatment of disease and the holistic wellbeing of individuals and communities, which serves as an intervention to poorer health outcomes.

There is scope for greater partnerships in public health by social enterprise in health education and promotion, nutrition, health improvement, tackling health inequalities and patient safety. The Department for Health recently launched a health promotion campaign, Change4Life, encouraging young families to eat better and move more (see also Chapter 8). In a joint letter by the chief medical officer and the chief nursing officer they solicited the support of all stakeholders in driving through its objectives.

Social enterprises have played and continue to play a crucial role in public health interventions. Some social enterprises engaged in public health and social care activities in the UK are Bikeworks, Metrosexual Health Limited, Nature Cure Clinic, One to One, Positive East, Ramal Health and Care, Stroke Care, HIV Training and Resource Initiative, Waltham Forest Mencap and Expert Patient Programme (SEL London, 2008). In the last three years, a number of NHS hospitals have metamorphosed into social enterprises, while several are in the process of transitioning into a social enterprise. The *Nursing Times* (December Issue, 2008) lists a few Primary Care Trusts (PCTs) that have become social enterprises, including Central Surrey Health and Principia, originally part of Rushcliffe PCT Nottingham, which started in 2006.

Box 14.1 Key facts about social enterprises

- The total turnover of social enterprises is estimated at £27 billion or 1.3 per cent of the total turnover of all businesses with employees. Their contribution to GDP is estimated to be £8.4 billion.

- There are over 55 000 social enterprises in the UK.
- Social enterprises work successfully with excluded, marginalised and vulnerable groups.
- They are proactive in their approach to community engagement and social action.
- Social enterprises are usually led by change agents and innovators.
- The vast majority of their income (around 50 per cent) is derived from trading activity (SBS, 2005).
- The largest representation of social enterprises (33 per cent) are in health and social care in the UK.
- 19 per cent of registered social enterprises exist to help people with disabilities.
- 24 per cent of registered social enterprises exist to help the communities in which they exist.
- London accounts for around a fifth (22 per cent) of all social enterprises, more than its share (14 per cent) of all UK businesses.
- Social enterprises are likely to be situated in areas of multiple deprivation.

(Sources: Office of the Third Sector, IFF (2005) research for the Small Business Service, Social Enterprise, London)

The benefits of social enterprises

Social enterprises provide several advantages to their stakeholders, including goodwill. Patton (2003) states that the standing of social enterprises has increased, and often they have what governments and corporations seek, notably credibility, expertise and public support. In the past most trust and philanthropic organisations provided funding to charities exclusively; they are now recognising the benefits of charitable trading and have developed programmes to fund social enterprises.

High staff motivation is a reflection of the intrinsic benefits and the job satisfaction most volunteers and employees get when working for social enterprises. Peattie and Morley (2008) reveal a trend known as 'downshifting' where highly-paid professionals opt for a less materially intensive lifestyle in search of quality of life. The social enterprise model may be the answer to the quality of life that many seek. Social enterprises can act as a human resource 'factory', churning out experienced and skilled labour for other sectors of the economy. Due to financial constraints and volunteering, most start-up social enterprises have high labour turnovers, which feed into the employment chain. Social enterprises have been key drivers of regeneration and optimum resource utilisation by taking over derelict and abandoned properties and community assets and putting them back into use, working with excluded people within the areas of high deprivation. It is clear that these businesses have demonstrated that there can be a clear break away from the funding dependency cycle, which most charities rely on.

Social enterprises are overtly innovative for various reasons: a lack of funding, a strong willingness to break even and run profitably and efficiently, a lack of adequate staff, and so on. A lack of resources has had an influence on their organisational culture by making them highly resourceful and inventive in the designing of systems, projects, programmes and community engagement activities. Most social enterprises are run by volunteers instead of staff, which the organisations may not be able to afford, although this may come with its own challenges. This innovative edge (competitive advantage) has made them thrive in the most adverse environments. Engagement with social enterprises now forms an important part of many organisations' corporate social responsibility strategy. Social enterprise adds colour to the supply chain diversity and corporate social responsibility agenda of many corporate organisations. This is achieved by these 'big buyers' procuring and working with them to develop the communities in which they operate.

Social businesses act as a catalyst to their host communities, facilitating community cohesion and development. An attractive proposition of social enterprises is lower set-up and running costs, due to various factors. Social enterprises are at the forefront of better and improved working practices, they give their staff the opportunity to work flexibly, enhancing their quality of life and improving their work-life balance.

Underpinning the operations of most social enterprises is a consciousness that the environment needs to be managed in a sustainable way. They are quick to adopt new ways of 'greening' their business and communities by driving through the ideals of environmental sustainability. Their innovative capacity is high, breaking new ground in markets that the public and private sector deem unprofitable.

Box 14.2 Case study: community development in Clays Lane, London Borough of Newham, UK

When a group of church planners were commissioned by their parent church to start a new mission, they identified a community estate known as Clays Lane. It was the second largest housing cooperative in Europe, providing one-room accommodation for single people. Clays Lane was situated in one of the most deprived areas in the London Borough of Newham. The group identified worklessness as a key issue during a mapping exercise. Unemployment figures were as high as 50 per cent among residents of the estate. Other issues identified were a high suicide rate, crime and anti-social behaviour. The volunteers decided to set up a social enterprise called the Clays Lane Advice and Training Centre (CLATC). This approach signified identification with the community and its people. The objective of this organisation was to tackle unemployment through training and community development activity, thus having a huge effect on other social problems.

They started out by designing and developing an ICT training project and internet suite. Their first training was in Oracle, HTML and later MS Office. This proved to be popular with the residents, mostly students who could not afford the cost of professional training and exams. The volunteer trainers were students who had graduated from local universities and were required to develop their skills and employment prospects by gaining work experience. The internet suite proved to be successful as it was a free service and also served as a community meeting place. Most of the computers and equipment used for the project were donated by members of the local church, and the equipment was refurbished by an in-house computer engineer. The project demonstrated resourcefulness, innovation and motivation on the part of the volunteers. As a result of running this pilot project the organisation was able to get a service level contract with the regional authority to run a one-year IT training project. CLATC went on to run various community projects such as a personal development conference tagged 'SMC' (Success and Motivation Conference), and a weekly youth meeting and counselling service. Most of the volunteers on the project gained relevant work experience and now work in various full-time capacities as managers. One of the volunteers working on the project was Gloria, the first administrator of the centre. She developed most of her skills at the centre and went on to work for a number of community organisations in a paid capacity. She now works as an administrative manager with a major NHS Trust.

One remarkable encounter occurred when an insurance broker visited the centre to sell public and employer's liability insurance. He was impressed by CLATC's entrepreneurial activities and commitment to the project and community. He later sent them a personal cheque for £250 to cover the cost of insurance.

Currently, the Clays Lane estate has ceased to exist as it has been subsumed into the London Olympic 2012 Park area; the organisation has also been relocated under the compulsory purchase order by the London Development Agency. CLATC is in the process of restructuring and has plans to set up youth and training projects nearby in the future. They recently acquired a property in Norfolk, which will serve as an investment vehicle and income generator for their social projects, once refurbished and rented. The CLATC case study goes a long way to show the benefits social enterprises bring to the development of people and communities, whether affluent or deprived.

The demerits of social enterprises

It would be unrealistic to conclude that social enterprises have no drawbacks. Like all other types of businesses, they have their challenges. Listed below are some disadvantages of social enterprises. This is not a blanket diagnosis however, as the disadvantages may vary across the sectors in which social enterprises operate.

A major factor that has affected the sustainability of many social businesses is a lack of finance. Social enterprises are often stereotyped as amateur in various circles. However, perspectives are gradually changing and social enterprises are taken more seriously. Slowness to respond to opportunities or threats due to the structures and governance requirements could impede sustainability. A lack of capacity to engage in high-level procurement opportunities due to buyer criteria has affected many social enterprises. For instance, the proportionality rule of most local authorities states that businesses can only tender for contracts valued at up to 25–30 per cent of their turnover. Most social enterprises are small and may not be able to tender where contract values are exponentially higher than 30 per cent of their turnover; this scenario raises the level of risk with commissioners.

Recent research has raised a number of factors that social enterprises face, such as a lack of capacity to tender for contracts, the concept of enterprise and aggressive competition within the context of ethics, territorialism and poor understanding of social enterprises by commissioners and buyers (Lyon, 2007). These can have profound effects on the vulnerable staff and volunteers who are gradually coming back into employment and wider social engagement. Generally, a lack of people management skills is identified as a gap in social enterprise training provision by Peattie and Morley (2008), who state that there is a single emphasis on entrepreneurship skills only, and not on skills needed to develop and run management teams.

Other issues are the implementation of governmental policies that may not be in the interest of some social enterprises. For example, a move towards commissioning and partnership could be a barrier to increasing supplier diversity and the varied aspirations of social enterprises, whose strategy may be to be less collaborative. It is also common knowledge in the third sector that only the most successful social entrepreneurs get recognition and rewards for their work, and this may discourage other social entrepreneurs as the cost of starting and managing a social enterprise comes with high personal and financial sacrifices. Lastly, governance is an area in need of robust development work, unlike the private sector business where governance is less rigid. For instance, it is mandatory for social enterprises to adhere to their constitution and articles of association; this may slow down their response to opportunities and changes in their micro and macro environment.

Social enterprises	Private businesses
Community ownership.	Owned by shareholders.
Profits reinvested in the organisation and community to fulfil objectives.	Profits shared or reinvested for shareholders' capital increase.
Goodwill from the public and government.	Goodwill will have to be built up over long periods through a corporate social responsibility strategy.
Driven by social needs.	Driven by wealth maximisation and enterprise.

Innovative and resourceful due to resource limitation.	Can develop a culture of inefficiency as the focus is mostly a profit and bonus driven culture: for example, the financial services sector in UK and the US.
Lower overheads and set-up cost.	Highly capital intensive.
Volunteering and staffing culture.	Staffing culture.
Employs simple and effective business processes.	Management systems can become complex and bureaucratic.
Capital is raised through grant funding, donations, loans, in-kind funding and trading activity.	Capitalisation through shareholder investment, loans, venture capital and initial public offering (IPO).

Table 14.1 Comparisons between social enterprises and private businesses

Activity 14.2 Reflective exercise: analysing the macro environment for social enterprises in public health in the UK

It is imperative that a social enterprise analyses its internal structure, the micro and the macro environment, so as to be able to implement an effective business strategy. Various analytical tools are used to understand organisations.

Responding tactically to the opportunities, threats and challenges presented is a key trait of successful enterprises. We will use the PESTLE analytical tool to consider the external environment of a social enterprise (see, for example, Burnes, 2006). It is called PESTLE analysis as it stands for Political, Economic, Social, Technological, Legal and Environmental factors in the macro environment that affect a business. The tool helps managers to understand their environment and respond accordingly. A picture is built up when intelligence is gathered and put under the relevant headings. Please note that the information outlined below is not exhaustive.

Political
- Government support and legislation in favour of social enterprise – the Third Sector Action Plan released £42.5 million earmarked to help social enterprises during the UK's economic downturn.

- The Office of the Third Sector is set up to support and fund social enterprises.
- The Department for Health sets up a pathfinders fund for social enterprises delivering health and social care services.
- The government appoints 20 Social Enterprise Ambassadors who champion and inspire upcoming social entrepreneurs and projects.
- The NHS is restructured to create social enterprises and internal markets.
- Funding is increased from the Department of Health for Social Enterprise in the Health sector.
- Staff in hospitals are encouraged to consider transitioning into a social enterprise through 'right to request'.
- A government £100 million wellness fund is set up for social enterprises to tap into.
- Social clauses such as Section 106 are factored into many major regeneration projects, encouraging large corporations to engage with community organisations and businesses.
- The Department for Health launches Change4Life, encouraging families to eat more healthily and move more, soliciting the support of all stakeholders including social enterprise.

Economic
- The NHS spends £4.2 billion a year on obesity and overweight-related themes (DoH online, 2008).
- Economic downturn favours the social enterprise model.
- An increase in unemployment; social enterprise could act as a pathway to employment.
- A robust financial structure is set up by banks and financial institutions to fund social enterprise.
- Royal Bank of Scotland sets up the SE 100 index to track growth and impact of social enterprise.
- Corporate social responsibility is high on the agenda of many large organisations.

Social
- There is a high percentage of volunteers in the UK.
- There is a long history of social action in the UK.
- Special employment schemes are set up to encourage employers to take on the unemployed.
- Faith-based groups are heavily involved in social enterprise activity.

- Growing numbers of ethnic minority people are involved in social enterprise.
- Ethical consumerism is growing.

Technological
- Knowledge transfer and innovation are high within the social enterprise sector.
- Social enterprises are highly innovative and inclusive technological structures are available.
- There is a high convergence of social action due to the advances in information and communication technology, making social action and collaboration across states attainable.

Legal
- Social enterprises can register under different forms such as community interest companies, friendly and provident societies, companies limited by guarantee and as charitable trading companies.
- Support structures and umbrella bodies are available at the centre, such as Social Enterprise Coalition and Social Enterprise London.
- Risk to directors in the event of liquidation is minimal.

Environmental
- Public awareness on global warming is high.
- The effect of global warming is being felt.
- Social enterprises are playing key roles in green action and environmental sustainability.
- Ethical consumerism is growing.
- Legislation is being passed in favour of environmental sustainability and the green agenda.

Think about the above in relation to your organisation.

Box 14.3 How can health commissioners support social enterprises without losing out?

- Develop effective procurement frameworks that foster supply chain diversity.
- Undertake a shift in attitude, as current policies and strategies may not be effective in engaging with social enterprises and it might require radical and new ways of thinking to reduce cost, improve performance and retain staff.
- Encourage capacity building for long-term benefit and reward; health commissioners should work with social enterprises to build capacity and reap incremental and sustainable service as a legacy.
- Encourage partnership working and consortium bidding.
- Avoid stereotyping and deal with each social enterprise on a case-by-case basis.

CONCLUSION

This chapter considered the scope of social capital and social enterprises and focused on the benefits for community development and social cohesion. Both have become pivotal to government thinking in public health. Social enterprises can play a vital role in public health intervention by developing and administering innovative solutions to the challenges currently being faced in public health.

Social enterprises should ensure that they are ready for the challenges ahead. They must understand that the expectations of stakeholders are growing constantly, and that learning, flexibility and innovation must be entrenched as core values if they are to attain and maintain the sustainability of their social, environmental and business goals. They must use their collective power as stakeholders, suppliers and buyers to address the various environmental pressures that they face. Social enterprises need to embrace new concepts through research, knowledge transfer and partnerships. Proper avenues for sharing best practice should be constituted. There is continued pressure to do more for less. However, social enterprises do not need to conform to unrealistic expectations, but to reform policies through engagement. Social enterprises must look deeper and understand that their competitive advantage is in their unique characteristics and they should use these traits to create income streams that defy convention and push them within the territories of independence. The challenge is to develop new concepts that build their capacity and influence policies, especially those affecting the marginalised.

Activity 14.3 Reflective exercise

- What is the implication of the social enterprise model in a free market economy driven by reward for enterprise?
- Design a project proposal for a public health social enterprise project. What are the implications of the project within the macro environment?

Further reading and useful websites

Alkhafaji, A. (2003) *Strategic Management Formulation, Implementation, and Control in a Dynamic Environment.* New York, London, Victoria (Au): Hawthorne Press

Paton, R. (2003) *Managing and Measuring Social Enterprises* (Chapter 2, p. 22). London: Sage Publications

ONS (2003) *Social Capital: Measuring Networks and Shared Values.* Online – available at: **www.statistics.gov.uk/CCI/nugget.asp?ID=314** (accessed 8 April 2009)

Divine Chocolate : **www.divinechocolate.com/about/story.aspx** (accessed 15 July 2009)

Grameen Bank: **www.grameen-info.org** (accessed 15 July 2009)

Office of the Third Sector: **www.cabinetoffice.gov.uk/third_sector.aspx** (accessed 15 July 2009)

Social Enterprise Coalition: **www.socialenterprise.org.uk** (accessed 15 July 2009)

Social Enterprise London: **www.sel.org.uk** (accessed 15 July 2009)

Chapter 15

Ethics in public health

Mandy Mitchelmore

This chapter will focus on the ways in which ethical issues relate to public health. First of all a review or revision of ethical principles will be provided and the implications that this has for public health will be examined. Then a more detailed analysis of public health issues including abortion and Human Immuno-deficiency Virus (HIV) will be considered.

Learning outcomes

In this chapter you will learn how to:

- relate ethical issues to public health;

- apply the implications of ethical issues to public health, providing examples;

- analyse ethical issues in public health, using the example of HIV.

INTRODUCTION

The reasons why we need to think about a framework for ethics could be debated but, in terms of promoting critical thinking, if we focus on moral philosophical standpoints we can use these as a framework for analysing what are quite often difficult situations or dilemmas. This is helpful in terms of making us more objective about an issue instead of only seeing it from our own moral perspective. Beauchamp and Childress (2001: 15) state that: 'Ethical theories should build on, systematise, and rationally reconstruct our ordinary action-guides and judgement'.

Ethical considerations may relate to professional practice for individuals, their colleagues and their clients. When we broaden this to professional practice in public health, it might be helpful to try to think what the differences and the similarities are. A useful definition is offered by Dickens and Cook (2007: 75) when they state that: 'Bioethical principles have been developed at the clinical or microethical level affecting relations among individuals, whereas public health ethics applies at the population-based or macroethical level'.

ETHICAL AND LEGAL RIGHTS

It does not matter if we focus on the clinical level or on a broader level such as in public health; there is always an association between ethical rights and legal rights. This is not to say that they are the same thing but legal solutions are sought when there is no clear way forward or in order to maintain a minimum standard.

Moral or universal rights are generally seen as rights that should apply to all people at all times, although these rights are often set in the context of the country in which we live. These rights are often referred to as human rights and there is the Human Rights Act 1998 in this country to encompass these. The Human Rights Act 1998 is being cited more and more in regard to decisions regarding the funding of treatments as well as the right to life and the right to privacy. An example of this was the nurse who went to court to demand that she be allowed the drug herceptin that, at the time, was only licensed for use in advanced breast cancer. She successfully argued that it was a violation of her human rights to deny her a potentially life-saving treatment (BBC, 2005).

Legal rights are often combined with moral rights to allow patients or clients to use the legal system if they are not satisfied with the care they have received. Legislation has allowed patients to have access to their medical records and generally there is a legal obligation to gain informed consent and to have documentation to that effect. However, in cases of a sudden outbreak of a contagious disease, the rights of the individual to give their informed consent might be overridden by the rights of the majority who need to be protected. With regard to the Public Health Act 1984, nobody is allowed to opt out of notification.

ETHICAL PRINCIPLES IN INDIVIDUAL PRACTICE AND PUBLIC HEALTH

Having briefly explored the relationship between rights and ethical decision-making, it is worth considering the principles that are most often cited, as these have relevance in both individual practice and in the broader area of public health. It does however mean that certain aspects of practice such as confidentiality and consent might be altered when moving from the individual level to the population level, and certain tenets might have to be overlooked in terms of the public interest. We often refer to four principles when discussing ethics, which are autonomy, beneficence, non-malificence and justice (Beauchamp and Childress, 2001):

- **Autonomy** is concerned with self-governance or the right to be self-directed. All of us should be able to choose options and be consulted on issues that have a direct bearing on our health or welfare. Autonomy is considered to be a key principle and one that guides others who we might need to consider (Newham and Hawley, 2007)
- **Beneficence** (or 'doing good'). It is appropriate that we should want the best for others and try to do good in all of our actions and thoughts. In trying to do good we would have to consider what the person really wants i.e., their autonomy, otherwise our own idea of what might be good could be quite different from theirs.
- **Non-malificence** or not doing harm is not the opposite of doing good. Rather it is a recognition that we cannot always put something right but we should at least do no harm. An example of this would be Florence Nightingale, who talked about doing the patient no harm by making sure that they were cared for in sanitary conditions. The modern-day equivalent might be about preventing MRSA (*methocillin resistant staphylococcus aureus*) or the so-called hospital super bug. Patients should not be harmed just because they have been in hospital.
- **Justice** is concerned with advocacy in terms of representing the patient's or client's views if they are unable to put them forward themselves. There may, of course, also be justice in the legal sense if the case goes to court but justice is also concerned with the allocation of resources. This is relevant in a system where we know that there is rationing and that there are inequalities in terms of treatments that are accessible. How do we ensure that we treat all of our patients or clients with the same justice when as human beings we are bound to make judgements? (Hoban, 2006)

Kant, Bentham and Mill

There are different schools of thought on these principles and two notable names associated with ethics are Emmanuel Kant (1734–1804) and Jeremy Bentham (1748–1832). Slightly later, John Stuart Mill (1806–1876) added to the work of Bentham.

Emmanuel Kant proposed that it is not the end or consequences of an act which make it right or wrong but the moral intention of the agent. His philosophical thinking is known as Deontology. 'Deon' comes from Greek and means duty (Fletcher, *et al.*, 1995). With regard to autonomy Kant would argue that all people have unconditional worth and therefore are worthy of respect in terms of their right to make choices or be self-directed.

Utilitarianism or consequentialism is a doctrine suggested by Jeremy Bentham, and later by John Stuart Mill, which is commonly quoted as that which proposes that an action is morally good if it produces the greatest amount of good for the greatest number of people and that the end justifies the means. 'All's well that ends well' might be seen as a utilitarian statement. With respect to autonomy John Stuart Mill discussed the individuality of action and thought and the need not to interfere with freedom. Achieving the greatest good is often cited when decisions regarding funding or allocating resources are being considered. A utilitarian would say that the costly intensive care bed should go to the person with the best chance of recovery, but the deontologists would say that the duty of care is the same for all patients, regardless of their chances of recovery. In reality both schools of thought come into play and individual health care professionals need to exercise their judgement in deciding how to allocate precious resources.

John Stuart Mill would value autonomy as much as Kant but the reasons for doing so would be different. Kant would see it as a duty and part of unconditional regard that you would do your utmost to allow the person to be self-directed. Whereas John Stuart Mill would not see it so much as duty but rather as the right of individuals to exercise their right to freedom and to make choices. Both theories support autonomy and recognise its importance but from different perspectives. There is, however, agreement that this principle has a bearing on all the others and that it should be upheld whenever possible.

In reality we probably need a bit of both as it can be difficult to know if we are always doing good and, equally, carrying out utilitarianism to the letter might not always be beneficial. Sometimes we want to achieve happiness for people who might not be of the greater number. For example, there are some very rare medical conditions only affecting a small number of people. Should we not bother with them? A recent example of this was the decision by the National Institute for Health and Clinical Excellence (NICE) not to fund a cancer drug for a rare type of kidney cancer affecting 2 000 people, which would extend life by 12 to 18 months. A successful campaign was fought by leading oncologists who argued that, although the cost of this drug is currently £25 000 per patient, the number needing the drug was comparatively small and the overall cancer bill was nothing like the bill for coronary heart disease, and that these factors should be considered as well as the cost of the drug in question (Cancer Research, 2008; Medscape, 2008). This is a clear scenario where we can see that a utilitarian view would not be helpful if you happened to be in a minority where your length and quality of life is not being given any consideration.

Activity 15.1 Reflective exercise: ethics in practice

Consider an issue that you have dealt with recently that you think had an ethical component to it. Apply all four of the principles outlined above to the situation. Think about how each of them came into play and your own role in promoting justice or autonomy or how you know that you did 'good' in that particular situation.

ETHICS AND AUTONOMY

As we discussed earlier, autonomy is about self-government or autonomous decision-making. Most of us expect to make choices in our lives, whether it is which house or neighbourhood we live in, which schools we select for our children or which supermarket we buy our food in. We make choices and, although some days we wish someone could decide things for us, by and large we would not want to lose control over our own lives and destiny.

The challenge we have in public health is promoting independence and yet, at the same time, making sure that the choices that individuals make are not detrimental to themselves or others. An example of this might be vaccination. As vaccines are given to healthy children they need to have a very high safety profile in order to limit harm (Lachmann, 1998). Recent scares about outbreaks of measles (Eaton, 2009) have been attributed to the lower uptake of vaccination linked to adverse publicity concerning the MMR vaccine. If parents have been worried about possible links with autism and have not vaccinated their child, they are relying on the fact that most other parents will have had their children vaccinated and that the overall risk of contracting measles is low. It is obvious that the child themselves does not have the ability to consent and so it is the autonomous choice of the parents that decides whether the child will be vaccinated and against which diseases. Another recent example has been the debate about whether people should be able to buy cheap alcohol from supermarkets, which is under review in Scotland (Scottish Intercollegiate Group on Alcohol, 2009). The debate is whether people should be trusted to drink responsibly or a standard price for alcohol should be used as a means of making sure that it is relatively expensive in both pubs and supermarkets. Would this price rise penalise the majority who do drink sensibly?

Autonomy and consent

One of the key aspects of autonomy is consent. We get informed consent so that the person has a say in what is going to happen to them. There is also a clear obligation to get consent for medical research. The Nuremburg Trials revealed how prisoners of war were being experimented on without consent. It was decided that this sort of inhumane treatment should never happen again and that people should not be experimented on in terms of drug or other treatments without informed consent. This is governed by the (1964) Declaration of Helsinki (*British Medical Journal*, 1996).

Activity 15.2 Reflective exercise: autonomy

In which situations might we not respect autonomy? Make a list.

Thinking about autonomy

In most societies suicide is not thought of as a good thing and the reduction of suicide and mental health problems has been the focus of previous and current public health policy. It is always assumed that the person might not be making a sound judgement at the time of trying to commit suicide.

In cases where the person is unconscious, perhaps after a road traffic accident, and is brought into the Accident and Emergency (A&E) Department then decisions regarding emergency surgery or medical interventions would be carried out without consent. This would only be acceptable in emergency situations.

In sudden outbreaks such as *E.coli, salmonella* and meningitis, for example, it is not possible to always gain consent and it is considered that nobody has the right to opt out of notification.

Complete autonomy is not given to children on the basis that they are not mature enough to understand all of the options. A child may not choose to go to the dentist but a parent would normally consider that it was important for their dental health and would make the choices for their child. There is, however, wide-ranging legislation designed to protect children, both in this country and internationally. The Children's Act 1989 gives children the right to be listened to and to make certain choices that they are capable of making.

We know that certain groups of people are not necessarily given the right to complete autonomy. Mental health patients who are sectioned under the Mental Health Act 2007 do not have the right to choose whether they receive treatment. However, there are other mental health patients who are able to make choices and whose condition could be made worse if these options were taken away from them. For example, a person with depression might not be able to cope but if the depression was treated then they might be able to resume their usual life.

We know that people with learning disabilities are often not given the choices that they should be offered, particularly when they come into busy acute hospitals. Decisions regarding contraception might also be made for them and there have been cases where the courts have decided on whether sterilisation operations are appropriate (Fletcher, *et al.*, 1995).

Another problem with trying to respect autonomy is that it is not always static. It can change and for health care professionals this is difficult. With regard to public health then, we see that there are issues with people making autonomous choices. This is often cited in relation to sexual health where a person might be able to assert themselves in one sexual relationship but be unable to insist on safer sex in the next one. The issue of teenagers and sexual relationships has also been much debated as intellectual maturity is not always as developed as physical maturity. The recent pictures of a very child-like boy of 12 holding a baby allegedly conceived with a 15-year-old girl have disturbed many (*The Times*, 2009). Effective sexual education in schools is thought by many to be a relevant public health strategy, although the age at which this should start is often debated. Autonomous choices are affected by beliefs as to which conditions people consider themselves susceptible to, and this again can be influenced by the media. For example, the recent rise in the uptake of cervical smear tests has been attributed to a high-profile celebrity case. This has, however, had the effect of leaving some women more anxious as they are considered too young for the cervical screening programme and are not in the age category for the new vaccine. This has led to the Department of Health (DoH) reviewing women under the age of 25 for cervical cancer (DoH, 2009) and subsequently maintaining their position not to screen.

In summary, autonomy is important and should be respected in most situations. If a person is an adult and of 'sound mind' then they should be able to be self-governing. This is generally possible but, in public health, we cannot ignore the rest of society. An example of this might be a person who chooses to live their life in squalor but the consequences of this might be unacceptable to their immediate neighbours who may have to endure infestation by rodents, etc. (Lauder, *et al.* 2005).

Considerations in autonomy

Particular care needs to be given to groups of patients who are more likely to have their autonomy overridden. As discussed above, these might be children because of their immaturity or people with learning disability or mental health problems. Additionally there is quite a lot of evidence to suggest that elderly people are not given the respect and dignity that they should have and who might not be encouraged to make important choices (Age Concern, 2009; NMC, 2009).

There is also evidence to suggest that people from ethnic minorities may have a worse health status than the rest of the population (DoH, 2005). Written information is often seen as reinforcing the spoken word, especially as vulnerable patients do not necessarily hear everything that is being said to them. This information also needs to be translated into the appropriate languages as there are specific problems that might arise if there is a need for a translator and there is not one available. Family members may not present the facts in the same way and, again, informed consent may suffer as a consequence (Caress, 2003).

CONFIDENTIALITY

Confidentiality is enshrined in the Hippocratic Oath and it is part of all codes of conduct for health and social care professionals to:

- respect people's right to confidentiality; and
- ensure people are informed about how and why information is shared by those who will be providing the care.

(NMC, 2008)

In relation to ethics, discussion tends to focus on what would be the consequence of breaching confidentiality, rather than on the merit in maintaining confidentiality. This might be because it is generally believed to be a good thing and so the consequences of breaching confidentiality tend to be discussed in terms of deontology and the importance of being able to keep promises and perform your duty to the person. If the person is being afforded unconditional worth then it should follow that the same regard would be given to personal information concerning them.

Activity 15.3 Reflective exercise: confidentiality

Consider situations where you know that a breach of confidentiality occurred.
- How did it come to light?
- What were the consequences?
- How did it affect the patient/professional relationship?
- Consider if you have ever been in a situation where disclosure was necessary and how did you or the team decide that this was the only course of action?
- What were the consequences of the action (for you, the patient and others in the scenario)?

Downie and Calman (1994) provide us with a useful guide to exploring confidentiality. They suggest that people with whom information might be shared include:

- those who must know;
- those who should know;
- those who could know;
- those who should not know.

Consent like autonomy does not necessarily remain static. A person may withdraw consent at any time and this would need to be respected. The issue of whether consent can truly be informed, and whether it is always in patients' best interests to know everything, is debated.

ETHICAL DILEMMAS: ABORTION AND HIV

It is often stated that most ethical dilemmas centre around either start of life or end of life issues. There are many controversies surrounding start of life issues that are often associated with developments in new technologies, and do raise questions about what is desirable in society and whether there is an element of 'playing God' in some cases.

Abortion

Abortion is often hotly debated and is a key public health issue. Historically, deliberate termination of pregnancy was made illegal by the Offences Against the Person Act 1861. This was followed by The Infant Preservation Act 1929, which allowed abortion if the life of the woman was at risk but set a 28-week limit. The Abortion Act 1967 was not amended until 1990 by the Human Fertilisation and Embryology Act, which reduced the limit to 24 weeks.

The Abortion Act works by stating that a pregnancy can be terminated before 24 weeks if: 'Continuance would involve risk greater than if the pregnancy were terminated or injury to the physical or mental health of the pregnant woman or any existing children'.

Unsafe abortions occur mainly in developing countries (97 per cent) where contraception is not necessarily affordable or easily available (Dickens and Cook, 2007). Termination of pregnancy in developed countries is, in contrast, a very safe procedure. Abortion remains unacceptable to some individuals and groups and is defended by others in respect of choice and the alternative being a poor outcome for women's health.

Fertility treatment

Other start of life issues are concerned with fertility treatments, which are raised by couples using the Human Rights Act 1988 and citing the article on the 'right to found a family'. Involuntary infertility is psychologically disturbing for the people involved but this is not seen as a public health problem in the same way as the prevention of unwanted pregnancy and sexually transmitted infections.

In terms of justice it can be seen that not all couples will have access to assisted conception centres, the treatments can be very expensive and there is often rationing of this type of treatment within the health service. Currently there are 50 conditions that can be screened for in embryos to prevent conditions such as sickle cell or cystic fibrosis, and the Human Fertilisation and Embryology Authority (HFEA) recently increased this to include some later onset conditions. With regard to public health we have to be aware of how socially acceptable disability will be and if we should screen out conditions such as Downs Syndrome. If we do, how does that affect the person who is alive with that condition?

Human Immuno-deficiency Virus (HIV)

So far, we have touched on various examples where ethics has a bearing on public health issues, but it might be useful to now consider ethics in relation to one condition. HIV has been selected because it is a modern-day public health issue that is significant across all countries. The issue of whether developed countries are morally obliged to help developing countries with treatments, etc. is also debated (Bryan, 2002). The history of public health has been about stopping diseases such as TB and smallpox, and HIV is one of today's challenges. It is also looked at differently to other diseases and, as such, it is interesting in relation to consent and also to the fact that it falls under the remit of criminal law with regard to deliberate transmission.

According to Lachmann (1998) the principal focus of public health has generally been the need to control infectious diseases. In the past, this would have been anything from leprosy to epidemics associated with infected food or water. The spread of HIV has been largely attributed to the fact that people travel more frequently around the world and taboos regarding sexual relationships have changed (Bryan, 2002). When HIV was first diagnosed in this country there was a great deal of fear and apprehension, with a high degree of stigma attached to the disease. The fact that the disease also affected injecting drug users and homosexuals contributed to some of the very judgemental sentiments that were expressed (NAM, 2007).

The prevalence of HIV is recorded, along with other sexually transmitted diseases, to ascertain whether there is a high prevalence in certain areas and to look at trends. Testing for HIV has also involved gaining informed consent and providing counselling as to the result. This has changed in some respects now that it is seen as a routine test in some areas of health care.

An example of routine testing would be in maternity care where a woman would need to opt out of HIV testing rather than opt in (DoH, 2000). The justification for this is that treatments have advanced to the point where effective anti-retroviral drugs can be given in pregnancy, which would dramatically reduce the incidence of the child being born with HIV. According to the Department of Health (1998b) treatment given to an infected mother reduced the likelihood of their child being infected from one in six to one in a hundred. This is obviously a sensible public health measure but, at the individual level, there is still a problem if the woman does not share the fact that she is positive with her partner. Midwives have found themselves in difficult positions when treatment is being given to a newborn child and the father of the child has no idea why this is happening. This is again an example of individual autonomy in opposition to what is in the best interests of the population at large. If people do not know their HIV status they may inadvertently infect others and they are being denied access to treatment through ignorance.

The fact that deliberate transmission of HIV is considered a criminal offence under the Offences Against the Person Act 1861 has also, in some respects, created complications for the public health agenda with this disease. The Act was drawn up in 1861 but was invoked in relation to HIV at a time when there were dramatic headlines about people deliberately infecting as many people as possible, and at this time treatments were not available which led many to see it as giving someone a death sentence (The *Guardian*, 2001). The availability of effective treatments has changed the course of the disease and it is now not clear how the Act will be used in the future and in which situations. Some have argued that it is a deterrent to knowing your HIV status as you could not be said to be deliberately infecting partners with HIV if you did not know you definitely had the disease (NAM, 2007). This would obviously be counterproductive from a public health point of view. The fact that HIV comes under criminal law in this regard now has implications for confidentiality as well, which is an ethical concern. In the conviction of Stephen Kelly, for example, blood results from confidential research in prison were seized by police to prove that he did know his HIV status before his release (NAM, 2007).

CONCLUSION

This chapter has reconsidered the bio-medical principles of ethics, which are probably familiar to many at an individual level, and explored the ways in which these principles relate to public health. We have seen that individual confidentiality and consent might be overridden for the greater needs of society in sudden outbreaks of infectious diseases. Individual autonomy has been considered, as have the ways in which choices can affect others such as immunisation, sexual health. At the broader level ethical considerations should inform public health strategy as this will help to protect the vulnerable and contribute to a fairer and more equal society.

Further reading and useful websites

Beauchamp, T.L. and Childress, J.F. (2001) *Principles of Biomedical Ethics* (5th edn). Oxford: Oxford University Press.

Seedhouse, D. (2007) *Ethics: The Heart of Health Care* (2nd edn). Chichester: John Wiley and Sons.

Tingle, J. and Cribb, A. (eds) (2007) *Nursing Law and Ethics* (2nd edn). Oxford: Blackwell Science.

www.bma.org.uk/ethics/index.jsphttp:/www-ethics-network.org.uk
Research and publication on key ethical issues, including child protection in England and Wales, guidance on access to health care for asylum seekers and refused asylum seekers and prompts for doctors in making decisions about those who lack the mental capacity to do so themselves etc.

www.ethics-network.org.uk
to provide up to date and reliable information on ethical issues.

/intute.ac.uk/bioethicsweb
gateway to resources relating to biomedical ethics, including ethical, social, legal and public policy questions arising from advances in medicine and biology.

//nuffieldbioethics.org/go/ourwork/publichealth/introduction
concerned with how and when the government should intervene into our lives concerning health issues and the responsibilities for industry.

(all above websites last accessed 11 September 2009).

Chapter 16

Evidence-based practice

Ven Veeramah and Jill Stewart

This chapter outlines the development of socio-economic evidence-based practice and the types of evidence that can increasingly inform practice. We advise on where to source the best evidence, how to assess its rigour and how it might be applied to practice. At the time of writing, NICE was rolling out its new National Public Health Evidence Base and so this chapter in particular was constantly being overtaken by events.

Learning outcomes

In this chapter you will learn how to:

- define the development and application of evidence-based public health;

- rate hierarchies of evidence, and define research methods and their application to public health;

- appreciate the significance of systematic reviews and meta-analysis in summarising data;

- access, search and analyse public health research;

- assess gaps in published evidence and appreciate the need for practitioners to contribute to the evidence base;

- implement evidence-based public health strategies and interventions.

FROM EVIDENCE-BASED MEDICINE TO EVIDENCE-BASED PUBLIC HEALTH

Although evidence-based practice was initially developed for adoption in clinical medicine to improve the care for individual patients, more recently it has gradually found its way into public health practice (Muir Gray, 1997). The main reason has been the growing demand in public health to use scientific reasoning approaches to support informed decisions in regard to public health issues and policy development, as well as to provide effective public health programmes (Brownson, *et al.*, 2003). However, unlike evidence-based medicine where the main focus is usually on individual patients, evidence-based public health involves using the best available evidence to make informed public health practice decisions with respect to whole communities and populations. The main emphasis is on disease prevention, health maintenance and health promotion. This is aptly illustrated by Jenicek (1997: 187) who defines it as 'the conscientious, explicit, and judicious use of current best evidence in making decisions about the care of communities and populations in the domain of health protection, disease prevention, health maintenance and improvement'.

The strategy to be employed when implementing evidence-based public health necessitates a clear identification of the relevant question(s), a comprehensive search of the appropriate literature, a critical appraisal of the currently available evidence and how this can be applied to the situation at hand, and a balanced application of the conclusions to the public health problem (Guyatt and Rennie, 2002). It is important when implementing evidence-based practice to search for the best evidence available. This means that the quality of the evidence is of primary significance. However, there is general recognition that the quality of all research evidence on any topic of interest may not be equal in terms of its validity (Evans, 2003).

HIERARCHIES OF EVIDENCE

To help with the interpretation and evaluation of research findings, hierarchies of evidence have been identified. These hierarchies have used a range of different research approaches and classify the evidence generated according to its validity (Evans, 2003). One example of the hierarchy of evidence is given below in Box 16.1, with a brief description of study designs given in Box 16.2.

Box 16.1: Rating system for the hierarchy of evidence/levels of evidence

- Level I – Evidence from a systematic review or meta-analysis of all relevant randomised controlled trials (RCTs).
- Level II – Evidence obtained from at least one well-designed RCT.
- Level III – Evidence obtained from one well-designed controlled trial without randomisation.
- Level IV – Evidence from well-designed case-control and cohort studies.
- Level V – Evidence from systematic reviews of descriptive studies such as cross-sectional surveys or qualitative studies.
- Level VI – Evidence from a single descriptive or qualitative study.
- Level VII – Evidence from the opinion of authorities, case reports/studies and/or reports of expert committees.

(Adapted from Mazurek, M.B. and Fineout-Overholt, E. (2005: 10) *Evidence-based Practice in Nursing and Healthcare*. Philadelphia: Lippincott Williams and Wilkins.)

Box 16.2: A brief description of study designs

A **systematic review** is a synthesis of relevant primary research studies on a particular subject. It uses thorough methods to search for and include all, or as much as possible, research on the topic of interest. Only relevant studies, usually of a certain minimum quality, are included.

A **meta-analysis** is a statistical technique for combining data from several quantitative studies within a systematic review.

A **randomised controlled clinical trial** is a study where people are allocated randomly to receiving a particular intervention or not (this could be two different treatments or one treatment and a placebo). The aim of randomly allocating subjects to the two groups is to minimise the effect of any known and unknown confounding factors that could influence the results. It is considered the strongest design to establish a cause and effect relationship.

A **cohort study is a prospective study** that identifies a group of people and follows them over a period of time to see how being exposed to a particular risk factor affects the outcome. Usually, there is a comparison group that is not exposed to the risk factor but is followed in the same way as the exposed group with regard to their health status. This type of study is normally used to look at the effect of suspected risk factors that cannot be controlled experimentally on outcomes like, for example, the effect of smoking on lung cancer. Cohort studies are observational and not as reliable as randomised controlled studies, since the two groups may differ in ways other than in the variable under study.

Case-control studies are epidemiological studies that are often used to identify risk factors for a medical problem. This type of study compares a group of patients who have that condition with a group of patients who do not and looks back in time to see how the characteristics of the two groups differ. They often rely on medical records and patient recall for data collection. The study is concerned with the frequency and amount of exposure to the risk factor being investigated in the two groups.

Case series and **case reports** are a descriptive study of a group of people, usually receiving the same treatment or with the same disease. In this type of study, it is possible to describe characteristics or outcomes in a particular group of people, but not to determine how this compares with people who are not treated in the same way or do not have this condition. Because these are reports of cases and use no control groups with which to compare outcomes, they have no statistical validity.

Cross-sectional studies are epidemiological studies that describe characteristics of populations to include the presence or absence of disease or other health-related variables. They are 'cross-sectional' because data is collected at one point in time and then the relationships between characteristics are considered. Importantly, because such a study does not look at time trends, it cannot establish what causes what. This contrasts with longitudinal studies, such as cohort studies, that are followed over a period of time.

Qualitative research uses individual in-depth interviews, focus groups or questionnaires to collect, analyse and interpret data by observing what people do and say. It reports on the meanings, concepts, definitions, characteristics, metaphors, symbols and descriptions of things. It is more subjective than quantitative research and is often exploratory and open-ended. Small numbers of people are interviewed in depth and/or a relatively small number of focus groups are conducted.

(Adapted source: NHS Knowledge Service, which can be accessed online at: **www.nhs.uk/news/pages/newsglossary.aspx** [accessed 15 July 2009].)

The pros and cons of RCTs

A limitation of these hierarchies is that they have focused mainly on effectiveness of treatments and interventions (Evans, 2003). It is generally acknowledged and commonly accepted that the most significant and highest level of evidence is derived from randomised controlled trials (RCTs), especially multi-centre RCTs. The RCT is regarded as 'the gold standard' because of the methodological robustness of this particular research design. The findings constitute the best evidence that practitioners could rely upon to inform their practice in comparison with evidence from other research approaches. For example, the Cochrane Centre and the NHS Centre for Reviews and Dissemination at the University of York were created so that health care professionals working within the NHS could be provided with updated research evidence from RCTs. Recently, systematic reviews are beginning to replace the RCT as the best source of evidence (NHMRC, 1995).

The consensus appears to be that evidence from RCTs or systematic reviews of RCTs should be considered the best evidence for the evaluation of the effectiveness of various treatment modalities. However, this type of evidence may be limited in scope in terms of its application to health, public health and social care which encompass a more holistic approach, and many of the problems investigated may not always be related just to the effectiveness of therapeutic interventions. More importantly, as pointed out by Evans (2003), there exist many valid approaches to research but they are often ranked at a lower level than the RCT, despite the fact that each approach provides its own unique perspective. For example, the traditional scientific approach dismisses the experience of the individual and views of people as merely reacting and responding to the environment (Cormack, 1991).

The heavy reliance on evidence from RCTs, systematic reviews and meta-analysis suggests that quantitative research methods provide a stronger evidence base than interpretive or qualitative research methods (Blomfield and Hardy, 2000). But, as Mead (2000: 114) argues, '. . . the perceived hierarchy of evidence may have inflicted considerable harm on the notion of evidence-based practice, particularly for the "softer" professions, such as nursing, whose work may not always lend itself comfortably to the evaluative framework of an RCT'. It can be added that this applies to public health as well. This is supported by Rodgers (1998) who argues that RCTs may not necessarily be the most appropriate method at times to study a problem in health care. More importantly, for many disciplines allied to medicine including public health that use a more eclectic and holistic approach, other forms of research are considered as relevant and rigorous. The view is that a combination of evidence based on the traditional scientific methods and qualitative research methodologies is advocated. This is supported by the Task Force on the Strategy for Research in Nursing, Midwifery and Health Visiting (DoH, 1993).

The rationale for using evidence from RCTs as well as observational studies such as cohort and case-control studies with regards to evidence-based public health is provided by Muir Gray (1997). He argues that, given public health is mainly concerned with the improvement of health through the organised efforts of society – social interventions – many of these interventions cannot be undertaken by individual members of the public or individual clinicians. These include:

- screening programmes;
- immunisation;
- environmental protection.

Screening and immunisation programmes are simple interventions that are not different to those in clinical practice, hence the effectiveness of these programmes should be evaluated by RCTs and systematic reviews of trials. On the other hand, environmental protection policies are social interventions targeted to remove or reduce risk. In order to evaluate these interventions, it is necessary first to establish that a specific factor or set of factors increases the risk of a disease and then to determine whether the policies to reduce risk are feasible, effective and affordable. Evidence to evaluate these policies can be obtained from epidemiological research in which cohort and case-control studies are an integral part and which are specifically designed to identify and quantify risk factors. These are referred to as observational studies. As Mant (1999: 73) puts it, 'Case control and cohort studies come into their own when the question involves harm'.

Therefore, the main sources of research evidence to support a number of public health strategies to promote the health of specific populations and communities are obtained from cohort, case-control and cross-sectional studies rather than RCTs. For example, it is not practically and ethically feasible to assess the degree of risk that people might experience when exposed to factors that could produce harmful outcomes such as heavy smoking and lung cancer, contraceptive pills and breast cancer, lack of exercise and cardiovascular problems. It must be acknowledged though, when using evidence from these observational studies to inform practice, that the evidence may be biased and at greater risk of systematic error than the RCTs as it is very difficult to control for confounding factors (Miller, *et al.*, 1989). Also, it is not possible to establish causation between exposure and outcome. All that can be inferred from the findings is that there is a relationship between the risk factor and the outcome. The strength of this relationship could have been confounded by factors other than the risk factor under investigation. Hence, this could lead to either an underestimation or overestimation of the level of risk between the exposure and outcome (Mulrow and Oxman, 1997).

Qualitative research

Evidence from qualitative research is also placed fairly low down the hierarchy. Qualitative research has traditionally been considered to be inferior to quantitative research. However, many people will argue that this comparison is not appropriate. Evidence from qualitative research is simply different from that obtained from quantitative research. Sackett and Wennberg (1997) argue strongly that the research question should determine the research design. Hence, the answers to the questions practitioners might be seeking to inform their practice could be more appropriately obtained from research studies using a qualitative design. Qualitative research designs are very appropriate when trying to understand the perceptions, motives and actions of individuals and organisations (Boulton and Fitzpatrick, 1997). Evidence from qualitative research is derived from observation, interviews, or verbal interactions and focuses on the meanings and interpretations of the participants (Holloway and Wheeler, 1995). The focus is mainly on personal experiences, attitudes and beliefs and how situations are perceived by people (Seers, 1999).

SYSTEMATIC REVIEWS

Systematic reviews are increasing in popularity and, as mentioned earlier, are beginning to replace single RCTs as the best source of evidence. In fact, it has been argued that the findings from systematic reviews provide more rigorous and robust evidence in comparison with those from other research designs and constitute the best evidence to use when evaluating the effectiveness of care (Evans, 2003).

A systematic review is defined as 'the application of scientific strategies that limit bias to the systematic assembly, critical appraisal and synthesis of all relevant studies on a specific topic' (Greener and Grimshaw, 1996: 27). Evans and Pearson (1998) maintain that there has been a rapid growth in the use of systematic reviews and many health care decisions are being underpinned by research evidence from these reviews. One possible explanation could be that the increasing number of health-related journals on the market and the generation of an ever-expanding amount of research projects from the UK and other countries has led to what a number of authors have termed an 'information overload' (Closs and Cheater, 1994). This has made it difficult, if not impossible, for health care practitioners to keep up to date with new developments in their respective specialities. Given the large volume of research information being generated in some areas, the time and the high level of skill necessary to search and critically appraise this information, systematic reviews and meta-analysis have been suggested as a way forward (Rodgers, 2000).

Meta-analysis is a technique of combining the results of multiple studies on a particular topic using a number of statistical procedures in the construction of systematic reviews. However, the use of meta-analysis depends on the nature and quality of the studies included in the review. When this is not possible, a narrative summary to describe the pooling of the data is normally given (Pearson, 2004).

There is an increasing availability of high-quality systematic reviews to health care professionals. A list of a number of international databases relevant to public health and which can be accessed through the internet is given in Box 16.3 below.

Box 16.3 Selected international databases relevant to public health

- **Centre for Reviews and Dissemination Databases** (University of York, UK) – a collection of searchable databases for systematic reviews, economic evaluations and health technology assessments from around the world.
- **Cochrane Library, Abstracts** (Cochrane Collaboration) – a searchable database of abstracts from the Cochrane Collaboration, an international non-profit and independent organisation that produces and disseminates systematic reviews of health care interventions and promotes the search for evidence in the form of clinical trials and other studies of interventions. Since 1999, public health now has its own 'Cochrane Health Promotion and Public Practice' branch of the Cochrane collaboration (see: **www.vichealth.vic.gov.au/en/research/cochrane-collaboration. aspx**). The aim of the group is to compile systematic reviews of effectiveness of health promotion and public health interventions.
- **EPPI (Evidence for Practice and Policy Information) Centre** (Social Science Research Unit, Institute of Education, University of London, UK) – a collection of searchable databases of reviews related to health promotion and intervention.
- **Evidence-Based Health Promotion** (Victoria State Government, Department of Human Services, Australia) – a series of reviews containing current evidence and critical appraisal related to several public health topics.
- **Health Evidence Bulletins Wales** (Duthie Library, University of Wales College of Medicine, Cardiff, UK) – a collection of published documents outlining current clinical evidence for several health topics.
- **Health-Evidence.ca** (Canadian Institutes of Health Research) – a searchable collection of systematic reviews for topics in health promotion and public health interventions (in both French and English).
- **Public Health Evidence Briefings** (Centre for Public Health Excellence, National Institute for Health and Clinical Excellence, UK) – a collection of detailed reports on the existing evidence available (for example, systematic reviews and meta-analyses) for public health and health improvement, with a particular focus on health inequities.

Until fairly recently systematic reviews have, in the main, consisted of the synthesising and summarising of the results from randomised (RCTs) and non-randomised controlled trials and other studies using a quantitative methodology, while excluding, as much as possible, results from descriptive and interpretative studies (Pearson, 2004). There is an argument that systematic reviews comprising the findings from all forms of rigorous research including RCTs should be made available to health care practitioners (Evans and Pearson, 1998). More importantly, knowledge generated by qualitative research has been largely absent. One possible explanation offered by Pearson (2004) is that the efforts put in by quantitative researchers in the appraisal and synthesis of the evidence generated by such methodologies has not been matched by their counterparts with expertise in qualitative research. However, there are signs that the picture is changing and that a more comprehensive view of evidence is being acknowledged. More and more appraisal and synthesis of the results from qualitative research, referred to as 'meta-synthesis', is being attempted, with a view to incorporating the findings and recommendations within systematic reviews to be made available to health care practitioners. Several attempts to synthesise the results of similar qualitative studies are well documented in the literature (see, for example, Sandelowski, *et al.*, 1997). A number of authors have also reported on evidence generated using qualitative research methodologies (see, for example, Barroso and Powell-Cope, 2000). Furthermore, the Cochrane Qualitative Methods Group, which came into being in 2002, has explored the feasibility of incorporating qualitative research into Cochrane reviews (Pearson, 2004). There is every indication that more and more qualitative evidence will be incorporated into systematic reviews in the future and be made available to practitioners (Pearson, 2004).

SEARCHING PUBLIC HEALTH LITERATURE

Having identified a specific public health problem, the next stage within evidence-based public health practice is to search for the relevant evidence relating to the question. A guide to searching the public health literature is provided in Box 16.4 below.

Box 16.4 A guide to searching the public health literature

A seven-step process can be used for searching the evidence-based public health literature.

- **Step 1**: Determine the public health problem and define the question.
- **Step 2**: Select information sources.
- **Step 3**: Identify key concepts and terms.
- **Step 4**: Conduct the search in subject-appropriate databases.
- **Step 5**: Select documents for review.
- **Step 6**: Abstract relevant information from the documentation.
- **Step 7**: Summarise and apply the literature review.

Source: Adapted from Brownson, R. C., Baker, E. A., Leet, T. L. and Gillespie, K.N. (2003: 128) (eds) *Evidence-Based Public Health*. New York: Oxford University Press.

ANALYSE THE EVIDENCE

It is not sufficient to just identify the current best available evidence by searching through the various databases and journals relevant to public health. It is also necessary to appraise the soundness and strengths of this evidence in terms of its validity, reliability and applicability to the public health problem. There are a number of frameworks you can use to critically appraise research findings available in the literature. Box 16.5 below provides a set of questions that can be used to appraise the reported public health research results.

Box 16.5 A guide to evaluating the quality and methodology of public health research results

The following set of questions can be used to assess reported research results.

- What are the results?
    - Were the results similar from study to study?
    - What are the overall results of the review?
    - How precise were the results?

- ♦ Can a causal association be inferred from the available data?
- Are the results valid?
  - ♦ Did the review explicitly address the public health question?
  - ♦ Was the search for relevant studies detailed and exhaustive? Is it likely that important, relevant studies were missed?
  - ♦ Were the primary studies of high methodological quality?
  - ♦ Were assessments of studies reproducible?

- How can the results be applied to public health practice and interventions?
  - ♦ How can the results be interpreted and applied to public health?
  - ♦ Were all important public health outcomes considered?
  - ♦ Are the benefits worth the costs and potential risks?

Sources: Guyatt, G. and Rennie, D. (2002: 159) *User's Guides to the Medical Literature: A Manual for Evidence-Based Practice*. Chicago: American Medical Association. Brownson, R. C., Baker, E. A., Leet, T. L. and Gillespie, K.N. (2003: 47) (eds) *Evidence-Based Public Health*. New York: Oxford University Press.

ESTABLISHING A PUBLIC HEALTH EVIDENCE BASE

The *Wanless Report* (Wanless, 2004) reported that, although there was a plethora of public health information, there was insufficient information on sustainable solutions and a lack of evidence of their effectiveness. He also identified a paucity of funding for public health research and gaps in knowledge around the cost-effectiveness of many policies, which lacked clear objectives and quantifiable outcomes.

It can be difficult for public health practitioners to locate valid public health and health promotion research to inform their strategies and much evidence remains unpublished (Howes, *et al.*, 2004). Research has traditionally been published and disseminated on the basis of its academic rigour in scientific journals (assessed through peer review), rather than at the level of successful practitioner implementation (HDA, 2004a and 2004b).

Can evidence of health gain help?

The concept of health gain was first pioneered by the Welsh Health Planning Forum in 1989 (NHS Wales, last updated 2006) and refers to identifying the health outcome(s) arising from the 'effectiveness of intervention', rather than defining the health (care) input. It represents added value in 'non-health' policies (DoH, 1999b; NICE, 2006). Health gain relies on setting evidence-based targets specific to a particular subject area and recognises the need for partnership-based working in achieving health improvements (Gabbay and Stevens, 1994). In order to be fully effective, health gain measures need to be founded on valid evidence to establish specific current health status, needs and outcomes and this area is developing. There needs to be increasing attention given to evaluating the impact of a given policy as well as the systematic collation and dissemination of the best evidence of effectiveness, with reference to addressing health inequalities (Macintyre, 2003).

Despite the range of research evidence available, there is relatively little longitudinal evidence of health gain arising from interventions. Quantitative data needs to be supported by qualitative data about what is working, how and why. A sound evidence base should be contemporary, valid and reliable and based on a consolidation of sound research and good practice that should help deliver high quality and effective approaches in the longer term. It needs to be continually developing and revisable as new data is presented (Trinder, 2000); made readily accessible; and regularly evaluated so that its use is maximised in relevant interventions (Muir Gray, 2000). For practitioners, evidence needs to be readily available and in suitable format.

NICE and the National Public Health Evidence Base

Since 2005, the National Public Health Evidence Base has fallen under the auspices of the National Institute for Health and Clinical Excellence (NICE) (it was previously the responsibility of the Health Development Agency). This is an independent organisation responsible for providing national guidance on promoting good health and preventing and treating ill health. NICE produces guidance in three areas of health, including public health to support the promotion of good health and the prevention of ill health for those working in the NHS, local authorities and the wider public and voluntary sector (see: **www.nice.org.uk** and **www.nice.org.uk/page.aspx?o=aboutnice** [accessed 15 July 2009]).

At the time of writing, NICE was publishing and disseminating 'How to put NICE guidance into practice to improve the health and wellbeing of communities' (NICE, 2008) as a guide for chief executives, senior officers and others in local authorities leading on health and wellbeing. The purpose of this is to disseminate quality-assured evidence to be incorporated into priorities identified through Joint Strategic Needs Assessments and delivered through Local Strategic Partnerships and Local Area Agreements (see also Chapters 5 and 18). The NICE website provides a range of guidance to help local authorities to plan, deliver and evaluate more effective public health services. The NICE guidance requires that organisations adopt the following key principles of implementation:

- support from the chief executive and clear leadership (including from officers, elected members, stakeholders, etc.);
- dedicated resources (a NICE manager is recommended, to effectively lead progress and be responsible for receiving and acting on NICE e-alerts and other guidance);
- support from a multi-agency group (probably part of the LSP, linking to JSNA, LAA and commissioning groups);
- a systematic approach to commissioning and financial planning, implementation and evaluation (to develop value-for-money approaches to improve health and reduce inequality through rigorous business cases for implementing guidance; auditing and evaluation).

There is also an emphasis on sharing good practice and the website will be developing as this book is published.

CONCLUSIONS

Evidence-based practice in contemporary public health remains a rapidly evolving policy area and one that is subject to much debate on what constitutes 'acceptable' evidence, its research base and rigour, and how it can be best applied in practice to improve health at local, national and international level. There are also issues relating to accessing, searching and analysing public health research. There remain significant gaps in some areas of public health and there is a need for further rigorous research, but there is also a need for practitioners, in particular, to publish and thereby disseminate their work and its outcomes at local level.

Useful websites

Shared Learning: **www.nice.org.uk/usingguidance/
sharedlearningimplementingniceguidance/shared_learning_
implementing_nice_guidance.jsp** (accessed 15 July 2009)
This provides guidance on the 'Shared Learning' scheme developed by
NICE.

NHS Evidence: **www.nice.org.uk/nhsevidence**
'NHS Evidence' was launched in 2009 and includes public health (non-clinical) evidence.

Chapter 17

Globalisation and public health

Jill Stewart and Yvonne Cornish

This chapter presents some of the contested definitions of globalisation and explores the concept of globalisation in relation to public health. It sets this in the context of the WHO Commission on the Social Determinants of Health (2008) and the Chief Medical Officer's report: 'Health is Global: Proposals for UK government-wide strategy' (DoH, 2007a). It looks at some international public health issues and comparisons before turning to some of the domestic effects of globalisation, with particular reference to environmental health in public health.

Learning outcomes

In this chapter you will learn how to:

- appreciate the global context of health issues and some of the health differences in the developed and developing world;

- define globalisation and appreciate its contested definitions, particularly in the context of public health;

- appreciate the importance of acting on global health issues, and apply the principles of leading WHO and UK documents;

- understand and provide examples of the emerging risks in a rapidly globalising world and the domestic effects of globalisation.

GLOBAL PUBLIC HEALTH ISSUES: AN INTRODUCTION

There have been major improvements in health status seen in the developed countries over the last century or so. However, these have not been shared equally within or between countries. For example, life expectancy at birth ranges from 81.4 years for women in the established market economies of Western Europe, Japan, Australia and New Zealand to 48.1 years for men in sub-Saharan Africa (Beaglehole, 2003: 33). The global burden of disease is such that (WHO, 1995):

- more than 12 million children under five die in the developing world every year;
- 40 per cent of the world's 51 million deaths are caused by communicable diseases;
- smoking kill six people a minute worldwide;
- circulatory diseases kill 10 million a year;
- cancers kill six million a year;
- approximately 600 people die each day because of unsafe working conditions.

The burden of disease and death differs in developed and developing countries as summarised in Table 17.1 below.

Developed countries	Developing countries
Ischemic heart disease.	Ischemic heart disease.
Cerebrovascular disease.	Cerebrovascular disease.
Cancers of the trachea, bronchus and lung.	Lower respiratory infections.
Lower respiratory infections.	HIV/Aids.
Chronic obstructive pulmonary disease.	Perinatal conditions.
Colon and rectum cancers.	Chronic obstructive pulmonary disease.
Stomach cancer.	Diarrhoeal diseases.
Self-inflicted injuries.	Tuberculosis.
Diabetes mellitus.	Malaria.
Breast cancer.	Road traffic accidents.

Table 17.1 Leading causes of death: developed and developing countries (source: adapted from Beaglehole, 2003: 35)

The *WHO Health Report* 1995 identified that the world's population is currently 5.6 billion, with 4.4 billion living in the developing world. The average life expectancy is 78 years in most developed countries but only

43 years in the least developed countries, with declining life expectancy in lower income countries. Half the world's population still lacks access to treatment for common diseases and essential drugs. The major causes of death in lowest 'Healthy Life Expectancy' countries are HIV/AIDS with HIV/AIDS now surpassing other infectious diseases such as malaria, TB, diarrhoeal disease, acute respiratory infections and other infections of childhood (for example, measles and neo-natal tetanus). In richer countries, there are differences in tobacco use, HIV/AIDS and the quality of health care systems (WHO, 1995).

The nature and extent of poverty differs between developed and developing countries and poverty is the world's leading cause of death (WHO, 1995). Extreme poverty results in: babies not being vaccinated; a lack of clean water and sanitation; high rates of maternal and neonatal mortality; difficulty in accessing health care and drugs; reduced life expectancy; increased disability; and mental health problems, stress, suicide, substance misuse and family disintegration. Poverty is not only experienced in 'poor' countries but has different consequences than in richer countries, i.e. absolute or 'extreme' poverty including a lack of basic amenities such as food, water and shelter. Developed countries are more likely to experience 'relative' poverty, an important cause of health inequalities.

DEFINING GLOBALISATION

Globalisation is a highly contested topic, and the subject of much debate (Lee, 2005). Although the term is used extensively, there is surprisingly little consensus as to its meaning, and no precise, widely-agreed definition. Globalisation has been predominantly associated with economic processes, particularly the observed increase in cross-border trade and investment (World Bank, 2001) and the increasing liberalisation of trade (DoH, 2007a), but its meaning is by no means confined to economics. The social theorist Anthony Giddens, who has written extensively on this topic, has argued that the concept has taken an almost routine place in current literature, but that there remain dichotomous views as to its meaning and application, creating multiple new pressures (Giddens, 1999). The sense of globalisation as interdependency is gaining importance in public health circles. A good example can be found in Orme *et al.* (2003: 210) who describe it as '. . . growing interdependence between different peoples, religions and countries in the world' and 'social and economic relations that stretch worldwide and will continue to do so . . .'.

Pomerleau and McKee (2005) add another dimension, referring to globalisation as a set of processes that alter the nature of human interaction by intensifying cross-border interactions that previously divided individuals and populations. These eroding boundaries, they argue, are spatial, temporal and cognitive boundaries, leading to new forms of interaction. Spatial boundaries are concerned with changes in the way we experience and perceive geographical boundaries (including national boundaries). Temporal boundaries include changes in the actual and/or perceived timescale of human interactions and communications. Cognitive boundaries refer to changes in how we think about the world and about ourselves within it. Globalising forces are therefore:

- economic;
- political;
- social;
- cultural;
- technological; and
- environmental.

The question for those involved in public health is: what impact will globalising forces have on the health of populations?

WHY ACT ON GLOBAL HEALTH?

Dr Brundtland, Director General, WHO (quoted in Griffiths and Hunter, 1999: 17) argues that: 'Many of our health problems are of a global nature and are closely related to economic development, the environment and other challenges. They can therefore only be overcome by intensified global cooperation, where strong, efficient and forward-looking international institutions must underpin our common efforts'.

Public health challenges do not respect international boundaries, with people relocating and taking with them local disease and changes in their own immunity resulting from a new living area, lifestyles and behaviours (good and bad, existing or new as coping mechanisms), cultural norms that no longer 'fit' or may not feel (or be) welcome (anomie) – and the list goes on. The public health challenges are not confined to individuals and communities; there are also threats arising from wider environmental factors such as climate change and refuse disposal, including toxic and hazardous waste (some of which are addressed in Chapter 6). Some of the emerging risks include: communicable disease; non-communicable disease; food and nutrition; environmental health; delivery of health care and public health policy, and these are summarised in Box 17.1.

Box 17.1 Emerging risks in public health

- In communicable disease, there are both new and newly emerging diseases, including HIV/AIDS, Ebola, nvCJD and SARS. There has also been a re-emergence of 'old' infectious disease, including malaria (in areas where it had been eradicated), TB (including the emergence of resistant strains), plague and cholera.
- Non-communicable disease has become a major cause of death in developed countries, notably cardiovascular disease (CHD/Strokes), cancers and respiratory diseases. These are also affecting developing countries, as is a worldwide increase in tobacco-related diseases.
- Factors in environmental health include the impact of global environmental change, bringing with it risks for public health including natural disasters (flood, famine, etc.), a change in the pattern of vector-borne diseases (for example, malaria), and the impact of climate change on 'tropical' diseases.
- In food and health, there are concerns about the globalisation of production, distribution and consumption of food linked to the industrialisation of farming: increasing concern about trans-border food-borne disease (for example, avian flu) and an increasing incidence of obesity (mainly, but not exclusively, in higher-income countries).
- Changes in the delivery of health care include: the opening up of health care systems to international markets; the influence of initiatives such as 'evidence-based' practice; the movement of health care workers between countries; and developments such as 'telemedicine' and 'teleconsulting' across national boundaries.

(Source: adapted from Lee, 2000.)

SUSTAINABLE ENVIRONMENTS AND PUBLIC HEALTH

A sustainable environment is paramount for public health and there are many and unbalanced challenges to our environment arising from current lifestyles in both the developed and developing world. Chapter 6 defined sustainability, is concerned with issues such as climate change, and should be read in conjunction with this chapter. Table 17.2 below summarises some impacts of environmental change on global health.

Worldwide	Europe /UK
One third of the world's population faces water scarcity or poor water quality and this figure is increasing.	Hazardous waste is primarily produced by the developed world and is often exported for disposal.
More people will be at risk from vector-borne diseases as global temperatures increase.	The 2003 Europe heatwave led to 27 000 deaths, including 2 000 in England and Wales.
In 2000 climate change caused 154 000 deaths; outdoor air pollution caused 1.6 million deaths.	By 2050 UK heat-related deaths could increase to around 2 800 cases per year, with an extra 5 000 cases of skin cancer.
60 per cent of life-supporting resources are being degraded or non-sustainably used.	Up to 13 000 children's deaths are caused by outdoor air pollution with particulate matter.
1.7 million deaths are caused by unsafe water, hygiene and sanitation, mostly in children.	The EC estimates that air pollution kills 370 000 annually and may cost the EU more than £290 billion.
150 million tonnes of hazardous waste is produced every year.	

Table 17.2 The impact of environmental change on global health (source: adapted from DoH, 2007a: 31)

There is a need to (re)build local public health systems in collaboration with regional and global level efforts, accommodating a wider range of stakeholders. There is also a need to improve the evidence base for public health practice and improve decision-making at all levels. This is particularly highlighted in two key documents, the *WHO Commission on the Social Determinants of Health* (WHO, 2008) and the UK's *Health is Global: Proposals for a UK Government-wide Strategy* (DoH, 2007a), and these are now explored below.

The *WHO Commission on the Social Determinants of Health*

The *WHO Commission* (2008) emphasised the importance of social justice and focused on the way in which this affects how people live and the consequences of this for illness and the risk of premature death. In particular, it emphasised avoidable health inequalities due to the circumstances in which people grow, live, work, age and in their health systems and how these are shaped by political, social and economic forces. It also pointed to the importance of an integrated global approach to address health inequalities. The report's recommendations were derived from the principle of improving daily life and, as such, to:

- improve the daily living conditions – circumstances in which people are born, grow, live, work and age;
- tackle the inequitable distribution of power, money and resources – the structural drivers of those conditions of daily life – globally, nationally and locally; and
- measure and understand the problems faced – evaluate action, expand the knowledge base, develop a workforce trained in the social determinants of health, raise public awareness and assess the impact of action.

Health is Global: Proposals for a UK government-wide strategy

In the Foreword to the report *Health is Global: Proposals for a UK Government-Wide Strategy*, Sir Liam Donaldson, Chief Medical Officer, stressed the need to consider health in the context of a globalised world with health trends, poverty and prosperity affecting populations worldwide. He emphasised that infectious diseases – just as narcotics, unhealthy lifestyles and chemical and biological pollutants – cross borders. He argued that solutions required cooperative partnership actions, including from departments with no direct health remit. He emphasised the need to build on the positive achievements to date in global health and stressed the need to continue to work toward a robust UK government global health strategy (DoH, 2007a; 2008c).

The report argued that there were five key reasons for the UK to engage with the global health agenda, and that the strategy would need to navigate an economically and ethically acceptable route though what may be diverse and conflicting areas. The reasons are summarised as follows:

- it is important for world security, protecting domestic health and safeguarding health and the economy;
- it is central to work on sustainable development;
- health is a valuable commodity to trade in;
- health is a global public good; and
- health is a human right.

These two reports help situate domestic policy and strategy in addressing emerging public health risks.

THE DOMESTIC EFFECTS OF GLOBALISATION

Globalisation has led to many changes in domestic health and has many public health implications for improving health and addressing inequality. Many of these changes are concerned with migrant workers', asylum seekers' and refugees' occupational and living conditions, but there are also wider effects in terms of issues such as climate change and environmental challenges – some of which are addressed in Chapter 6 – and also new social exclusions (see, for example, Chapter 7's example of prostitution). The next section is concerned mainly with living arrangements and the subsequent health effects experienced by some of the most marginal communities in the UK.

Migrant workers

A migrant worker is someone who voluntarily moves from their homeland to a new country in search of employment. The Home Office has estimated that some 750 000 migrants have arrived from Eastern Europe, mostly Poland, since 2004, although the figure may be higher, and migrant workers may bring some £40 billion to the Treasury (cited in Spear, 2008). This has lead to a range of issues including occupational health and safety, overcrowded and multiple-occupant housing and other living accommodation such as caravan sites, concerns around social cohesion and different public health implications for urban and rural areas.

Migrant workers currently working on the 2012 Olympics projects have led to a range of new public health concerns. Steve Miller, Chief EHO at London Borough of Newham – where the Olympic Village will be largely constructed – (cited in Spear, 2008) has reported a range of pest invasions such as bed bugs and cockroaches resulting from overcrowding, bed hopping (to enable 24-hour working) and new overseas pests, such as ghost ants. There has also been a rise in prostitution (see Chapter 7) (cited in Spear, 2008).

In more rural areas, different issues are faced arising from caravan sites and seasonal labour, and Hope Bradbury, Environmental Health Manager in Private Sector Housing Kerrier District Council (cited in Spear, 2008), reported that health and safety issues in agricultural working include a lack of portable toilets, no hand-washing facilities and a lack of personal protective equipment. The Cornwall Strategic Partnership and Cornwall Migrant Workers Group have been proactive in supporting the needs of migrant workers and have helped ensure that migrant workers are integrated into the local community by addressing barriers such as language and culture and equality of access to, and support and information around, services such as education, housing, skills and training. There is an ethos of tolerance, inclusivity and understanding and they are developing an information base in the community to help ensure good practice at local level, which is being delivered by partnership working, led by Inclusion Cornwall, and based on consultation and participation. For further information, see the Cornwall Migrant Worker Site at:

www.cornwallstrategicpartnership.gov.uk/index.cfm?articleid=10653 (accessed 13 March 2009).

The Building and Social Housing Foundation (BSHF) recently coordinated consultation on migrant workers' housing conditions and sought to provide a new perspective in this area. It made recommendations to address current and future issues affecting both migrant workers and existing communities in the following areas:

- improving accommodation options and addressing homelessness;
- improving accommodation conditions and the enforcement of required standards;
- building stronger communities; and
- delivering change.

Migrant workers' often poor and overcrowded housing accommodation presents important implications for local authority housing strategies and, in particular, for environmental health practitioners (EHPs) responsible for the private housing sector and caravan sites, formal or otherwise. The BSHF website (**www.bshf.org/published-information/publication. cfm?thePubID=2EED9E14-15C5-F4C0-998CFFEC3D54FF93** [accessed 15 July 2009]) provides a downloadable summary specific to environmental health departments (see also BSHF, 2008; Williams, 2008). Further information on private sector housing conditions can be found in Chapter 20.

The Health Protection Agency (HPA, 2006) (see also Chapter 9) recently published its first report on infectious diseases affecting migrants using surveillance data from England, Wales and Northern Ireland for 2004. It highlights the fact that migrants have a range of health needs, not just infectious disease, and refers to the general health needs of migrants, providing a resource for public health practitioners and others to help improve the health of UK migrant communities and contribute to domestic communicable disease control.

The Gangmasters Licencing Authority (GLA)

The GLA is a government agency established to protect workers from exploitation in agriculture, horticulture, shellfish gathering and food processing and packaging. It was set up following the deaths of 23 Chinese cockle pickers in Morecambe Bay in 2004 (Spear, 2008). Most workers in these industries are from countries including Romania, Poland, Slovakia, Hungary, Bulgaria, Lithuania, Latvia, India, Pakistan and Portugal. The GLA has licensed over 1200 labour providers and is involved with the prosecution of those operating without a licence (**www.gla.gov.uk/** [accessed 15 July 2009]).

The GLA launched Operation Ajax in June 2008 to instigate a programme of unannounced raids to help protect workers and uncover rogue gangmasters. One of its programmes, covering Lincolnshire and Lancashire, identified complaint gangmasters, but also many unacceptable activities such as working without contracts, payment below the minimum wage, working without sick or holiday pay, long days without supervision or the absence of transport in isolated areas.

Numbers of migrant workers remain unclear nationally, but the Local Government Association is urging better statistics through health care services and National Insurance numbers to calculate population trends (cited in Spear, 2008).

Box 17.2 Immigration into the UK – 2004 figures

- There were 0.3 million UK-based refugees by the end of 2004.
- Over 40 000 people applied for asylum in the UK – 43 per cent were Africans.
- 51 000 illegal migrants had enforcement action initiated against them.
- Overseas residents in UK doubled between 1984 and 2004 to 27.8 million.
- In 2004, 145 000 people were granted settlement in the UK, excluding European Economic Area nationals.

(DoH, 2007)

Food production and availability

The effect of globalisation on food and health is wide and varied, bringing positive benefits such as a wider range and availability of foodstuffs (and a side effect of contributing to rising obesity globally), but conversely a range of negative factors arising from an increasingly liberalised free market in food production and distribution. In response to this the Codex Alimentarius Commission – a Food and Agriculture Organisation and WHO body – sets standards, codes of practice, guidelines and recommendations for food quality and safety, and is led in the UK by the Food Standards Agency (FSA) (DoH, 2007a).

One of the more unacceptable factors of the globalisation of food is that of illegal imports into the UK. Illegal imports of bush meat (which includes species such as gorilla, chimpanzee, cane rat and land snails) have been documented as responsible for spreading disease globally and, as such, have major implications for public health (Manzano, cited in Stewart, Bushell and Habgood, 2005). Partnership approaches have helped in addressing some of the more negative effects of globalisation in food safety and control in the UK, and environmental health practitioners have worked with other health agencies, such as Port Health Officers, Customs and Excise, DEFRA and the FSA.

Positive features of globalisation on food choices include the fact that we have information and knowledge more freely available and can choose to purchase food based on informed ethical considerations. One example of a social response in food production is the Divine Chocolate Company, a fair-trade social enterprise (see Chapter 14). The company was set up in 1998 to assist the 'Kuapa Kokoo' cocoa farmers of Ghana (West Africa) with vertical integration into the UK chocolate market, which is worth £4 billion. This strategy has assisted the farmers to get a fair price for their cocoa beans produce. The effect of this intervention has been an exponential increase in the farmers' standard of living and quality of life through community ownership of the business and a sustainable approach to addressing poverty and dependency. It demonstrates a non-dependent strategic intent to break away from a total reliance on long-term funding and grant aid models that may restrict their objectives owing to funding and investment variables. In responding to global health, this is an important development in helping to sustainably combat local poverty in the developing world. Readers should also refer to Chapter 19 on food, health and wellbeing.

Asylum seekers and refugees

An asylum seeker is someone who has arrived in the UK, often fleeing war, persecution or torture and seeking refugee status. An asylum seeker has limited rights and temporary residence only. A refugee normally has rights to residence, work and benefits. In terms of public health, asylum seekers and refugees many have specific needs and may be destitute, alone, have language and cultural barriers, and may have specific health and social care needs arising from trauma such as war, torture and rape.

Many asylum seekers therefore have complex and specific health and social care needs and all asylum seekers are offered health assessment and TB screening. The Department of Health (DoH) is developing guidance for commissioners and providers on mental health services for asylum seekers, refugees and victims of torture. Many areas with high numbers of asylum seekers have dedicated asylum health teams aimed at meeting their needs (DoH, 2007a).

Tuberculosis

Some 4 000 people die each year in the UK from tuberculosis (TB) or related complications (see TB Alert website at: **www.tbalert.org/** [accessed 15 July 2009]). The homeless (including 'rejected and hidden' asylum seekers and migrant workers) are particularly at risk, and poor quality and overcrowded accommodation provides ideal conditions for the disease to spread. Those arriving from warmer climates, particularly if stressed and with weakened immune systems, are more likely to develop TB in the UK and nearly three quarters of those with TB were not born in the UK. Successful treatment requires decent, secure housing accommodation, completion of courses of antibiotics and related health and social care. Mobile screening services and temporary accommodation during treatment, as part of wider partnership working, have been found to be successful in reaching out to those at risk of, and suffering from, TB (Brandon, 2008).

The Health Protection Agency has a role in supporting the DoH and NHS in contributing toward eliminating TB in England. The HPA TB programme coordinates control activities across its departments, including the Centre for Infections, Local and Regional Services, the Regional Microbiology Network and the Centre for Emergency Preparedness and Response. Its roles include local and national surveillance, laboratory services, population disease control, partnership working and research see: **www. hpa.org.uk** [accessed 15 July 2009]). The HPA's (2008b) publication,

Tuberculosis in the UK: Annual Report on Tuberculosis Surveillance in the UK, refers to the scale of the problem, drug resistance and treatment outcomes. It reports that TB numbers and rates have remained relatively stable since 2005 and 8 417 TB cases were reported in the UK in 2007. Most cases occurred in England (92 per cent) and, proportionally, most of these were in London (39 per cent UK cases). Some 72 per cent of cases were born outside of the UK, with the highest rates among black African and Indian/Pakistan/Bangladeshi groups. Treatment outcomes were provided for 93 per cent of cases, which was an increase on previous years, and the proportion completing treatment remained at 79 per cent. See also Chapter 9.

Activity 17.1 Reflective exercise: globalisation and public health

Globalisation is not necessarily a recent phenomenon – some commentators argue that it is a relatively recent term for a process that has been going on for some time.

- How relevant is this to public health?
- What impact will these 'globalising forces' have on the health of populations?

CONCLUSIONS

Globalisation is a 'contested concept', both in terms of its meaning and its impact. There are many definitions of globalisation arising from different disciplines and viewpoints. Rigorous debate continues around the impact of globalising forces, as both positive and negative.

Improvements in global health status have been accompanied by a widening health gap between and within countries. People in poorer countries have a lower life expectancy and spend more time living in poor health. Developing countries are experiencing a 'double burden' of disease, with the incidence of both old and new infectious diseases (including TB, HIV/Aids, etc.) remaining relatively high. There have also been increasing rates of non-communicable disease (CHD, stroke, cancers, diabetes and so on).

Globalisation has numerous impacts on public health domestically. The most obvious effects include climate change; living and working conditions facing migrant workers, asylum seekers and refugees; and the positive and negative effects of food availability and controls.

Useful websites

WHO world health reports: **www.who.int/whr/previous/en/index.html** (accessed 15 July 2009)
Use this site to access all WHO world health reports since 1995.

Part Three: Environmental Health in Public Health

Chapter 18

Environmental health practice

Ian Gray, Rachel Flowers and Tony Lewis

This chapter provides an overview of the changing role of environmental health practitioners within the wider public health workforce (see also Chapter 5). The chapter also covers training opportunities and requirements, and the ways in which environmental health engages with health and social care services.

Learning outcomes

In this chapter you will learn how to:

- briefly describe the role of the environmental health practitioner and their changing role in the public health workforce;

- identify new and developing education and training requirements for environmental health practitioners;

- identify the skills and competencies environmental health practitioners are able to bring to public health organisations in the delivery of public health strategies at local level.

INTRODUCTION

Environmental health practitioners (EHPs) in general, and local authority environmental health officers (EHOs) in particular, have always engaged with the public health agenda. Environmental health is public health and in recent books such *Environmental Health as Public Health* (Stewart, Bushell and Habgood, 2005) and the introduction to the latest edition of *Clay's Handbook of Environmental Health* (Flowers, Gray and MacArthur, 2004), the environmental health contribution to public health throughout our 150-year history is robustly demonstrated.

Environmental health practitioners are one of the fundamental professional groups involved in public health and have a range of roles in integrating their wide social, economic, scientific, technological and legal knowledge and skills base in improving health. Their role has traditionally been in local government as law enforcers in disciplines including housing, food, health and safety and pollution control. However, their roles are rapidly changing now as many are taking up new public health career opportunities in other organisations and agencies such as Primary Care Trusts (PCTs), the Food Standards Agency, the Health Protection Agency and academic posts. Wherever they are based, the EHPs' work is fundamentally about protecting human health in relation to the environment, and there has been a recent move toward, and emphasis on, sustainable approaches to reducing health inequality and psychosocial health.

EHPs are therefore very well placed to be involved in the new public health strategies. Strategic partnerships include Local Strategic Partnerships and Community Strategies and EHPs are frequently involved in such partnerships to deliver health improvement, including enhancing the quality of life at community level. In this way, national and global concerns can be addressed through local needs-assessed action and through integrated initiatives with maximised health impact.

There are important opportunities and challenges that EHPs and EHOs need to take into account in the way that modern public health is practiced. The capacity and capability of the wider public health workforce was addressed in Chapter 5. This chapter largely focuses on the requirements for education and training of the modern environmental health practitioners and the agenda and structures that direct how public health is delivered effectively and efficiently.

ENVIRONMENTAL HEALTH: A KEY PARTNER IN DELIVERING THE PUBLIC HEALTH AGENDA

The publication of *Environmental Health 2012: A Key Partner in Delivering the Public Health Agenda* (Burke, *et al.*, 2002) described the project carried out by the former Health Development Agency, with the Chartered Institute of Environmental Health (CIEH), to support the environmental health profession in developing a strategic vision for its contribution to health development and wellbeing. It captured challenges, constraints and ideas from mixed groups of environmental health, public health and health improvement professionals from local authorities, the NHS, organisations, environment, voluntary and community.

The vision for environmental health by 2012 is well summarised in Figure 18.1 below. This should be read in conjunction with Chapter 5. It clearly identifies the sphere for environmental health, the knowledge base of health determinants and environmental stressors required by practitioners, and the operational skills including inspection and audit, enforcement, advocacy and research that environmental health practitioners possess.

The '2012 Vision' Model of Environmental Health

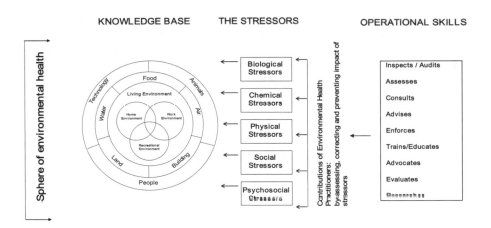

Figure 18.1 The scope of environmental health (reproduced with kind permission from CIEH)

This vision statement was formally adopted by the CIEH and has been highly influential in focusing future training and practice on maintaining and improving public health.

ENVIRONMENTAL HEALTH EDUCATION AND TRAINING

The process for becoming an EHP is set out in detail on the website of the CIEH (**www.cieh.org**) (accessed 18 July 2009) and the key requirements are summarised below.

Education, training and maintaining competence

Environmental health is a graduate profession, requiring a degree accredited by the CIEH. This academic study, work-based learning, and professional examinations create the fully-qualified environmental health practitioner or EHP. Competence is maintained through reflective practice and a process of continuous professional development.

The academic curriculum

Following the publication of *Environmental Health 2012* (Burke, *et al.*, 2002), the CIEH conducted a radical overhaul of the core curriculum for accredited university degree courses. 'Curriculum 2003' broadened the focus of environmental health education and training to equip today's EHPs with the knowledge and skills to enable them to play a full role within the new public health agenda and engage effectively in health partnerships.

The curriculum of both BSc and MSc courses offers in-depth studies of food safety, occupational health, environmental protection, public health and housing. Other studies put science in a social, economic and legal context. There is an emphasis on developing skills in general management, communication, negotiating, analysis and evaluation. Students learn how to intervene, educate and ensure legal compliance – a feature of environmental health practice that distinguishes it from other areas of public health practice.

Experiential learning

The academic study is reinforced by work-based learning, through completion of an experiential learning portfolio, and followed by professional examinations. On successfully completing all elements of the qualification process, the student is a fully qualified environmental health practitioner, and can be awarded the Certificate of Registration by the Environmental Health Registration Board, a professional qualification that is recognised and respected throughout Europe and in many parts of the world.

Reflective practice

One of the key objectives of the academic programme is to develop the Reflective Practitioner, who regularly and actively reviews their professional actions in a critically evaluative manner as part of an ongoing process of continuous professional development through experiential learning.

Maintaining competence

Continuing professional development (CPD) both validates and supports the environmental health profession by acting as a quality assurance scheme for the competency of practitioners. CIEH required that EHPs complete the standard requirement of 20 hours of CPD per year, with Accredited Associate members doing the lesser amount of 10 hours and members holding Chartered status doing 30 hours.

Future developments

The adoption of Curriculum 2003 has satisfactorily met the need to re-engage environmental health practice with the modern public health agenda. However, over the last two or three years, there have been other substantial and growing pressures on the ability of the CIEH education system for EHPs to manage itself (Lewis, 2008).

Of all of the drivers for change impacting upon environmental health, the emergence of the government's focus on competence is without doubt the most powerful. Born out of a financial imperative, the drive for 'competence not qualifications' has swept across central government departments and is now cascading down into government agencies. From January 2009, the first competence framework covering all persons engaged in health and safety regulation will become operational and will prescribe a level of knowledge, skills and competencies for all persons who wish to obtain a full warrant to enforce the Health and Safety at Work etc. Act 1974. It would be unthinkable for the profession to knowingly produce graduates who were not given an opportunity to meet that framework or, indeed, the other frameworks that are currently under development and are likely to follow over the next few months, which include health protection, public health and port health and may well extend to food safety, housing and aspects of environmental protection.

'Curriculum 2007'

The 2007 curriculum for environmental health embraces the redesigning of the base level qualification to reflect the changes being generated by the emergence of competence frameworks but to also, where possible, address the other drivers for change that are impacting on the qualification process. It sees the future education of student EHPs modelled as a 'daisy' and is known as 'Curriculum 2007' (see Figure 18.2).

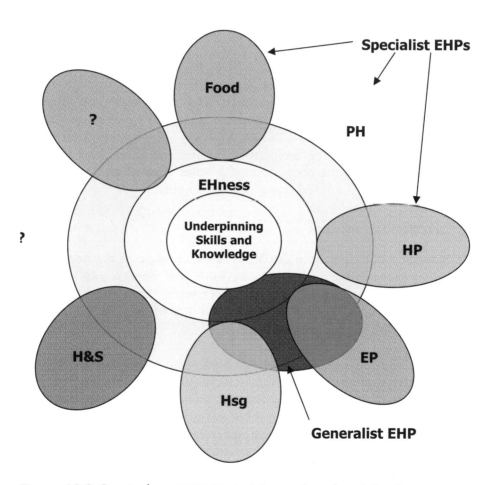

Figure 18.2 Curriculum 2007 'Daisy' (reproduced with kind permission from CIEH)

All students will begin their education in environmental health by developing underpinning knowledge and skills. They will then go on to undertake studies that have been bracketed under the somewhat unusual term 'EHness'. In a sense, 'EHness' can best be described as the way of approaching problems that is unique to EHPs. 'EHness' represents the ability to look at problems and to generate solutions that reflects the holistic public health position. However, in terms of real world teaching and learning, this means that students develop this approach from within a framework of studies that include such staples as pest control, drainage, nuisance, anatomy, physiology, food safety, air quality and occupational health and safety, etc. In essence, students are given a thorough grounding in all key aspects of environmental health.

Having developed 'EHness', student EHPs and, indeed, universities will be faced, for the first time, with some choices. They can choose to continue their studies in the traditional broad manner with the goal of becoming or producing general practice EHPs. Alternatively, they can opt to complete their studies by 'in-depth' consideration of one or more aspects of environmental health, with the intention of qualifying with deep knowledge, extensive skills and verified competencies such that at least one competence framework will have been met in full.

Over and above providing a solution to the issue of competence frameworks, Curriculum 2007 reflects current practice within many of the organisations that are delivering an environmental health service and it increases the numbers of qualified EHPs by widening the number of organisations that can take student EHPs on placement. However, above all else, the chosen solution gives student EHPs, and the universities, choice and will, in time, allow employers in all sectors to select practitioners to meet their specific needs.

International developments

In 1998, the International Federation of Environmental Health (IFEH) commissioned the International Faculty Forum (IFF) of environmental health educators to develop an international curriculum for environmental health. In commissioning such a curriculum, IFEH implicitly recognised and sought to address the ongoing issues of professional identity, status and the transportability of qualifications for EHPs.

A draft model for an international curriculum, based on competence, has been proposed (Brennan, *et al.*, 2008) and was developed and supported by IFF members when they met in May 2008 in Brisbane, Australia. Development of the model and its underpinning concept of 'environmental healthness' ('EHness') has already been completed. 'EHness' is defined as those abilities/skills that are uniquely possessed and focused on in professional practice by EHPs. The draft international curriculum details 'EHness' by the specification of core knowledge, skill and competencies to be attained and maintained by EHPs during the initial qualification process and via lifelong professional development and learning.

A draft curriculum has been developed which represents these elements as a curriculum 'daisy' where knowledge, skills and the resultant competencies – or 'EHness' – sit at the daisy's centre and the additional knowledge, skills and competencies deemed necessary to be held by competent practitioners within each nation, state or region assume the position of the daisy's petals. This model ensures that, irrespective of their location within the world, all EHPs will be educated to the same 'core' curriculum but with divergence taking place via the 'daisy' petals.

ENVIRONMENTAL HEALTH ENGAGING WITH HEALTH AND CARE SERVICES

During the last decade there have been significant changes to the organisations, policies and culture that deliver health and care services. The impact of these changes not only affects those increasing numbers of EHPs who are working within the NHS and other health services, but it also affects the way that EHPs work within local authorities and other sectors, not least in their relationship to their local PCTs and other key agencies such as the Health Protection Agency and the Health and Safety Executive.

The reader should note that the key features of these changes outlined below have occurred in England, but there are similar systematic changes taking place within Northern Ireland, Scotland and Wales. In all cases, the significance and scale of the modernisation agenda of health services, and the shift from a procuring to a commissioning culture, need further reading in order to gain a proper appreciation of their extent and impact.

NHS modernisation

At the start of this dramatic change process a key document *The NHS Plan: A Plan for Investment, a Plan for Reform* (DoH, 2000b: 15) set out the vision of a health service designed around the patient. This document not only allocated additional resources for the NHS, it also set out a modernisation and improvement agenda which shifted the axis of decision-making from Whitehall to local settings:

> For the first time social services and the NHS will come together with new agreements to pool resources. There will be new Care Trusts to commission health and social care in a single organisation. This will help prevent patients – particularly old people – falling in the cracks between the two services or being left in hospital when they could be safely in their own home. (DoH, 2000b: 15).

The government's aim is to devolve power to neighbourhoods and create a more patient-focused NHS. In line with this remit, the Public Health White Paper: *Choosing Health: Making healthy choices easier* (DoH, 2004), reinforced the principles of patient choice, of resources following patient choice and of greater autonomy for local professionals. *Our Health, Our Care, Our Say: A New Direction for Community Services* (DoH, 2006), developed this strategy further, with the 'move towards fitting services round people, not people round services'.

The improvement agenda was shaped and formed over the subsequent years with a series of documents including *Creating a Patient-led NHS – Delivering the NHS Improvement Plan* (DoH, 2007b: 5) which stated:

> The NHS now has the capacity and the capability to move on from being an organisation which simply delivers services to people to being one which is totally patient-led – responding to their needs and wishes.

> The ambition for the next few years is to deliver a change which is even more profound – to change the whole system so that there is more choice, more personalised care, real empowerment of people to improve their health – a fundamental change in our relationships with patients and the public. In other words, to move from a service that does things to and for its patients to one which is patient led, where the service works with patients to support them with their health needs.

Commissioning and providing

The major means for delivering the required changes is through the process of commissioning. Commissioning is the process by which the NHS ensures that health and care services are provided most effectively to meet the needs of the population. It is a complex process with responsibilities ranging from assessing population needs and prioritising health outcomes, to procuring products and services, and managing service providers.

Although traditionally associated with the NHS and social care, over recent years the 'commissioning' rather than 'procuring' agenda is starting to cascade across what have previously been uncharted parts of local government. It has even been reported from one London Borough that all council services, including environmental health, could be 'outsourced' as part of a process to turn the council into a commissioning body (Wall, 2009).

The Department of Health (DoH) has made changes to develop commissioning throughout the whole NHS system (Crisp, 2005), including the functions of PCTs and strategic health authorities where their main remit has become:

- promoting health improvement and reducing inequalities;
- securing safe and high-quality services for their population;
- emergency planning.

World class commissioning

The commissioning process is so fundamentally important to the way that health and care services are to be provided that a 'world class commissioning programme' has been established to deliver a more strategic and long-term approach to commissioning services, with a clear focus on delivering improved health outcomes.

Local government modernisation

While the NHS has been undergoing its modernisation programme, there has also been a modernisation agenda being implemented for local government, some aspects of which directly relate to its involvement in the provision of health and care services.

The policy agenda has been to shift the focus for local government on to the needs of the local community and to make partnership working a necessity. This is being achieved, in part, by the introduction of the Local Strategic Partnership (LSP), Joint Strategic Needs Assessments and Local Area Agreements. For definitions and scope, see Box 5.2 in Chapter 5.

The New Performance Framework for Local Authorities and Local Authority Partnerships: Single Set of National Indicators

The Local Government White Paper, *Strong and Prosperous Communities*, (Department for Communities and Local Government, 2006) promised greater freedom for local government to set local priorities. It replaced an estimated 1 200 measures for assessing performance with a single set of just 198 indicators, which represented what the government believes should be the national priorities for local government, working alone or in partnership.

The new indicators are intended to strengthen the incentives for closer partnership working between key local agencies to deliver joined-up outcomes, including the PCT. The headline definitions for the 198 indicators are contained in the document *The New Performance Framework for Local Authorities and Local Authority Partnerships: Single Set of National Indicators* (Department of Communities and Local Government, 2007).

Bringing it all together – joint working on local targets

In each local authority area, targets against the set of national indicators will be negotiated through new Local Area Agreements (LAAs). Each LAA will include up to 35 targets from among the national indicators, complemented by 17 statutory targets on educational attainment and early years. In addition, each LSP can, if they wish, negotiate with central government to include their own local indicators – i.e., indicators that were not part of the national indicator set. It is important for the LSP to be able to demonstrate to central government that their chosen indicators have been selected by a robust consultation process involving partners and local communities.

Healthy Communities

The aim of the Healthy Communities Programme is to build capacity in councils to improve local health and to tackle health inequalities. It is part of the Government's current agenda of NHS reform, the wider remit of the modernisation of public services and the requirement for the seamless integration and joining up of services across the public, private and voluntary sectors. It is funded by the DoH and is due to run until 2011.

Healthy Towns

A Healthy Towns initiative has recently been announced and supported through a coalition called *Change4Life* (see also Chapters 8 and 14), which is backed by the government, food retailers, charities and community groups. These towns will share additional funding from the government to encourage healthy lifestyles through increasing the opportunities for their population to be more physically active and make healthy food choices. They will help residents to live healthily through a holistic approach to promoting physical activity both in the community and the infrastructure of the town. The 'towns' included are Dudley, Halifax (Calderdale), Sheffield, Tower Hamlets, Thetford, Middlesbrough, Manchester, Tewkesbury and Portsmouth.

New inspection regimes

Comprehensive Area Assessment

From April 2009, the Comprehensive Performance Assessment (CPA), which was an assessment only of a council's performance, will be replaced by the Comprehensive Area Assessment (CAA). This will be a cross-inspectorate approach looking at how well people are served by all their local public services, not just their councils. The CAA will be composed of two basic components:

- an area assessment – focusing on the delivery of improvements on the issues that matter to people in the locality;
- an organisational assessment – focusing on the individual public bodies within an area, to ensure they are accountable for quality and impact.

LAAs will be at the centre of the new assessment criteria and the CAA will therefore assess whether partnerships are achieving their aims for an area.

Care Quality Commission

The Health and Social Care Act 2008 paved the way for the establishment of a new integrated health and adult social care regulator, the Care Quality Commission (CQC). From April 2009, the CQC will take over the functions of the Healthcare Commission, the Commission for Social Care Inspection and the Mental Health Act Commission. Whatever the care setting, the CQC will be able to require that services are safe, people are not put at risk of harm, and that essential levels of service quality are maintained. These requirements, which will be set out in secondary legislation, will be monitored and enforced by the CQC.

So what does this mean for the EHP?

For EHPs to make their valuable contributions to maintaining and improving public health it is important that they understand how this modernisation agenda is increasingly determining what gets done, how and by whom. An example of this is shown in Box 18.1 and demonstrates how an EHP, now working as a Consultant in Public Health, has been able to bring their expertise to the forefront of partnership working in addressing cardiovascular disease in Newham.

Box 18.1 Case study: Partnership working around cardiovascular disease

I work in the London Borough of Newham, an area of the country with one of the highest rates of problems with heart health, with many people experiencing poor quality of life and premature death. To put this into context, the average age of the people in cardiac support groups in Newham, i.e. people who have survived a heart incident, is 44 and at the beginning of 2009 I met a heart attack survivor aged 26 – this was a young man who had non-congenital heart disease.

As the PCT's lead person on heart health I am expected to provide strategic leadership, ensure that all partners are engaged, provide public health expertise, ensure that there is community engagement and involvement, and ensure that all services are quality assured and performance monitored. These are all skills I learnt as an EHP and have developed and enhanced over my career.

I am supported in my task in that the Local Strategic Partnership agreed National Indicator 121 *Mortality rate from all circulatory diseases at ages under 75* as one of its Local Area Agreement (LAA) indicators. Each quarter I have to provide an update on progress achieved against this target and the actions and interventions being taken to assist in Newham meeting this target.

In March 2008, I was given a lead role to co-author a multi-agency bid to the British Heart Foundation (BHF) for funding to support the work that was being undertaken in Newham. The bid had to be submitted by 11 April – one thing about public health bids is that frequently you have to compile them quickly, so time management and work prioritisation is essential if you wish to have a good

---

work-life balance. Over the next few weeks I convened a multi-agency steering group and provided leadership to develop a seven-strand, three-year, multi-million pound bid. I remember that, as a newly qualified EHP, my first bid was for £500 but, in many ways, the principles are the same. I needed to prepare a plan, develop a budget, negotiate with others to secure their agreement around their roles in the project, establish what the baselines were and how I would measure outputs and outcomes in terms of improved health. I also had to develop a communication plan to let people know what was going to take place and the positive publicity that I would aim to achieve. An important thread running through the whole programme was establishing a monitoring and performance framework. This was not only to measure its effectiveness but to potentially inform a business case to commission all or part of the programme after the funding ceases.

The British Heart Foundation did award Newham the first of its Localities Funding Programme awards. The funding is for three years and has the potential to substantially impact positively on heart health by improving heart health promotion and cardiac rehabilitation.

(Case study provided by Rachel Flowers, Consultant in Public Health.)

The resources for public health are increasingly being provided through organisations that have been reshaped and reformed as commissioning bodies. The commissioning agenda itself is continuously expanding and can include services traditionally considered to be part of local public service provision such as health visiting, district nursing, many aspects of social care and maybe even environmental health and other regulatory functions within local authorities. Although many EHPs may be unfamiliar with these arrangements there may be models elsewhere, including within the environmental health field, that we may learn from.

Coupled with this shift towards a commissioning culture, there are also clearly defined ways in which organisations are now expected, and even statutorily required, to work in partnerships. These partnership relationships are subject to performance monitoring along with agreed local targets, with local communities playing a key role in identifying the improvement agenda for their area.

The challenge for EHPs working at local level in the NHS, local government, business or voluntary sectors is to understand how these changes can impact on their work and the way they work and establish what their role is, or could be, now and for the future.

CONCLUSIONS

This is a very challenging and exciting time for environmental health. There are changes in the traditional local authority roles of environmental health officers, but far wider opportunities are also becoming available for environmental health practitioners in NHS organisations, and for becoming involved in public health strategies across organisations.

Useful websites

Commissioning: **www.dh.gov.uk/en/Managingyourorganisation/ Commissioning/index.htm**

Comprehensive Area Assessment: **www.audit-commission.gov.uk/ localgov/audit/caa/index.asp**
and
www.idea.gov.uk/idk/core/page.do?pageId=8680506

Healthy Communities Programme: **www.idea.gov.uk/idk/aio/6936706**

Joint Strategic Needs Assessment: **www.dh.gov.uk/en/ Managingyourorganisation/JointStrategicNeedsAssessment/index.htm**

Local Area Agreements: **www.communities.gov.uk/localgovernment/ performanceframeworkpartnerships/localareaagreements**

Local Strategic Partnerships: **www.neighbourhood.gov.uk/page. asp?id=531**
and
www.idea.gov.uk/idk/core/page.do?pageId=7890619

Practical Guidance on using LSPs and LAAs: **www.idea.gov.uk/idk/ core/page.do?pageId=1174195**

Local Strategic Partnerships and Local Area Agreements: **www.beacons. idea.gov.uk/idk/core/page.do?pageId=8042050**
A website on the Beacon Scheme for Excellence in local government (the Beacon Scheme) is jointly supported by the DCLG and the IDeA.

This site contains both guidance and case studies on the effective use of LSPs and LAAs.

www.emphasisnetwork.org.uk/news/downloads/
FSAEMLAAGuidancefinal.pdf
A useful guide is this joint publication from the Food Standards Agency and LACoRS, *Local Area Agreements – Guidance on Food and Health*.

http: //ideatest.conseq.org.uk/idk/aio/4607203
A very useful example of Stockport's LAA submission, *Working Together for a Better Stockport*, March 2006 submission.

NICE Guidance: www.nice.org.uk/media/5AA/EE/
NICEGuidanceLAATargets090209.pdf
Very recent advice on how NICE guidance can help achieve Local Area Agreement targets and Multi Area Agreement priorities.

EHPs: www.cieh.org/ehp/crossing_the_line.html
A recent article on EHPs now working in the NHS in public health. (Websites all accessed 18 July 2009.)

Chapter 19

Food, health and wellbeing

Nargis Kayani

This chapter discusses health and wellbeing; food security; food sovereignty and the change revolution. It explores the relationship between health determinants and their relationship to food, and the need for major and sustainable changes across political, cultural and practical levels to address the many modern dilemmas and challenges in food, health and wellbeing.

Learning outcomes

In this chapter you will learn how to:

- explore the correlation between health determinants, food policy and practice;

- consider the need for change on a political, cultural and practical level to meet deep-rooted and modern health challenges.

INTRODUCTION

Food is essential for human survival. The right to food is enshrined in the United Nations (1948) Universal Declaration of Human Rights, which states that: 'Everyone has the right to a standard of living adequate for the health and well-being of himself and his family, including food . . .' (Article 25.1). The right to food imposes obligations on states to respect, protect and fulfil the right to food for citizens (Ziegler, 2004).

The UK food and drink industry undoubtedly plays an important role in the food chain and is also the country's single largest manufacturing sector, yielding a turnover of £7.37 billion (DEFRA, 2006c).

The quantity, quality, composition, nutritional value, availability and cost of food are all factors that determine good and bad health. The health divide, for many disadvantaged and low-income households, is often-compounded by their inability to access adequate food, due to a host of fiscal, practical, environmental, cultural and social barriers.

In recent years, there has been a marked change in attitudes to and perceptions of food and health (Lang, 2005). Traditional 'food fears' of past years regarding food-borne illnesses, malnutrition and food poverty have become interchanged with newer anxieties about 'super' and 'pure' foods, with their perceived health benefits and nutritional claims (FSA, 2007). Wider ranging issues such as food miles, junk food, organic and locally sourced food, loss of local shops and supermarket monopolies, along with conflicting issues of national and global food security, have added to the melee of confusion.

Meanwhile, inequalities in health outcomes persist between socially disadvantaged and affluent groups, between males and females and people from different ethnic groups. Many of these gaps are significant and, in some cases, the disparity is greater now than 20 years ago (DoH, 2002b).

Despite ten years of policy statements on holistic public health partnerships, there remains a dogmatic compartmentalisation of health practitioners' roles into those who seek to prevent ill health, through the provision of safe food, and those who deal with the ill health consequences of unsafe food.

HEALTH AND WELLBEING

Humans clearly have a complex relationship with food. Food consumption is only partly associated with assuaging hunger. Eating and drinking fulfils a number of social, cultural and emotional needs and rituals (Kayani, 2006). The impact of food on physical, mental and emotional health is well documented, along with its societal impacts (see Table 19.1). There is consensus among medical experts that obesity is the single most significant post-war health challenge facing the UK. The links between type 2 diabetes and obesity are firmly established. Currently more than 66 per cent of adults and over 33 per cent of children are considered overweight or obese. According to prediction models, if trends continue, 60 per cent of men, 50 per cent of women and 25 per cent of children could be obese by 2050 (Government Office for Science, 2007). If diets matched nutritional guidelines in terms of increased fruit and vegetable consumption and reduced salt, saturated fat and added sugar consumption, then 70 000 premature deaths per annum could be avoided (Cabinet Office, 2008).

Physical	Mental and emotional	Social, cultural and religious
Malnutrition. Obesity. Diarrhoea. Low birth weight. Food allergy. Dental caries. Heart disease and stroke. Type 2 diabetes. Cancers: postmenopausal breast cancer, ovary and colon cancer. Hypertension. Gall bladder disease. Osteoarthritis. Sleep apnoea. Breathing problems. Lower back pain. Pregnancy complications. Increased surgical risks.	Psychosocial and social problems: reduced self-esteem, increased risk of depression and social isolation. Suicidal tendencies. Self-harming. Bulimia. Anorexia. Hyperactivity. Attention deficiency disorders. Aggression/violence. Anxiety.	Vital for adherence to social customs/social inclusion. Part of cultural norms/ religious practice: can lead to feelings of isolation, inequality and social exclusion. Eating certain foods/ eating out part of social aspirance.

Table 19.1 Effects of food on health and wellbeing (source: based on FHF, 2008; Kayani, 2003; Petersen, 2005; Wanless, 2004).

Adequate nutrition is not just necessary for survival, growth and development, but is a central component of brain development, and intrinsic to emotional and mental security. The phrases 'mood food' and 'comfort food' are part of everyday common parlance, used to describe food that induces feelings of happiness and wellbeing, and generally makes us feel better. The concept of 'mood food' is often employed by purveyors of unhealthy foods, as part of subliminal marketing strategies. Consumers are encouraged to make positive associations with certain foods even before consuming them. While these foods may be accessible in terms of immediate availability and cost, and may meet daily calorie quotas, they may not provide the required, specific nutrients necessary for good health (Kayani, 2007).

There is an abundance of research confirming the correlation between what we eat and how we feel and think, with foods such as oily fish, fruit and vegetables supporting positive mental health, and alcohol, caffeine and high sugar, fat and additive laden food recognised as stressors, negatively impacting on moods (Geary, 2002). In countries where recorded seafood consumption levels per capita are high, rates of major depression, bipolar and post-partum depression and homicide levels have been found to be considerably lower (Food and Health Forums, 2008). There is also a wealth of evidence of the association between nutritional status and cognitive function in older people (Greenwood, 2003). In other experimental research on the impact of diet on anti-social, violent and criminal behaviour, supplementing the diet of prison inmates with the omega-3 fatty acid DHA was found to greatly decrease hostility and aggression (Benton, 2007).

Body image and self-esteem

On average, children in the UK are exposed to between 20 000–40 000 television adverts each year, along with daily exposure to ambient advertising, often leading to stress and conflict between parents and children. By the age of ten the average child will recognise almost 400 brands and, by the age of three, 70 per cent of children are able to recognise the McDonalds sign (Compass, 2007; FSA, 2004). For 27 per cent of 15–17 year olds, the media is one of the earliest influences on beauty and body image (Etcoff, *et al.*, 2006). The stigmatising of overweight or obese children and even adults in such a hostile cultural climate perpetuates negative feelings of self-esteem. Fasting, starving, binging and avoiding certain food groups, coupled with obesogenic environments, can create conditions where, for some individuals, a preoccupation and obsession with food and its consumption can develop. In many instances an erratic food relationship, surrounding issues of control or lack of control about food, can develop into eating disorders. It is estimated that at least 1.1 million people in the UK are directly affected by eating disorders, with those between the ages of 14–25 years old at greatest risk (Beating Eating Disorders, 2007).

Religious and cultural issues

Food has enormous cultural significance. While fish and chips are quintessentially English, for minority ethnic groups other foods are imbued with similarly powerful associations. For some groups, access to religiously appropriate food is part of spiritual observance and cultural identity. Yet access to safe, nutritious, culturally appropriate food can be as disparate as the chasm between the health inequalities of minority groups and the general population.

Children of Pakistani and Bangladeshi origin are among those at greatest risk of poverty (DWP, 2008). Bangladeshi men are almost four times as likely to be diagnosed with diabetes, and the rates are almost three times as high for Pakistani and Indian men than the general population. Black Caribbean and Black African women are more likely to have an increased waist to hip ratio and raised waist circumference than the general population (Randhawa, 2007). The reality of food access is that discerning pet owners can obtain high quality, healthy food more effortlessly than some individuals. The major high street supermarkets all stock varieties of organic pet food, yet there is no provision for organic kosher or halal food, with only one Soil Association certified organic halal meat supplier in the country.

FOOD SECURITY

Food security is a complex issue. The much lauded, but complex definition announced at the World Food Summit in 1996 defines food security as:

> When all people, at all times, have physical and economic access to sufficient, safe and nutritious food to meet their dietary needs and food preferences for an active and healthy life. (Food and Agriculture Organization, 1996: 1).

Food antonyms

Discussions around food security can be confusing, not only because food security means different things for developed economies when compared with less industrialised economies, but also because it has become an all-encompassing phrase that can mean all things to all people. Table 19.2 examines how different aspects of food security can be interlinked but mean different things to health practitioners, individuals and policy-makers.

	Perceptions at national level – UK government	Perceptions at local level – health practitioners and individuals
Availability	Diversity of products and supply sources. UK has about 60 per cent market share.	Lack of independent shops with top four supermarkets dominating market share. High fat and sugar foods more readily available than fresh fruit and vegetables.
Access	Competitive retail structure. Sophisticated distribution system. 80–90 per cent of food consumption through retail sector, remainder through food services sector.	Physical barriers such as out-of-town shopping areas. Low car ownership. Poor transport infrastructure.
Affordability	UK has high per capita incomes. Real price of food has declined. Food a declining share of household budgets.	Promotional practices of supermarkets can often make less healthy food cheaper than healthy food. For low-income households food costs are relatively high.
Nutrition and quality	UK suffers from calorie excess, not deficient nutrition. Widespread assurance schemes.	Nutritional content of supermarket own and value brands lower than more expensive foods. High fat and sugar foods deliver instant feelings of satiety. Fast food outlet chains consistently meet consumer expectations of quality and taste.

Safety	Food Standards Agency, EU and international laws and codes. Occasional food scares. Private assurance and traceability.	Marketing and targeting of children by purveyors of unhealthy foods. Ready availability/low cost of unhealthy food. Distrust of health fascists.
Resilience	Scope for demand and supply-side substitution in response to particular shortages. Retailers pro-actively managing supply chains.	Food interventions need to be sustainable to achieve lasting health benefits. Conflicting priorities for basic living requirements.
Confidence	Consumers have confidence in retailers but have high expectations of food supply. Occasional panic-buying of essentials.	Inconsistent health messages for cash- and time-strapped families. Lack of cooking and budgeting skills. Readily available unhealthy foods meet adequate calorie requirements.

Table 19.2 Summary of food security perceptions at national and local level (adapted from Table 10.1: Annex A, DEFRA, 2006c and Kayani, 2003, 2007)

Threats to national food security are of increasing concern for policy-makers, with mounting unease about the ratio of domestic production to consumption, falling self-sufficiency, reliance on agricultural imports, and the potential for disruption to domestic food supplies from threats of bioterrorism (DEFRA, 2008d; Food and Agriculture Organization, 2008).

Despite the UK's relatively affluent status, government figures reveal that 13 million people were living below the poverty line in 2006/07 (DWP, 2008). For health practitioners, global economic depressions compound the difficulties of ameliorating food access for low-income households less able to implement self-sufficiency measures. Cheap food imports rather than locally sourced food through a supermarket network can be a means of providing food security for households by making sufficient affordable food available, but this clearly raises several food antonyms.

FOOD SOVEREIGNTY

Food sovereignty is likely to be the single most important food and agricultural policy issue of the twenty-first century. The notion of food sovereignty, much like food security, is multifaceted. The phrase was first coined by La Via Campesina: routinely referred to as a peasant movement of small scale producers, farmers, agricultural workers, rural women and indigenous communities. In reality, the highly organised movement has 149 member organisations from 56 countries, including groups such as the National Family Farm Coalition in America and National Farmers Union of Canada (La Via Campesina, 2008).

La Via Campesina achieved international prominence during the 1996 World Trade Summit, which members attended with the express purpose of influencing the World Trade Organisation to promote changes to international trade agreements, taking into full account the interests of peasants and small farmers (La Via Campesina, 1996). Within four years, the campaign had evolved into a well supported network made up of 2 000 Non-Governmental and Civil Society Organisations (NGO/CSO) and social movements, leading to the creation of a Food Sovereignty International Planning Committee (IPC). The IPC's audacious objective enshrined in its official declaration defines food sovereignty as (NGO/ CSO Forum for Food Sovereignty, 2002: 2):

> the right of peoples, communities, and countries to define their own agricultural, labor, fishing, food and land policies which are ecologically, socially, economically and culturally appropriate to their unique circumstances. It includes the true right to food and to produce food, which means that all people have the right to safe, nutritious and culturally appropriate food and to food-producing resources and the ability to sustain themselves and their societies.

A primary aim of the food sovereignty movement is to reclaim sovereignty over decision making on agricultural and food security issues (Ziegler, 2004). Clearly, food sovereignty is based on a core political ideology but, for others, it is an idiom largely interchangeable with food security, with similar associations. The FAO's (1996) declaration clearly recognised that food security would only be achieved by nations taking diverse paths and by adopting strategies consistent with their resources and capacities to achieve individual goals; while cooperating regionally and internationally to organise collective global food security solutions.

Land and food

At a more social and individual level, the aspirational aspects of autonomy symbolised by food sovereignty hold an obviously romantic yet widespread appeal. Food sovereignty can be utilised to focus on national policies, and also oriented towards reducing rural and urban poverty, due to its ideological emphasis on issues of access to land for the hungry and malnourished. Land-based health initiatives have the added benefits of tackling sedentary behaviour patterns, a key contributor to rising obesity levels.

Three such land-based food and health initiatives are Capital Growth, Landfit and Landshare (see Table 19.3). Food growing schemes such as allotments and food co-ops are a recognised means of dismantling barriers to accessing healthy, affordable food. The difference with these projects is that they are interlinked and widely supported with a certain added kudos. The indirect involvement of health practitioners in the support and facilitation of the initiatives enables the scheme to retain grass-root ownership rather than becoming a 'nanny state' edict.

Capital Growth	Coordinated by London Food Link and supported by a grant from the London Development Agency, the project aims to transform London by creating 2 012 new food growing spaces in time for the 2012 London Olympics, improving health and making the capital's food sustainable as part of the wider London Food Strategy. See: **www.capitalgrowth.org** (accessed 18 July 2009).
Landfit	A London-based initiative working in tandem with Capital Growth; aimed at bringing aspirant gardeners together with unused gardens, for 'garden sharing' or 'open allotments'. See: **www.landfit.org** (accessed 18 July 2009).
Landshare	High-profile venture involving celebrity chef Hugh Fearnley-Whittingstall, Keo Films and Channel 4, based on the Capital Growth project, but reaching out UK-wide and using established networks such as Landfit and Totnes Transition Town 'garden share network'. See: **http://landshare.channel4.com** and **http://totnes. transitionnetwork.org/gardenshare/home** (accessed 18 July 2009).

Table 19.3 Land-based food and health projects

CHANGE REVOLUTION

Governments can often become preoccupied with changing and repackaging food ideology; from safe food, food poverty, food access and food deserts to food security and food sovereignty. Change, like food terminology, is subject to various interpretations. The concept of 'real' change in the context of food, health and wellbeing is not simply about changing one policy for another, but more about an all-encompassing and revolutionary approach, robustly addressing food antonyms. The call for a change revolution is a rallying cry for a synchronised 'big idea' to create a cultural shift at all levels, not necessarily reliant on top-down or bottom-up accepted strategies. It advocates a central approach of creative interventions by those holding a centre position within public sector organisations or those from independent and charitable sectors.

Obesogenic environments

Fiscal, practical, social and geographical barriers to food access have long been recognised as impacting adversely on the ability of individuals to attain healthy diets, particularly in areas of urban deprivation, and are synonymous with food deserts (Kayani, 2003).

The steep rise in obesity levels has added to these concerns and raised issues of wider detriments to society. There is an increased recognition of factors that reinforce deep-rooted social problems, creating obesity-prone hotspots. The phrase 'obesogenic environment' is used to describe such environmental factors, including socio-cultural, built and food environments, believed to promote obesity among individuals or populations (Lake, *et al.*, 2006).

Obviously, a pervasive culture of readily available high salt, sugar and high fat foods in public institutions, schools, workplaces, hospitals, canteens, shopping malls and high streets influence the shopping and eating choices of populations and individuals. In an economic downturn, lower quality and higher fat foods become even more readily available as organic and high end foods are replaced with value brands and cheaper, high sugar and high fat foods. This fact was highlighted by a National Consumer Council (2008) survey, which found that 54 per cent of supermarket promotions related to foods high in fat and sugar and only 12.5 per cent featured fruit and vegetables. There is also a clear consensus on the effect that food promotion has on children's preferences, purchase behaviour and consumption (Hastings, *et al.*, 2006).

Clearly, reducing the obesogenicity of environments, by using a variety of available techniques, is imperative for sustainable public heath interventions. Evidence suggests that social marketing interventions can improve diet and, to some lesser extent, food safety (McDermott, *et al.*, 2005). The proposed introduction of a Healthier Food Mark, for public sector food, identifying the availability of healthier and more sustainable food is also a positive step (Cabinet Office, 2008), as is the allocation of £20 million for a pilot project in two deprived areas to ensure that all school children receive at least one nutritious hot meal a day (DoH, 2008b). There is also a need for more groundbreaking policies, such as the London Borough of Waltham Forest's (2008) plan to use material planning considerations to restrict planning permission for hot food takeaway shops (pizza, burger and kebab shops), which fall within a ten-minute walking distance of schools, parks and youth facility boundaries.

Community food

Food sharing and redistribution schemes have been widely used since the 1960s by many industrialised countries to enable homeless and vulnerable groups to have access to vital food supplies. Although still not part of the mainstream, since the early 1990s similar UK schemes have become more prevalent.

The schemes, often widely supported by supermarket networks, enable corporations to enhance their social credentials; allowing them to dispose of surplus food, saving on landfill costs while simultaneously gaining tax breaks. Three UK food and health initiatives, coordinated by charities working closely with statutory agencies are Fare Share, The Food Bank and Food Share (see Table 19.4). The three charitable organisations vary in the way that they collect and distribute food, but all meet a variety of other health and social community needs.

Fare Share	Started as a project in 1994 as part of the homelessness charity Crisis. Since 2004, it has operated independently to distribute unwanted food taken from supermarkets (such as Marks & Spencer, Sainsbury and Tesco) to charities and homeless centres through eight regional warehouses. The regional centres work as franchises, taking food from local sources to provide cooked food for the homeless in 12 UK-wide locations. In 2007, food redistributed by the network contributed towards more than 4.5 million meals. The charity aims to open another 18 depots redistributing 20 000 tonnes of food through 2 500 community organisations and charities by 2011. **www.fareshare.org.uk** (accessed 18 July 2009)
The Food Bank	Started in 2000 by the Trussel Trust, a Christian charity, as a small operation in a shed, the Salisbury Food Bank has rapidly expanded as a franchise network of 35 UK-wide Food Banks providing food to over 12 000 people. Food Banks are entirely reliant on public donations of food and money to distribute emergency food boxes containing three days' worth of non-perishable food to those in crisis, usually referred to Food Banks through a voucher scheme by health professionals. **www.trusselltrust.org/content/foodbank/foodbank.htm** (accessed 18 July 2009)
Food Share	Started in 1994, CCP Food Share is an emergency food distribution service run by County Community Projects operating in the Cheltenham area. Reliant entirely on food donations from members of the public, churches, schools and businesses, they redistribute the donations in the form of over 500 annual food parcels, through health professional referrals. **www.ccprojects.org.uk/ccp-food-share.html** (accessed 18 July 2009)

Table 19.4 Food sharing and redistribution projects

Activity 19.1 Reflective exercise

Review a local food project and consider the influence of the obesogenic environment and its possible impact on the health gain objectives of the project.

This exercise examines the wider context of barriers to healthy eating, by analysing the role of small scale community/ food projects in securing lasting health gains.

- Should we be preventing or treating obesity?
- What are the causal factors of obesity at a local level?
- Will the provision of low-cost food outlets encourage fruit and vegetable consumption?
- Will banning junk food shops near schools, hospitals and in town centres encourage healthy food choices?
- How can food projects reduce contributory factors of obesity, such as sedentary lifestyles?

Activity 19.2 Reflective exercise: food security

Should the UK consider using import controls to reduce dependence on global food supplies, reduce food miles and encourage the consumption of seasonal/locally grown food to improve health? Should we be growing or buying?

This exercise examines food security in a global, national and local context. It raises a number of food antonyms, central to the health debate, such as:

- should we protect farmers and food producers from international competition?
- does free trade ensure national food security?
- can import tariffs and quotas encourage fruit and vegetable consumption?
- do current food policies ensure access to safe, nutritious and culturally appropriate food for all?

CONCLUSION

In an unequal society it is no surprise that access to adequate food sufficient for health and wellbeing remains inequitable. In a cultural climate dominated by corporate advertising, cheap mass-produced high fat and sugar foods readily available on every street corner, and in a society where most jobs are sedentary, are individuals really responsible for not buying or eating the right food?

Individuals are not the architects of obesogenic environments. They did not instigate the abolition of free school meals, nor are they responsible for the weekly purchase of 60 tonnes of chips by public sector organisations (DoH, 2007d). Neither did they create policies that mean that the average household income can only be achieved with two earners, leaving little time for inventive food security solutions.

It is not the choice of individuals to pile shelves high with cheap, value brand foods in times of economic instability or to withdraw 'better foods' to safeguard profit margins. More than ever health practitioners have a duty to safeguard the right to 'safe food' for all.

Useful websites

Abraham Natural Produce: **www.organic-halal-meat.com/index.php**
Soil Association-approved smallholding supplying organic, halal meat countrywide.

Food for the Brain: **www.foodforthebrain.org**
Useful evidence database for links between nutrition and mental health.

International Association for the Study of Obesity:
www.iaso.org/index.asp
Provides a global perspective on health and obesity.

Natural justice: **www.naturaljustice.org.uk**
Information on the role of nutrition in shaping social behaviour both in the community and in closed conditions.

Organic Inform: **www.organicinform.org**
Part-funded by DEFRA with useful information on organic farming, food and projects.

(Websites all accessed 18 July 2009.)

Chapter 20

The challenges for health and community in the private housing sector

Jill Stewart, Paul Mishkin and Russell Moffatt

This chapter identifies some of the links between health and housing and evaluates putting current policy into practice to optimum effect. It draws out the relationship between evidence-based policy, how this is implemented, professional roles and multi-agency partnerships involved in seeking to achieve sustainable results in the complex area of private sector housing interventions.

Learning outcomes

In this chapter you will learn how to:

- recognise the need for a private sector housing and health evidence base, particularly with regard to longitudinal evidence;

- understand the scope and potential of the Housing Health and Safety Rating System;

- appreciate the confounding factors in housing and health, including ongoing issues facing families in temporary accommodation;

- understand the roles of local authorities and their partners in addressing poor housing conditions and in area regeneration, empty homes and fuel poverty.

INTRODUCTION

Private sector housing (owner occupiers and the private rented sector) comprises the majority of UK tenure, and contains some of the most vulnerable households and highest levels of non-decent homes (DCLG, 2009). Policy interventions have sought to address conditions in the sector, largely through a range of enforcement and assistance regimes. More recently, there has been a marked shift back toward 'personal responsibility' for housing condition.

The main focus of this chapter is therefore on the traditional remit of the environmental health practitioner working in partnership with others in public health, and demonstrates some of the very positive interventions that can be possible through innovative and creative use of legislation and strategies to promote healthy housing and communities, particularly in the private housing sector. However, it is only relatively recently that government has attempted to realign health and housing policy and there remains a limited evidence base about good practice and what works in contemporary housing policy to improve health.

HOUSING AS A HEALTH DETERMINANT

Housing is a key health determinant (Dahlgren and Whitehead, 1991; Scott-Samuel, et al., 2001) and housing can affect health as both an internal and an external living environment (Health Education Authority (HEA), 2000; Krieger and Higgins, 2002; Ormandy, 2004; Thomson, et al., 2001 and 2002; Wilkinson, 1999). Housing is important in maintaining and improving public health as well as quality of life and wellbeing for all and, perhaps most of all, for those with disabilities and special needs who have particular design and facility requirements of their housing, for living and sometimes for working.

A problem is that there is a great amount of evidence about the relationship of housing to both physical and mental health, but impacts on health are complex and adaptive so direct evidence of effects on health are limited (Cave, et al., 2004; HEA, 2000; Lawrence, 2004; Thomson, et al., 2002; Wilkinson, 1999). Evidence of the health effects of interventions, including health gain, is lacking and a more holistic approach is necessary to respond to the complex issues in housing, health and deprivation (Thomson, et al., 2001). There is a need for flexible, innovative interventions as occupiers age and change health status, their housing conditions alter and they develop differing needs during the course of their lifetime (Lawrence, 2004). Appropriate housing interventions can help to reduce negative health impacts and thereby address health inequalities. However, it is difficult to accurately assess the impact of housing conditions on health, as health can result from wider socio-economic circumstance (HEA, 2000; Lawrence, 2004; Thomson, *et al.*, 2001; Wilkinson, 1999). Despite this, there is agreement that housing is important in maintaining and improving public health as well as quality of life and wellbeing (HEA, 2000).

Despite the wealth of information linking housing and health, partnerships have been difficult to establish and maintain. There are inconsistencies in how private sector housing is seen as a health determinant, in that views and evidence-based interventions are very fragmented and it is likely to be some time before housing practitioners will be able to influence the public health agenda more effectively (Stewart, Ruston and Clayton, 2006). This said, there are many examples of successful interventions although many go unreported and the information is often not successfully or widely disseminated by publication.

THE HOUSING HEALTH AND SAFETY RATING SYSTEM

The Housing Act 2004 introduced a completely new prescribed method of assessing and acting upon housing conditions, known as the Housing Health and Safety Rating System (HHSRS). HHSRS is a risk assessment-based approach to assessing housing and, specifically, its impact on the health of its occupants and their visitors. It looks at building defects and then rates, according to an evidence-based scale, the likelihood of a harmful health event, or hazard, occurring as a result of that defect. The likelihood is also rated against the potential health outcomes from that event and this produces a score. It is therefore a substantial change from the previous statutory standard relating to housing, which was a pass or fail test. The lack of a firm standard within the HHSRS is a deliberate move away from the prescriptive standard of the past to a risk-based system, common to other areas of environmental health such as food safety or workplace health and safety

There are 29 hazards that defects can be considered to contribute towards (see Box 20.1), although certain defects may contribute to more than one hazard. The resultant score for each hazard can then be compared on a linear scale, with higher scores representing higher risks. These can be placed into bands along this ascending scale from A–J, with A being the highest possible set of scores and J being the lowest. Those hazards that score in Bands A–C are classified as Category 1 Hazards and the local authority is under a legal duty to take action on those hazards. All other bands are classed as Category 2 Hazards and the local authority has discretion on whether or not to take action in these instances. Typically, the higher scoring Category 2 Hazards (in Band D for example) will usually be dealt with, although this varies upon the enforcement policy of each particular local authority. Local authorities have been able to use the HHSRS innovatively, and an example is given in Box 20.2.

Box 20.1 The 29 HHSRS hazards

A – PHYSIOLOGICAL REQUIREMENTS
Hygrothermal Conditions
1. Damp and mould growth.
2. Excess cold.
3. Excess heat.

Pollutants (Non-microbial)
4. Asbestos (and MMF).
5. Biocides.
6. Carbon monoxide and fuel combustion products.
7. Lead.
8. Radiation.
9. Uncombusted fuel gas.
10. Volatile organic compounds.

B – PSYCHOLOGICAL REQUIREMENTS
Space, Security, Light and Noise
11. Crowding and space.
12. Entry by intruders.
13. Lighting.
14. Noise.

C – PROTECTION AGAINST INFECTION
Hygiene, Sanitation and Water Supply
15. Domestic hygiene, pests and refuse.
16. Food safety.
17. Personal hygiene, sanitation and drainage.
18. Water supply.

D – PROTECTION AGAINST ACCIDENTS
Falls
19. Falls associated with baths, etc.

20. Falling on level surfaces, etc.
21. Falling on stairs, etc.
22. Falling between levels.

Electric Shocks, Fires, Burns and Scalds
23. Electrical hazards.
24. Fire.
25. Flames, hot surfaces, etc.

Collisions, Cuts and Strains
26. Collision and entrapment.
27. Explosions.
28. Position and operability of amenities, etc.
29. Structural collapse and falling elements.

(ODPM, 2004c)

Box 20.2 Case study: HHSRS and HIA in the London Borough of Islington (see also Chapter 11)

Environmental health practitioners in the London Borough of Islington conducted a Health Impact Assessment on their Private Sector Housing Strategy and looked at how HHSRS could be used strategically to meet objectives within this strategy based on locally relevant data.

The project evaluated what hazards typically have the most impact on residents, due to, for example, the frequency of their occurrence or the severity of their outcomes. The main focus was on the elderly and very young, who spend more time at home and may have comparatively weak or under-developed immune systems. The hazards that were studied were excess cold and its effects, overcrowding, security and accidents resulting from falls and fire.

A search for local data was sought for each hazard, using various statistics, which were then compared with both the London-wide and national data, where available. Where available, data was also broken down into ward level and then ranked numerically. This allowed various conclusions or educated inferences where clear trends were not immediately apparent.

Excess cold and its effects – Islington did not have a higher incidence of excess winter deaths than the London or England-wide figures, but it was still considered an important area to continue to work on.

Overcrowding – overcrowding had been rising in the social sector but decreasing in the private rented sector. Considering the increasing reliance on the private sector, there was a need to see this in terms of other hazards in the private sector arising from relocating tenants. The data also provided a ranking of the extent of the problem in each of the wards in the borough. However, there did not appear to be any major variation in the incidence.

Security – some robust data allowed a detailed picture to emerge. It identified that the entire borough had a higher crime rate than the London average and this could be used to easily justify action on this area.

Accidents – the data demonstrated some varying patterns across the borough. Four wards in particular showed significantly worse admission rates to hospital from falls than other areas. This could therefore allow a potentially more targeted response to the higher accident rates in those areas. It was also concluded that some updated data would have been useful to see if those trends still hold true.

Fire – the resulting data did not show any statistically worse scenario than elsewhere. However, when looking at the private sector stock profile from the most recently available private sector stock condition survey (from 2003, which was replaced by an updated survey report at the end of 2008) larger Victorian HMOs were identified as a particular risk category, although more commonly occupied by age groups outside of this study.

Recommendations included the need for regular updates to evaluate progress. Further detailed work could also be undertaken using local detailed maps, possibly with the use of GIS systems, with detailed information overlaid to help further identify local hot spots of problems.

A key recommendation was to further target vulnerable groups in non-decent homes. Some of these were already being implemented, for example via House Warming Islington, a joint working approach between the Residential Environmental Health Service and Islington Council's Green Living Centre, which has sought to make referrals between agencies that can assist vulnerable households. Environmental health practitioners were also undertaking promotional talks with other health professionals, social workers, police and voluntary agencies such as Age Concern. It was also anticipated that these meetings would initiate more joint visits between environmental health practitioners and officers from those organisations.

PRIVATELY RENTED HOUSING

Many choose to live in the private rented sector, yet for others it is not the tenure of choice and proves expensive and insecure. The English House Condition Survey (DCLG, 2009) reported that the private rented sector contains the poorest conditions. Environmental health practitioners face daily challenges of addressing conditions, while also working with landlords and tenants in an attempt to balance enforcement and other intervention activities.

One of the most vulnerable communities in society is lone parents with children in temporary accommodation, particularly bed and breakfast. The implications for poor health in bed and breakfast have been long established (Conway, 1988). The problem is not just one of a lack of joined-up working; it is mainly a problem of a lack of decent housing elsewhere. Many low-income families continue to be housed in such unsatisfactory accommodation, illustrating the disjointed policy of meeting immediate housing need, but failing to address parallel public health needs, particularly for children already faced with major social inequality. It can be difficult to break the cycle of inadequate access to health care services and other established welfare regimes (for discussion, see Stewart, Bushell and Habgood, 2005; Stewart and Rhoden, 2006). See also Box 20.3.

Box 20.3 Temporary accommodation and children's health

In 2004, the housing charity Shelter commissioned a report into what it termed 'the housing crisis', which specifically focused on the impact of poor housing on children. This report, called *Generation Squalor* (Minton, 2005), included findings from a series of expert panels held around the country to investigate how temporary accommodation affected children's health. An environmental health practitioner from the London Borough of Islington attended one of these panels and gave anecdotal accounts of extremely poor standards in bed and breakfast and other temporary accommodation and the resultant effects that these had on child occupants. Along with other evidence from tenants themselves, health visitors, MPs and other professionals it pointed to an increase in conditions such as asthma and other upper respiratory conditions as well as mental health issues such as stress and depression.

In addition, when these poor conditions were compounded with the fact of being overcrowded, the mental health effects were that much greater. Other effects such as feelings of social exclusion were also noted and there was a knock-on effect on educational attainment. A clear picture emerged of a vastly unsuitable method of housing, which, when children are present, can become even more hazardous in terms of health effects.

Reflective exercise
- What are the economic and social costs of temporary accommodation, and what is the evidence for this?
- What might be done at strategic level to help families with children to access decent, secure and affordable homes?

AREA REGENERATION

Regeneration areas have a geographical focus and are able to address the wider determinants of health and consequently improve public health. Regeneration principally aims to change the resources that are at people's disposal in a neighbourhood and the conditions in which people live. The extent and nature of community problems can vary considerably between one area and another. In some cases the key issue is worn-out housing and in others problems are associated with crime, social disorder or ill health. The worst areas have all of these.

The UK has at least 700 area-based regeneration projects, with as many as 75 operating in a single city at sub-regional, city-wide and neighbourhood levels, and an example is given in Box 20.4. These seek to tackle widespread socio-economic conditions through partnership working. Regional development agencies have taken over much of the responsibility and funding for regeneration, although delivery is primarily at a local government and neighbourhood level and some of the resources that have been available are summarised below:

- **Children's Fund**: education, health and social care partnership to support the wellbeing of school-age children and their parents.
- **Connexions**: partnerships to guide, inform and advise young people on training and other opportunities.
- **Employment Zones**: zones aiming to help long-term unemployed people into sustainable work and independence.
- **Education Action Zones**: zones aiming to raise educational standards through partnerships with local businesses, parents and the community.
- **Healthy Schools**: education and health partnerships to improve the health of the school community and enable children to make healthier choices.
- **Health Action Zones** (now disbanded): cross-cutting partnerships to improve health and address health inequalities between the better-off and the most deprived.
- **Healthy Living Centres** (New Opportunities Fund): community-led partnerships in the UK to improve the quality of life for people, especially the most disadvantaged.
- **Sure Start**: aims to support the physical, emotional, intellectual and social development of young children through the integration of early education, childcare, and health and family support services.
- **Sure Start Plus**: partnerships to support teenagers who become pregnant when they are aged 17 or under, or who may be at risk of becoming pregnant, and to improve health, wellbeing and learning for teenage parents.
- **New Deal for Communities**: regeneration partnerships to improve job prospects, reduce levels of crime, and improve educational achievement and health in some of the poorest areas.
- **Neighbourhood Renewal Fund**: fund aiming to enable the 88 most deprived local authorities to improve services, narrowing the gap between deprived areas.
- **Sports Action Zones**: zones aiming to bring the benefits of sport to deprived communities.

Box 20.4 Case study: Area regeneration in the London Borough of Newham

The London Borough of Newham has consistently used area-based regeneration as a method for improving the built environment and residents' wellbeing. Three neighbourhood renewal areas have been declared in the last decade, focused around Forest Gate. Before the Secretary of State makes the declaration, a neighbourhood renewal assessment (NRA) is completed, and this is used to diagnose the key issues and forms the evidence base for action.

The renewal has a ten-year areas life span, during which grant funding can be focused on particular areas through group repair schemes. Group repair has also been used to improve shop fronts located within a strategically important shopping area. At the same time larger one-off schemes have been prioritised to support enhanced community facilities, such as a library and health services. Paths, street lighting and other street furniture have also been upgraded.

Enforcement powers including compulsory purchase orders, control orders, enforcement notices, works in default and criminal prosecutions are focused on the worst landlords and property owners to force sustainable change. Prominent houses in multiple occupation have been targeted and licensed where appropriate.

Anti-social behaviour and crime hotspots where prostitution, drug dealing and rubbish dumping are commonplace have been targeted jointly by the police and the local authority. Where possible, the built environment has been redesigned to help prevent further problems. Alleyways are particularly vulnerable to undesirable behaviour and are a prime spot for intervention.

Area-based regeneration works well when all of the public services come together with local people to find lasting solutions. Managing expectation is important and can be difficult. It is therefore vital to have a balance between ambition and practicability. However one thing is clear, top-down area-based regeneration where the views of local people are ignored is certain to fail. Therefore it is crucial to communicate and consult with those who are affected.

In practice, working partnerships with the wide range of professionals, although very rewarding, can be difficult in the medium- and long-term as officer time for project work is scarce. By using any structured project management approach it is possible to fix in a commitment from agencies and services, focused on a particular outcome.

Underlying prospects for neighbourhood renewal often rely on influencing the nature and performance of the local property market, making disadvantaged areas more attractive to private investment. Prospects for renewal can hinge on making disadvantaged areas more attractive for doing business and for living. This often involves halting or reversing the trend of older dwellings being vacated by higher income groups and reoccupied by lower-income or benefit-dependent groups. The shift from single-family occupation to multiple occupations indicates a shift to lower-wage and higher-transience occupancy and is often identified as a driver of social decline.

Wider housing improvement programmes are thought to be especially cost-effective, not only because of direct health benefits but also indirect benefits in the form of better self-care and decision-making capacity by residents (Ambrose, 1996).

Empty homes and homelessness

Empty homes are a waste of a valuable resource, particularly where there are significant levels of unmet housing need. Moreover, empty properties can often become a target for vandals and squatters; they attract rubbish dumping, anti-social behaviour and crime and they become eyesores that affect the whole neighbourhood's wellbeing.

More than a Roof: A Report into Tackling Homelessness (ODPM, 2002) estimated that empty and commercial properties in England (including spaces above shops) have the potential for around 420 000 homes, taking into account the efficient operation of the property market. This represents housing for around 15 per cent of anticipated new households, highlighting the importance of unlocking the potential of empty property. However, vacancy turnover rates and the number of long-term empty properties can become excessively high particularly in poorer neighbourhoods as private investment leaves an area.

Intervention by the local authority can bring significant advantages to the community as a whole and can even act as a catalyst for wider regeneration. Advantages can be gained from dealing with the most prominent empty properties, including those on main arterial roads, and properties in the worst condition. A range of tools are available to turn properties around, ranging from developing a dialogue with the owners, through to financial incentives. Where other options fail local authorities are able to force empty property owners to take positive action, including compulsory purchase orders, empty dwelling management orders and a range of other enforcement measures.

LAAs: housing and health

Local Area Agreements (LAAs) (for definition and scope, see Chapter 5) present an opportunity to provide evidence-based holistic public health services. They promote the integration of organisations, particularly local authorities and Primary Care Trusts, around a priority issue. An example of this, within a health and housing context, was developed in Haringey, North London. The scheme integrated and structured home energy efficiency measures provided by the local authority, with home fire safety checks by the Fire Brigade and home safety checks by Age Concern. Services are coordinated as a package for vulnerable groups on a street by street basis, mainly in the owner-occupied and private-rented sectors. Intelligence gathered by each service is pooled and the information used to target hard to reach groups.

FUEL POVERTY

Fuel poverty arises where households are not able to afford sufficient heating due to a combination of low income, poor heating and inadequate thermal insulation. The links between fuel poverty and health are well documented, yet strategies remain discretionary and there are no statutory reporting requirements relating to the health gain arising from them. Fuel poverty is particularly acute in parts of the private housing sector as the sector can be 'hard to reach'.

The main problem is that fuel poverty strategies are discretionary. For this reason, they risk being short term, insufficiently funded and non sustainable, and therefore have to be championed largely by individuals within supportive organisations. Some local authorities have been very proactive in developing and implementing fuel poverty strategies. Luton Borough Council's Affordable Warmth Strategy tackles deprivation, poor housing, social exclusion and health. It has been successful as its partnership approach enables multiple health determinants to be addressed and the organisations involved have enabled a focus on health and not just income. However, despite being an award-winning strategy, it has proven difficult to quantify health gain arising at local level (Stewart and Habgood, 2008). In addition, the study reiterated the difficulty of focusing fuel poverty interventions in the private housing sector.

Sheffield First Partnership for Health and Wellbeing commissioned a Health Impact Assessment of its own housing stock's Decent Homes Programme (see also Chapter 11). It used the HHSRS to show how joined-up thinking could work in accounting for the wider health benefits of strategies. While this study focuses on social housing, important lessons can nevertheless be learnt for private sector housing about warmth and comfort without having to reinvent the wheel, and it suggests ways in which resources can be targeted to enhance health gain for residents. Such methods could be usefully adapted and applied in other areas to help turn around our inadequate impact on addressing fuel poverty to date (Green and Pugh, 2008).

PRIVATE SECTOR HOUSING: WHICH WAY NOW?

Despite some of the challenges presented, some partnerships are now working to develop local evidence bases to identify the cost effectiveness of possible interventions. Liverpool Primary Care Trust (PCT), for example, has recently funded some £3.9 million in a partnership between environmental health and the NHS. This is to fund additional inspections and enforcement in some of the worst private sector housing stock. An advantage of this partnership is to help facilitate environmental health access to GPs and the community health service, helping to reach some of the most marginal communities in tackling health inequalities. The PCT has estimated that this initiative could help prevent 200 deaths per year and up to 2 000 GP consultations over three years (Hatchett, 2008).

The Building Research Establishment (BRE) has very recently published a toolkit entitled *Good Housing Leads to Good Health* (BRE, 2008) that seeks to help practitioners with methodology, advice and case studies to demonstrate the value of proactive work in the private housing sector, as well as to provide evidence on the cost-effectiveness of interventions. It provides a HHSRS costs calculator that helps calculate the potential cost and therefore cost savings to the NHS arising from specified interventions. Anecdotal evidence to date suggests that many EHPs are finding this an invaluable resource in being able to justify the cost-effectiveness of their interventions, and that it is helping to demonstrate the importance of proactive housing interventions to wider health colleagues and to shift resources to this area.

A PRIVATE SECTOR HOUSING EVIDENCE BASE

One of the problems in attracting resources to private sector housing, as opposed to social housing, has been the lack of evidence of the effectiveness of interventions (see, for example, Stewart, 2009). This has been due in part to key players – most notably EHPs – not routinely disseminating the success of their work by publication. In order to address this, the CIEH and University of Greenwich have been working in partnership to develop an online evidence base with specific reference to the private housing sector. This will collate existing relevant published evidence and draw from 'grey literature' (i.e. unpublished sources) that are of sufficient rigour to be cited and accessed from the CIEH website, with a view to developing a culture of publication in the longer term. The website will also seek to be interactive and help form new working partnerships between practitioners and the academic community. It should be up and running by the time this book is published and it is hoped that the site will develop in the coming years through continued evaluation and application.

CONCLUSION

Housing is important in maintaining and improving public health as well as quality of life and wellbeing, but more longitudinal evidence is required. Interventions in the private housing sector prove particularly challenging as resources are withdrawn. Despite these challenges, many EHPs have been able to work with other agencies to deliver innovative approaches to private sector housing renewal and continue to work toward developing an evidence base to further champion their work.

Further reading and useful websites

Davies, A. (2007) *Cinderella Strikes Back: Strategic Housing and the Private Rented Sector*. Coventry: CIH: **www.cih.org/policy/cinderella. pdf** (accessed 20 February 2009).
Emphasises the strategic importance of the private rented sector as part of a wider housing function in regeneration and public health partnerships.

CIEH (2007) *Commission on Housing Renewal and Public Health Final Report*. London: CIEH: **www.cieh.org/library/Knowledge/Housing/Housing_renewal_report07.pdf** (accessed 20 February 2009). Identifies priority areas for housing and public health from an environmental health perspective.

Joseph Rowntree Foundation: **www.jrf.org.uk**

National HMO Network: **www.nationalhmonetwork.com**

Accreditation Network: **www.anuk.org.uk**
Professionals and organisations promoting accreditation in the privately rented housing sector.

Empty Homes Agency: **www.emptyhomes.com**

Building Research Establishment: **www.bre.co.uk**

Shelter: **www.shelter.org.uk**

National Energy Agency: **www.nea.org.uk**

Chartered Institute of Housing: **www.cih.org**

Chartered Institute of Environmental Health: **www.cieh.org**

Centre for Housing Policy: **www.york.ac.uk/inst/chp**

Centre for Urban and Regional Studies: **www.curs.bham.ac.uk**

Safe and Healthy Housing Unit, University of Warwick: **www2.warwick.ac.uk/fac/soc/law/research/centres/shhru**

(Websites all accessed 21 July 2009)

Chapter 21

Conclusions

Jill Stewart and Yvonne Cornish

As this book has demonstrated, the category of professional practitioner in public health includes a range of individuals, operating across a range of organisations from the highest strategic levels to the most loosely associated functions, but all of whom are crucial in addressing health inequalities and improving and protecting health. The roles of both professionals and practitioners have taken on a wider and more flexible remit in recent years, which requires new and complex skills in working in partnership to deliver public health in the postmodern world where factors such as information technology and globalisation continue to present new opportunities, but also new challenges.

Public health is so vast a subject, and with such a diverse workforce, that it is difficult to pinpoint where it starts and where it ends. This book has attempted to do justice to the major and fundamental subject areas by drawing from colleagues' expertise and both public and environmental health. These conclusions are therefore kept brief, to highlight some of the key issues arising that have been more thoroughly addressed in individual chapters by their specialist authors.

Public health is fundamentally about reducing health inequalities and improving health through evidence-based strategies and interventions, and the range and scope of organisations and workforce involved continues to develop apace. It has been increasingly important to demonstrate the effectiveness of interventions to help attract resources to where they are most needed and continually challenge conceptions around health and health inequality. Health needs assessment and health impact assessment have become increasingly pivotal in this process and have been able to help both develop and support partnership working so that strategic approaches can be optimised in securing resource and expertise and bringing an end to silo working. We are helped in these processes by being able to readily access online material helping to guide us through practices and processes, but must ensure that what we access is the most up-to-date and rigorous information. Websites such as PHOs and NICE help us in this process, and we need to continue to add to the evidence base, particularly in seeking to publish and thereby disseminate our own interventions. Some of these factors are summarised in Table 21.1.

Strategic question	Application/process	Considerations
Where are we now?	HNA, JSNA.	• Sustainable, long-term approach, not short-term fix. • Regard to continuing change (postmodernism). • Adaptation (local, national, global) and response to new challenges. • New roles of state, organisations, professionals, communities working together. • Constant learning and evaluation. • Ethical and equitable interventions.
Where do we want to be?	HNA, JSNA, HIA.	
How are we going to get there?	LSP, CS, LAA, other local strategies and interventions; new service commissioning.	
How are we going to review our success?	Use of EBP, CAA, audit, evaluation, performance monitoring, qualitative reports, etc.	

Table 21.1: Summary of public health strategic processes. Source: adapted from Goss and Blackaby (1998)

Environmental health has been a major focus of this book and environmental health practitioners (EHPs) have been identified as the key public health practitioners working in local government in assessing and correcting environmental stressors. While many EHPs are now working in high-profile roles in the NHS delivering public health, we should not be complacent and there is still a long way to go in promoting the role of the environment in improving health. There is a particular need for some areas, notably housing and regeneration as structural health determinants, to be strongly promoted, as there is a risk that these areas may lose out to lifestyles issues, such as obesity and smoking. However, environmental health has come a long way in public health and we need to continue our efforts in this area.

There still remain challenges to tackle and there is a need to address entrenched inequalities. What is needed is a continued focus on sustainability of approach so that the issues identified are addressed in a comprehensive and long-term manner, not just seen as a short-term or high-profile fix. There is a particular need to ensure that community development is enhanced and that social capital and social enterprise are sensitively nurtured at very local level, so that marginalised communities can move forward with appropriate support and can be helped to attract funding for their own local initiatives through new commissioning roles of statutory organisations in partnership with the not-for-profit sector.

We can all recognise how far we have come in public health, but must not be complacent and must ensure that our efforts are focused where they are most needed: in delivering public health interventions to some of our most deprived and marginal communities, so that everyone is offered a fair chance to reach their potential and can live a healthy life.

References and Bibliography

Acheson, D. (1988) *Public Health in England: Report to the Committee of Inquiry into the Future of the Public Health Function*. London: HMSO

Acheson, D. (1998) *Independent Inquiry into Inequalities in Health Report*. London: HMSO

Adshead, F., Thorpe, A. and Rutter, J. (2006) 'Sustainable development and public health: A national perspective'. *Public Health* 120 (12): 1102–05

Age Concern (2007) *Older People in the United Kingdom: Key Facts and Statistics 2007*. London: Age Concern

Age Concern (2008a) *The State Pension*. Online. Available at: **www.ageconcern. org.uk/AgeConcern/fs19.asp** (accessed 3 January 2009)

Age Concern (2008b) *Age Discrimination*. Online. Available at: **www. ageconcern.org.uk/AgeConcern/ageism.asp** (accessed 3 January 2009)

Age Concern (2009) *Ageism in the Health Service and Social Care*. Online. Available at: **www.ageconcern.org.uk/AgeConcern/ OE4DC476ED22451BB66ABDF52COB2** (accessed 16 March 2009)

Ajzen, I (1991). 'The theory of planned behavior'. *Organizational Behavior and Human Decision Processes*, 50: 179–211

Ajzen, I., and Driver, B. (1992) 'Application of the theory of planned behaviour to lecture choice'. *Journal of Leisure Research*, 24: 207–24

All Women Count (2008) *Packed Meeting in Parliament Backs New Zealand's Decriminalization*. Online. Available at: **www.allwomencount.net/EWC%20 Sex%20Workers/PackedMeeting16Jan08.htm** (accessed 30 January 2009)

Al-Osaimi, A. (2008) 'Securing health and human rights: Sandwell's Community Health Network'. *Medicine, Conflict and Survival*, 24 Suppl 1: S94–103

Ambrose, P. (1996). *I Mustn't Laugh too Much: Housing and Health on the Limehouse Fields and Ocean Estate in Stepney*. University of Sussex: Centre of the Urban and Regional Research

Anable, J, Lane, B and Kelay, T (2006) *An Evidence Based Review of Public Attitudes to Climate Change and Transport Behaviour for the Department for Transport*. Online. Available at: **www.dft.gov.uk/pgr/sustainable/ climatechange/iewofpublicattitudestocl5730.pdf** (accessed 6 March 2009)

Andrews, M. M. and Boyle, J. S. (1995) *Transcultural concepts in nursing care* (2nd Ed). Philadelphia, USA: JB Lippincott Co.

Armitage, C. J. and Conner, M. (2001) 'Efficacy of the theory of planned behaviour: A meta-analytic review'. *British Journal of Social Psychology*, 40: 471–99

Armstrong, D. (1993) 'Public health spaces and the fabrication of identity'. *Sociology* 27 (3): 393–410

Arnstein, S. R. (1969) *A Ladder of Citizen Participation*. Originally published as Arnstein, Sherry R. 'A ladder of citizen participation'. *JAIP*, 35 (4) July 1969: 216–24. Online. Available at: **http://lithgow-schmidt.dk/sherry-arnstein/ladder-of-citizen-participation.html** (accessed 17 February 2009)

Arrdondo, A. and Najera, P. (2008) 'Equity and accessibility in health? Out of pocket expenditures on health care in middle income countries: Evidence from Mexico'. *Cad Saude Publica*, 24(12): 2819–26

Assai, M., Siddiqi, S. and Watts, S., (2006) 'Tackling social determinants of health through community based initiatives'. *British Medical Journal*, 333: 854–6

Auletta, K. (1982) *The Underclass*. New York: Random House

Baggott, R. (2004) *Health and Health Care in Britain* (3rd Ed). Basingstoke: Palgrave

Bago, d'Uvat, Jones, A.M. and van Dooslaer, E. (2008) 'Measurement of horizontal equity in health care utilization using European panel data'. *Journal of Health Economics* (Epub ahead of print)

Baldwin, R. (1995) 'Rules, discretion, and legitimacy', in Hill, M. (ed) (1997) *The Policy Process: A Reader*, pp. 364–8. London: Prentice Hall Harvester Wheatsheaf

Bardsley, M. (2000) *Developing Health Assessment for the Black and Minority Ethnic Group: Analyzing Routine Health Information, Summary*. London: Health of Londoners' Project

Barker, C. (1996) *The Health Care Policy Process*. London: Sage Publications

Barroso, J. and Powell-Cope, G. (2000) 'Metasynthesis of qualitative research on living with HIV infection'. *Qualitative Health Research*, 10: 340–53

Baum, F. (1999) 'Social capital – is it good for your health? Issues for a public health agenda'. *Journal of Epidemiology and Community Health*, 53: 195–6

Baum, F. E. and Saunders, D. (1995) 'Can health promotion and primary health care achieve health for all without a return to the more radical agenda?'. *Health Promotion International*, 10: 149–60

Baum, J. (2000) 'Social capital, economic capital and power: further issues for a public health agenda'. *Journal of Epidemiology and Community Health*, 54: 409–10

BBC (2005) *Nurse Wins Breast Cancer Drug Row*. Online. Available at: **http://news.bbc.co.uk/1/hi/England/somerset/4304586.stm** (accessed 16 March 2009)

BBC News (2007) *How Worried Should People Be?*, Tuesday, 20 November 2007. BBC. Online. Available at: **http://news.bbc.co.uk/1/hi/business/7103940.stm** (accessed 29 January 2009)

Beaglehole, R. (ed) (2003) *Global Public Health: A New Era*. Oxford: Oxford University Press

Beating Eating Disorders (2007) *Something's Got to Change*. Norwich: Eating Disorders Association. Online. Available at: **www.b-eat.co.uk/Publications/Reports** (accessed 12 December 2008)

Beattie, A. (1991) 'Knowledge and control in health promotion: A test case for social policy and social theory', in Gabe, J., Calnan, M. and Bury, M. (eds) (1994) *The Sociology of Health Service*. London: Routledge

Beauchamp, T. and Childress, J. (2001) *Principles of Biomedical Ethics* (5th Ed), Morality and Ethical Theory: Chapter 1, pp. 1–24. Oxford: Oxford University Press

Beck, U. (1999 [2005]) *World Risk Society*. Cambridge: Polity Press

Belfast Healthy Cities (2004) *Community Health Impact Assessment Pilot Project Report*. Online. Available at: **www.belfasthealthycities.com/admin/editor/assets/6205%20bhc%20(chia%20report).pdf** (accessed 17 February 2009)

Benner, P. (1984) *From Novice to Expert*. California: Addison Wesley

Benton, D. (2007) 'The impact of diet on anti-social, violent and criminal behaviour'. *Neuroscience Biobehavioral Reviews*. Presentation to the Associate Parliamentary Food and Health Forum, 18 April 2007. Online. Available at: **www.fhf.org.uk/meetings/inquiry2007/2007-04-18_benton.pdf** (accessed 12 December 2008)

Berkman, L. F. and Syme, S. L. (1979) 'Social networks, host resistance, and mortality: A nine-year follow-up study of Alameda County Residents'. *American Journal of Epidemiology*, 109 (2):186–204.

Blair, S. and Brodney, S. (1999). 'Effects of physical inactivity and obesity on morbidity and mortality: Current evidence and research issues. *Medicine and Science in Sports and Exercise*, 31 (suppl.): S646–62

Blane, D., Brunner, E. and Wilkinson, R. (1996) *Health and Social Organisation: Towards a Health Policy for the 21st Century*. London: Routledge

Blaxter, M. (1995) 'What is health?', in Davey, B., Gray, A. and Seale, C. (1995) *Health and Disease: A Reader* (2nd Ed), pp. 26-32. Buckinghamshire: OU Press

Blum, H. L. (1981) *Planning for Health: Generics for the Eighties* (2nd Ed). New York: Human Sciences Press

Booth, C. (1903) *Life and Labour of the People of London*. London: Macmillan

Boulton M. and Fitzpatrick R. (1997) 'Evaluating Qualitative Research'. *Evidence Based Health Policy and Management*, 1 (4): 83–5.

Boynes-Watson, C. (2005) Community is Not a Place But a Relationship: Lessons for Organizational Development Public Organization Review: A Globel Journal 5: 359–74.

Bradby, H. and Chandola, T. (2007) *Ethnicity and Racism in the Politics of Health: Social Context and Action*. London: Open University Press McGraw-Hill Education

Bradshaw, J. (1994) 'The conceptualisation and measurement of need – a social policy perspective', in Popay, J. and Williams, G. (eds) Researching the People's Health. London: Routledge

Brandon, S. (2008) 'An ill wind'. *Inside Housing*, 5 December 2008: 26–7

Braveman, P. (2006) 'Health disparities and health equity: Concepts and measurements'. *Annual Review of Public Health*, 27: 167–94

BRE (2008) *Good Housing Good Health, a Toolkit for Environmental Health Practitioners*. London: CIEH

Brennan, M., Konkel, S. and Lewis, A. (2008) 'One road . . . many paths – A competence based curriculum for environmental health'. Paper presented to the 2008 International Federation of Environmental Health World Congress held in Brisbane, Australia

Bridgen, P. (2004) 'Evaluating the empowering potential of community-based health schemes: The case of community health policies in the UK since 1997'. *Community Development Journal*, 39 (3): 289–302

British Medical Journal (1996) *Declaration of Helsinki. British Medical Journal* (313) (7070): 1448–9

Brownson, R. C., Elizabeth, A., Baker, E. A., Terry, L., Leet, T. L., Kathleen, N. and Gillespie K. N. (2003) *Evidence-Based Public Health*. New York: Oxford University Press

Brumwell, S. (2005) *White Devil: A True Story of Savagery and Vengeance in Colonial America*. Cambridge, Mass: De Capo Press

Bryan, C. (2002) 'HIV/AIDS and bioethics: historical perspective, personal retrospective'. *Health Care Analysis*, (10): 5–18.

BSHF (2008) *Home from Home: Addressing the Issues of Migrant Workers' Housing*. Online. Available at: **www.bshf.org/published-information/publication. cfm?thePubID=2EED9E14-15C5-F4C0-998CFFEC3D54FF93** (accessed 13 March 2009)

Bulkeley, H. and Walker, G. (2005) 'Environmental justice: A new agenda for the UK'. *Local Environment*, 10 (4): 329–32

Burke, S., Gray, I., Paterson, K., and Meyrick, J. (2002) *Environmental Health 2012: A Key Partner in Delivering the Public Health Agenda*. London: HDA

Burnes, B. (2006) *Managing Change*. London: Prentice Hall

Buse, K., Mays, N. and Walt, G. (2005) *Making Health Policy*. Maidenhead: Open University Press

Cabinet Office (2008) *Food Matters: Towards a Strategy for the 21st Century*. Online. Available at: **www.cabinetoffice.gov.uk/strategy/work_areas/food_ policy.aspx** (accessed 5 December 2008)

Calman, K. (1998) *Chief Medical Officer's Project to Strengthen the Public Health Function – Report of Emerging Findings, Sir Kenneth Calman, Chief Medical Officer in 1998* (para 18, p. 17). Online. Available at: **www.dh.gov.uk/en/ Publicationsandstatistics/Publications/PublicationsPolicyAndGuidance/ DH_4121567** (accessed 18 January 2009)

Campbell, C. and McLean, C. (2002) 'Social capital, social exclusion and health: factors shaping African-Caribbean participation in local community networks', in Swann, C. and Morgan, M. (eds) *Social Capital: Insights from Qualitative Research*. London: HDA

Cancer Research UK (2008) *NICE Decision on Kidney Cancer Drugs*. Online. Available at: **http://scienceblog.cancerrearchuk.org/2008/08/06/nice- decision-on** (accessed 16 March 2009)

Caress, A, (2003) 'Giving information to patients'. *Nursing Standard*, 17 (44): 47–54

Carlisle, D. (2008) 'We have to narrow health inequalities'. *Society Guardian in association with IDeA, the LGA and Department of Health*, 19 November 2008: 2

Carr, S., Lhussier, M., Wilkinson, J., Gleadhill, S. (2008) 'Empowerment evaluation applied to public health practice'. *Critical Public Health*, 18 (2): 161–74

Carter-Pokras, O. and Baquet, C. (2002) 'What is health disparity?'. *Public Health Reports*, 117: 426–34

Castles, S. (1984) *Here for Good: Western Europe's New Ethnic Minorities*, London: Pluto Press

Cattrell, V. and Herring, R. (2002) 'Social capital, generations and health in east London', in Swann, C. and Morgan, M. (eds) *Social Capital: Insights from Qualitative Research*. London: HDA

Cave, B and Curtis, S. E. (2001a) 'Developing a practical guide to assess the potential health impact of urban regeneration schemes'. *Promotion and Education*, 8:1: 12–6

Cave, B and Curtis, S (2001b) *Health Impact Assessment for Regeneration Projects, Volume III Principle East London and the City Health Action Zone*. Online. Available at: **www.bcahealth.co.uk/docs/download/east_lon_guide_vol_3. pdf** (accessed 17 February 2009)

Cave, B., Molyneux, P., and Coutts, A. (2004) *Healthy Sustainable Communities: What Works?* Milton Keynes and South Midlands Health and Social Care Group

Chilton, M. (2004) 'Ideologies and pathologies of power: Two books that contribute to the cause of innovative public health theory, practice, and promotion'. *Health Promotion Practice*, October 2004, 5: 372.

Chiu, L. F. (2008) 'Engaging communities in health interventions'. *Critical Public Health*, 18 (2): 151–9

Climate Change Act 2008. Chapter 27. London: HMSO

Closs, S. J. and Cheater, F. M. (1994) 'Utilization of nursing research: culture, interest and support'. *Journal of Advanced Nursing*, 19: 762–73

Cobie-Smith, C., Thomas, S. B., George, D. M. (2002) 'Distrust, race and research'. *Archives of Internal Medicine*, 162: 2458–63

COI (2006) *A Coordinated Prostitution Strategy and a Summary of Responses to Paying the Price*. London: Home Office

Coker, R., Pomerleau, J., and McKee, M. (2005) *The Changing Nature of Infectious Major Determinants of Health*, Chapter 7, pp. 149–72. Maidenhead: Open University Press

Communities and Local Government Select Committee (CLG) (2007) *Communities and Local Government Committee Coastal Towns: Second Report of Session 2006/7*. London: House of Commons

Compass (2007) *The Commercialisation of Childhood*. Online. Available at: **www.compassonline.org.uk/publications/** (accessed 25 November 2008)

Connelly, J. and Worth, C. (1997) *Making Sense of Public Health Medicine*. Oxford: Radcliffe Publishing Ltd

Conner, M., Sheehan, P., Norman, P., and Armitage, C. J. (2000) 'Temporal stability as a moderator of relationships in the theory of planned behaviour'. *British Journal of Social Psychology*, 39: 469–93

Conway, J. (ed) (1988) *Prescription for Poor Health: The Crisis for Homeless Families*. London: London Food Commission, Maternity Alliance, SHAC and Shelter

Cooper, R. (1984) 'A note on the biological concept of race and its application in epidemiological research'. *American Health Journal*, 108(3 Part 2): 715–22

Cormack, D. F. S. (ed) (1991) *The Research Process in Nursing* (2nd Ed). Oxford: Blackwell Scientific

Cornwall, A., Lall, P. and Owen, F. (2003) 'Putting partnership into practice: Participatory wellbeing assessment on a south London housing estate'. *Health Expectations*, 6: 30–43

Cornwall Migrant Worker Site, Cornwall Strategic Partnership: Cornwall Migrant Worker Site. Online. Available at: **www.cornwallstrategicpartnership.gov. uk/index.cfm?articleid=10653** (accessed 13 March 2009)

Crawford, M., Rutter, D., Manley, C., Weaver, T., Bhui, K., Fulop, N., Tyrer, P., et al. (2002) 'Systematic review of involving patients in the planning and development of health care'. *British Medical Journal* 2002: 1263–1325

Crawley, L. M., Ahn, D. K. and Winkleby, M. A. (2008) 'Perceived Medical Discrimination and Cancer Screening Behaviors of Racial and Ethnic Minorities'. *Cancer Epidemiology Biomarkers and Prevention*, 17(8):1937–44

Crawshaw, P. (2007a) 'For a multidisciplinary critical public health'. *Critical Public Health*, March 2007; 17 (1): 1–2

Crawshaw, P. (2007b) 'Implementing the "new scientific spirit": A response to de Leuuw *et al*'. *Critical Public Health*, 18 (2) June 2008: 135–7

Crisp, N. (2005) *Commissioning a Patient–led NHS*. Cmnd 6268. Department of Health Gateway reference number: 5312. Letter: 28 July 2005

CRWRC (2004) *Defining Community Development*. USA Michigan. CRWRC

Curtis, S. (2003) *Health and Inequality: Geographical Perspectives*. London: Sage Publications

Curtis, S. (2008) 'How can we address health inequality through healthy public policy in Europe?'. *European Urban and Regional Studies*, 15: 293

Dahlgren, G. and Whitehead, M. (1991) *Policies and Strategies to Promote Social Equity in Health*. Stockholm: Institute for Futures Studies

Dailey, D. E. (2008) 'Conceptualizing perceived racism and its effects on the health of African Americans: Implications for practice and research'. *J Natl Black Nurses Assoc*, 19 (1):73–80

Darr, K. (1991) *Ethics in Health Management* (2nd Ed), London: Health Professions Press

Davies, T. D. (2008) 'The obesity epidemic: a holistic approach'. *Journal of Community Nursing*, 22 (22): 18–20

DCLG (2005). *Sustainable Communities: People, Places and Prosperity*. Cmnd 6425. London: HMSO

DCLG (2006) *Strong and Prosperous Communities: The Local Government White Paper*. London: HMSO

DCLG (2007) *The New Performance Framework for Local Authorities and Local Authority Partnerships: Single Set of National Indicators*. West Yorkshire: Communities and Local Government Publications

DCLG (2008) *Understanding Digital Exclusion Research Report*. London: HMSO

DCLG (2009) *English House Condition Survey 2007 – Headline Report (29 January 2009)*. London: DCLG. Online. Available at: **www.communities. gov.uk/housing/housingresearch/housingsurveys/englishhousecondition/ ehcsreports/** (accessed 18 March 2009)

DECC (2009) ACT ON CO$_2$ Calculator. Online. Available at: **http://actonco2. direct.gov.uk/index.html** (accessed 6 March 2009)

DEFRA (2005) *Securing the Future. The UK Government Sustainable Development* Strategy. CM 6467. London: HMSO

DEFRA (2006a) *Climate Change. The UK Programme 2006.* CM 6764. London: HMSO

DEFRA (2006b) *UK Food and Drink Manufacturing: An Economic Analysis. Food and Drink Economics branch.* Online. Available at: **https://statistics. defra.gov.uk/esg/reports/FDM%20paper%2019%20May%202006.pdf** (accessed 20 January 2009)

DEFRA (2006c) *Food Security and the UK: An Evidence and Analysis Paper. Food Chain Analysis Group.* Online. Available at: **https://statistics.defra. gov.uk/esg/reports/foodsecurity/foodsecurity.pdf** (accessed 2 November 2008)

DEFRA (2007) *The Air Quality Strategy for England, Scotland, Wales and Northern Ireland.* Volume 1. CM 7169. London: HMSO

DEFRA (2008a) *Sustainable Development Indicators in Your Pocket 2008.* London: DEFRA Publications (published annually)

DEFRA (2008b) *National Sustainable Development Indicators.* Online. Available at: **www.defra.gov.uk/sustainable/government/progress/national/index. htm** (accessed 6 March 2009)

DEFRA (2008c) *UK Climate Change Programme: Annual Report to Parliament,* July 2008. London: DEFRA Publications

DEFRA (2008d) *Ensuring the UK's Food Security in a Changing World.* A DEFRA Discussion Paper. Online. Available at: **www.defra.gov.uk/foodrin/ policy/pdf/Ensuring-UK-Food-Security-in-a-changing-world-170708.pdf** (accessed 2 November 2008)

DfT (2008) *Transport Statistics Great Britain: 2008 Edition.* London: HMSO

DoH (1992) *Health of the Nation.* London: HMSO

DoH (1993) *Report of the Taskforce on the Strategy for Research in Nursing, Midwifery and Health Visiting 04/93.* London: DoH

DoH (1998a) *Green Paper: Our Healthier Nation: A Contract for Health.* London: HMSO

DoH (1998b) *Antenatal Testing for HIV.* Online. Available at: **www.dh.gov. uk/en/publications and statistics/lettersandcirculars** (accessed 16 March 2009)

DoH (1999a) *White Paper: Saving Lives: Our Healthier Nation.* London: HMSO

DoH (1999b) *Health Impact Assessment: Report of a Methodological Seminar.* London: DoH

DoH (2000) *Shifting the Balance of Power.* London: HMSO

DoH. (2000a) *HIV Testing as Part of your Antenatal Care: Better for your Baby.* Online. Available at: **www.dh.gov.uk/en/publications** and statistics/ lettersandcirculars (accessed 16 March 2009)

DoH (2000b) *The NHS Plan: A Plan for Investment, a Plan for Reform.* Cmnd 4818-I. London: HMSO

DoH (2000c) *Coronary Heart Disease: a national service framework for coronary heart disease – modern standards and service models.* London: DoH

DoH (2001a) *The Report of the Chief Medical Officer's Project to Strengthen the Public Health Function*. London: DoH

DoH (2001b) *The National Service Framework for Older People*. London: DoH

DoH (2001c) *Annual Report of the Chief Medical Officer 2001*. London: HMSO

DoH (2002a) *Getting Ahead of the Curve: A Strategy for Combating Infectious Diseases (Including other Aspects of Health Protection)*. London: DoH

DoH (2002b) *Tackling Health Inequalities; 2002 Cross-cutting Review*. Online. Available at: **www.dh.gov.uk/en/Publicationsandstatistics/Publications/PublicationsPolicyAndGuidance/DH_4098280** (accessed 2 November 2008).

DoH (2004*) Choosing Health: Making Healthier Choices Easier*. CM 6374. London: HMSO

DoH (2005) *Public Attitudes to Self Care: Baseline Survey*. Online. Available at: **www.dh.gov.uk/en/index.htm** (accessed 18 March 2009)

DoH (2006) *Our Health: Our Care, Our Say: A New Direction for Community Services*. Cmnd 6737. London: HMSO

DoH (2007a) *Health is Global: Proposals for UK Government-Wide Strategy*. London: DoH

DoH (2007b) *Creating a Patient-led NHS – Delivering the NHS Improvement Plan*. London: HMSO

DoH (2007c) *Foresight Tackling Obesities Future Choice Project*. London: DoH

DoH (2007d) *On the State of the Public Health: Annual Report of the Chief Medical Officer 2004*. Online. Available at: **www.dh.gov.uk/en/Publicationsandstatistics/Publications/AnnualReports/Browsable/DH_4117035** (accessed 2 November 2008)

DoH (2007e) *The NHS in England: The Operating Framework for 2008/9*. Online. Available at: **www.dh.gov.uk/en/Publicationsandstatistics/Publications/PublicationsPolicyAndGuidance/DH_081094** (accessed 1 November 2008)

DoH/HPA (2008) *Health Effects of Climate Change in the UK 2008: An Update of the Department of Health Report 2001/2002*. London: DoH

DoH online (2008) *DH website*. Online. Available at: **www.dh.gov.uk/en/Publichealth/index.htm** (accessed 13 February 2009)

DoH (2008a) *The Health Impact of Climate Change: Promoting Sustainable Communities. Guidance Document – April 2008*. London: DoH

DoH (2008b) *Health Inequalities: Progress and Next Steps*. Online. Available at: **www.dh.gov.uk/en/Publicationsandstatistics/Publications/PublicationsPolicyAndGuidance/DH_085307** (accessed 18 February 2009)

DoH (2008c) *Health is Global: A UK Government Strategy 2008–13*. Online. Available at: **www.dh.gov.uk/en/Publicationsandstatistics/Publications/PublicationsPolicyAndGuidance/DH_088702** (accessed 18 February 2009)

DoH (2008d) 'New £20m free school meals pilot'. Press release, Wednesday 24 September 2008 11:44. Online. Available at: **http://nds.coi.gov.uk/environment/fullDetail.asp?ReleaseID=379579&NewsAreaID=2&NavigatedFromDepartment=False** (accessed 13 January 2009).

DoH (2009) *Cervical Screening Age – Experts to Review Evidence.* Online. Available at: **www.dh.gov.uk/en/index.htm** (accessed 16 March 2009)

Dines, A. and Cribb, A. (1993) *Health Promotion Concepts and Practice.* Oxford: Blackwell Science

Dickens, B. and Cook, R. (2007) 'Reproductive health and public health ethics'. *International Journal of Gynaecology and Obstetrics*, 99 (1): 75–9. Online. Available at: **www.sciencedirect.com/science?-ob=articleURL&-udi=B6T7M-4PON27B-5** (accessed 27 February 2009)

Donaldson, L. (2001) '125 years of public health in the UK'. *The Journal of the Royal Society for the Promotion of Health*, 2001: 121, 146

Donaldson, L. (2007) *Health is Global: A Report from the UK's Chief Medical Adviser.* London: DoH

Donaldson, R. J. and Donaldson, L. J. (2003) *Essential Public Health* (2nd Ed). Plymouth: Petroc Press

Dovidio, J. F., Penner, L.A., Albercht, T. L., Norton, W. E., Gaertner, S. L. and Shelton, J. N. (2008) 'Disparities and distrust: The implications of psychological processes for understanding racial disparities in health and health care'. *Soc Sci Med* 67 (3): 478–86

Downie, R. and Calman, K. (1994) *Healthy Respect: Ethics in Health Care.* Oxford: Oxford University Press

Doyal, L. and Gough, I (1991) *A Theory of Human Need.* Basingstoke: Macmillan Press

Dressler, W. W., Oths, K. S. and Gravelee, C. C. (2005) 'Race and ethnicity in public health research: Models to explain health disparities'. *Annual Review of Anthropolology*, 34: 231–52

Dunn, J. R. and Hayes, M. V. (2000) 'Social inequality, population health and housing: A study of two Vancouver neighbourhoods'. *Social Science and Medicine*, 51: 563–87

DWP (2005) *Opportunity Age: Meeting the Challenges of Ageing in the 21st century.* London: DWP

DWP (2008) Households Below Average Income 1994/95 to 2006/07. Online. Available at: **www.dwp.gov.uk/asd/hbai/hbai2007/contents.asp** (accessed 12 December 2008)

Eagleton, T. (1991) *Ideology.* London: Verso

Eaton, L. 'Measles cases in England and Wales rise sharply in 2008'. *British Medical Journal*, 10 February 2009, 338: 377. Online. Available at: **www.bmj.com/cgi/citmgr?gca=bmj,338/feb10-1/b533** (accessed 16 March 2009)

EEC (1985) *Council Directive of 27 June 1985 on the assessment of certain public and private projects on the environment.* Online. Available at: **http://ec.europa.eu/environment/eia/full-legal-text/85337.htm** (accessed 18 February 2009)

Elliott, E. and Williams, G. (2004) 'Developing a civic intelligence: local involvement in HIA'. *Environmental Impact Assessment Review*, 24(2): 231–43

Elliott, P., Briggs, D., Morris, S., de Hoogh, C., Hurt, C., Kold Jensen, T., Maitland, I., Richardson, S., Wakefield, J. and Jarup, L. (2001) 'Risk of adverse birth outcomes in populations living near landfill sites'. *British Medical Journal*, 323 (7309): 363–8

Engebretson, J., Mahoney, J. and Carson, E. D. (2008) 'Cultural competence in the era of evidence-based practice'. *Journal of Professional Nursing*, 24(3): 172–8

End Child Poverty (2009) *Key Facts*. Online. Available at: **www.endchildpoverty. org.uk/why-end-child-poverty/key-facts** (accessed 20 January 2009)

English Collective of Prostitutes (2004) *Criminalisation: The Price Women and Children Pay*. London: Cross Roads Books

English Heritage and Urban Practitioners (2007) *An Asset and a Challenge: Heritage and Regeneration in Coastal Towns in England. Final Report, October 2007*. London: English Heritage

Environment Agency (2005) *Better Environment, Healthier People*. Online. Available at: **http://publications.environment-agency.gov.uk/pdf/ GEHO0905BJOV-e-e.pdf** (accessed 6 March 2009)

Environment Agency (2008) *Contaminated Land*. Online. Available at: **www. environment-agency.gov.uk/research/library/data/34403.aspx** (accessed 6 March 2009)

ESRC (2001) *Global Environmental Change Programme. Environmental Justice: Rights and Means to a Healthy Environment for All. Special Briefing No. 7*, University of Sussex. Online. Available at: **www.foe.co.uk/resource/reports/ environmental_justice.pdf** (accessed 6 March 2009)

Etcoff, N., Orbach, S. Scott, J. and D'Agostino, H. (2006) B*eyond Stereotypes: Rebuilding the Foundation of Beauty Beliefs*. Findings of the 2005 Dove Global Study Commissioned by Unilever. Online. Available at: **www. campaignforrealbeauty.com/DoveBeyondStereotypesWhitePaper** (accessed 14 January 2009)

European Commission (2004) Joint Report on Social Exclusion. Online. Available at: **http://ec.europa.eu/employment_social/soc-prot/soc incl/ final_joint_inclusion_report_2003_en.pdf** (accessed 8 January 2009)

European Union (2001) *Directive 2001/42/EC of the European Parliament and of the Council on the assessment of the effects of certain plans and programmes on the environment*. Online. Available at: **http://ec.europa.eu/environment/ eia/full-legal-text/0142_en.pdf** (accessed 18 February 2009)

Evans D. (2003) 'Hierarchy of evidence: a framework for ranking evidence evaluating healthcare interventions'. *Journal of Clinical Nursing*, 12: 77–84

Evans, D. and Pearson, A. (1998) 'Systematic reviews: gatekeepers of nursing knowledge' *Journal of Clinical Nursing*, 10: 593–9

Ewles, L. and Simnett, I. (1999) *Promoting Health: A Practical Guide*. Edinburgh: Harcourt

Faculty of Public Health (2006) *Newsletter ph.Com*, June 2006, ISSN 1472-7501. Online. Available at: **www.fph.org.uk/resources/newsletters/phcom/ archive/2006/phcom_june06.pdf** (accessed 18 January 2009)

Faculty of Public Health (2006) *Public Health: Specialise in the Bigger Picture*. London: Faculty of Public Health

Faculty of Public Health (2008) *What is Public Health*. Online. Available at:

www.fph.org.uk/about_faculty/what_public_health/default.asp (accessed 26 November 2008)

Fairburn, J., Butler, B. and Smith, G. (2009) 'Environmental justice in South Yorkshire: locating social deprivation and poor environments using multiple indicators'. *Local Environment*, 14 (2): 139–54

Fletcher, N., Holt, J., Brazier, M. and Harris, J. (1995) *Ethics Law and Nursing*. Manchester: Manchester University Press

Flowers, R., Gray, I. and MacArthur, I. (2004) 'Introduction to environmental health', in Bassett, W. H. (ed.) *Clay's Handbook of Environmental Health* (19th Ed), Part One: Environmental Health – Definition and Organization, Chapter 1, pp. 3–21, London: Spon Press, Taylor and Francis Group

Food and Agriculture Organization (1996) *Rome Declaration on World Food Security and World Food Summit Plan of Action. WFS 96/3*, Italy. Online. Available at: www.fao.org/docrep/003/w3613e/w3613e00.htm (accessed 12 December 2008)

Food and Agriculture Organization (2008) *State of Food Insecurity in the World 2008. High Food Prices and Food Security – Threats and Opportunities*, FAO: Italy

Food and Health Forum (2008) *The Links Between Diet and Behaviour – The Influence of Nutrition on Mental Health: Report of an Inquiry Held by the Associate Parliamentary Food and Health Forum January 2008*. Online. Available at: www.fhf.org.uk/meetings/inquiry2007/FHF_inquiry_report_diet_and_behaviour.pdf (accessed 12 December 2008)

Food Standards Agency (2004) *Food Promotion and Marketing to Children – Views of Low Income Consumers: Qualitative Research Report*. Online. Available at: www.food.gov.uk/foodlabelling/researchandreports/209948 (accessed 12 December 2008)

Food Standards Agency (2007) *Review and Analysis of Current Literature on Consumer Understanding of Nutrition and Health Claims Made on Food*. Online. Available at: www.food.gov.uk/news/newsarchive/2007/jul/healthconfuse (accessed 12 December 2008)

Foods Standards Agency (2009) Report published following inquiry into 2005 outbreak of E.coli in Wales. Online. Available at: www.food.gov.uk/news/newsarchive/2009/mar/ecoliwales (accessed 10 September 2009)

Fudge, N., Wolfe, C. and McKevitt, C. (2008) 'Assessing the promise of user involvement in health service development: ethnographic study'. *British Medical Journal*, 336 (7639): 313

Gabbay, J. and Stevens, A. (1994) (Editorial) 'Towards investing in health gain'. *British Medical Journal*, 308 (1117–1118) Online. Available at: www.bmj.com/cgi/content/full/308/6937/1117 (accessed 17 November 2006)

Gangmasters Licencing Authority, *GLA Home page*. Online. Available at: www.gla.gov.uk/index.asp?id=42 (accessed 13 March 2009)

Gaster, L. and Taylor, M. (1993) *Learning from Consumers and Citizens*. Luton: Local Government Management Board

Geary, A. (2002) *The Food and Mood Self-help Report. A Survey of Dietary and Nutritional Self-help Strategies Used to Improve Emotional and Mental Health, The Food and Mood Project*. Online. Available at: www.mind.org.uk/foodandmood/info/survey.htm (accessed 10 January 2008)

George, V. and Wilding, P. (1988) *Ideology and Social Welfare*. London: Routledge

Giddens, A. (1984) *The Constitution of Society: Outline of the Theory of Structuration*. Cambridge: Polity

Giddens, A. (1999) *Transcript of BBC Radio 4 Homepage, 1999 Reith Lecture on Globalisation*. Online. Available at: **http://news.bbc.co.uk/hi/english/static/events/reith_99/week1/lecture1.htm** (accessed 5 July 2007)

Gillam, S., Yates, J. and Badrinath, P. (eds) (2007) 'Health protection and communicable disease control', pp. 165–82, in *Essential Public Health*. Cambridge: Cambridge University Press

GLA (2006) *Sustainability Appraisal of the Draft Further Alterations to the London Plan (Spatial Development Strategy for Greater London)* (Reissued April 2007). Online. Available at: **www.london.gov.uk/mayor/strategies/sds/further-alts/docs/sa-nts.pdf** (accessed 5 April 2009)

Godin, G. and Kok, G. (1996) 'The theory of planned behaviour: A review of its applications to health-related behaviours'. *American Journal of Health Promotion*, 11 (2): 87–98

Gollwitzer, P. M. (1999) 'Implementation intentions: Strong effects of simple plans'. *American Psychologist*, 54: 493–503

Goode, W. J. (1960) 'Encroachment, charlatanism and the emerging professions, psychology, sociology and medicine'. *American Sociological Review*, 22: 194–200

Goss, S. and Blackaby, B. (1998) *Developing Local Housing Strategies: A Good Practice Guide*. Coventry: CIH and LGA

Goulbourne, H. (1998) *Race Relations in Britain Since 1945*. New York: St. Martin's Press

Government Office for Science (2007) *Future Choices – Modelling Future Trends in Obesity and Their Impact on Health* (2nd Ed), Foresight, Department of Innovation Universities and Skills. Online. Available at: **www.foresight.gov.uk/OurWork/ActiveProjects/Obesity/Obesity.asp** (accessed 13 January 2009)

Gray, A. (2001) *World Health and Disease*. Buckingham: Open University Press

Grey, M., Studden, M. and Sarangi, J. (2007) 'Protecting the public's health', in Orme, J., Powell, J., Taylor, P. and Grey, M. (eds) *Public Health for the 21st Century* (2nd Ed), Part 3: Major contemporary themes in public health, Chapter 13, pp. 223–48. Maidenhead: Open University Press, McGraw Hill Education

Greenwood, C. E. (2003) 'Dietary carbohydrate, glucose regulation, and cognitive performance in elderly persons'. *Nutrition Reviews*, 61, Supplement 1, 1 May 2003: 68–74(7), International Life Sciences Institute

Guardian (The) (2001) *HIV Man Jailed for Knowingly Infecting Lover*. Online. Available at: **www.guardian.co.uk/uk/2001/mar/17/aids.world** (accessed 18 March 2009)

Graham, H. (2007) *Unequal Lives*. Buckingham: Open University Press

Graham, H. and Kelly, M. (2004) *Health Inequalities, Concepts, Frameworks and Policy*. London: HDA

Graves, J. L. Jr. (2002) *The Emperor's New Clothes: Biological Theories of Race at the Millennium*. New Brunswick: Rutgers' University Press

Green, G. and Pugh, P. (2008) *Better Homes, Better Health: Health Impact Assessment of Sheffield Housing Strategy*. Sheffield: Sheffield Hallam University

Green, M. (2007) *Voices of People Experiencing Poverty in Scotland. Everyone Matters?* Online. Available at: **www.jrf.org.uk/bookshop/eBooks/2020-experiencing-poverty-scotland.pdf** (accessed 8 January 2009)

Greener J. and Grimshaw J. (1996) 'Using meta-analysis to summarise evidence within systematic review'. *Nurse Researcher*, 4: 27–38

Griffiths, S. and Hunter, D. (eds) (1999) *Perspectives in Public Health*. Abingdon: Radcliffe Medical Press

Guyatt, G. and Renie, D. (2002) *User's Guides to the Medical Literature: A Manual for Evidence-Based Practice*. Chicago: American Medical Association

Hagger, M. S., Chatzisarantis, N. L. and Biddle, S. (2002) 'A meta-analytic review of the theories of reasoned action and planned behaviour in physical activity: Predictive validity and the contribution of additional variables'. *Journal of Sport and Exercise Psychology*, 24 (1): 3–23

Hall, L. and Marsh, K. (2000) *Professionalism, Policies and Values: A Reader*. London: University of Greenwich

Hanlon, G. (1998) 'Professionalism as enterprise: Service class politics and the redefinition of professionalism'. *Sociology*, 32 (1) 43–63

Hargreaves, A. (2000) 'Four ages of professionalism and professional learning'. *Teachers and Teaching: History and Practice*, 6 (2) 151–82

Harris, M. (1968) *The Rise of Anthropological Theory: A History of Theories of Culture*. New York: Crowell

Hastings, G., McDermott, L., Angus, K., Stead, M. and Thomson, S. (2006) *The Extent, Nature and Effects of Food Promotion to Children: A Review of the Evidence. Technical Paper Prepared for The World Health Organization*. Online. Available at: **www.ism.stir.ac.uk/projects_food_description.htm** (accessed 10 January 2009)

Hatchett, W. (2008) Liverpool PCT to fund £9.3m health and housing drive. *Environment Health News*, 23rd May 2008. Online. Available at: **www.cieh.org/ehn/ehn3.aspx?id=11504** (accessed 10 September 2009)

Hausmann, L. R., Jeong, K., Bost, J. E. and Ibrahim, S. A. (2008) 'Perceived discrimination in health care and health status in a racially diverse sample'. *Medical Care*, 46(9): 905–14

Hayes-Bautista, D. and Chapa, J. (1987) 'Latino terminology: Conceptual basis for standardized terminology'. *American Journal of Public Health*, 77 (1). 61–8

Hazelwood, N. (2004) *The Queen's Slave Trader: John Hawkyns, Elizabeth I and the Trafficking in Human Souls*. New York: William Morrow

HDA (2004a) *The Evidence of Effectiveness of Public Health Interventions – and the Implications: Briefing No. 1, June 2004*. London: HDA

HDA (2004b) *The Learning from Effective Practice Standard System (LEPSS): Outline Programme 2004–2007*. London: HDA

HEA (2000) *Health Update, Environment and Health: Housing*. London: Health Education Authority

Hebert, P.L., Sisk, J.E., and Howell, E. A. (2008) 'When Does a Difference Become a Disparity? Conceptualizing Racial and Ethnic Disparities in Health'. *Health Affairs*, 27(2):374–82

Helman, C. (2007) *Culture, Health and Illness* (5th Ed). Hodder Arnold

Hester and Westmarland (2004) *Tackling Street Prostitution: Towards an Holistic Approach*. London: Home Office

Hill, M. (1997) *The Policy Process in the Modern State* (3rd Ed). London: Prentice Hall Harvester Wheatsheaf

HM Government (2006) *Reaching Out: An Action Plan on Social Exclusion*. London: Cabinet Office

HM Government (2008a) *UK National Report on Strategies for Social Protection and Social Inclusion 2008–10*. Online. Available at: **www.dwp.gov.uk/publications/dwp/2008/socialprotection/ uknationalstrategyreport12-9-08.pdf** (accessed 3 February 2009)

HM Government (2008b) *Preparing for our Ageing Society: A Discussion Document*. London: DWP

HM Treasury, DWP, Department for Children, Schools and Families (2008) *Ending Child Poverty: Everybody's Business*. London: HM Treasury

Hoban, V. (2006) 'Do you judge your patients?'. *Nursing Times*, 10 (4): 14–5

Hofstadter, R. (1992) *Social Darwinism in American Thought*. Boston: Beacon Press

Hogston, R. and Simpson, P. (2002) *Foundations of Nursing Practice: Making the Difference* (2nd Ed). Basingstoke: Palgrave

Hogwood, B. and Gunn, L. (1984) 'Why perfect implementation is unattainable', in Hill, M. (ed) (1997) *The Policy Process: A Reader*, pp. 217–25. London: Prentice Hall Harvester Wheatsheaf

Holland, K. and Hogg, C. (2001) *Cultural Awareness in Nursing and Health Care*. London: Arnold Publishers

Holloway I. and Wheeler S. (1995) 'Ethical issues in qualitative nursing research'. *Nursing Ethics*, 2 (3): 223–32

Home Office (2004) *Paying the Price: A Consultation Paper on Prostitution*. London: Home Office

Honigsbaum, M. (2008) *Living with Enza: The Forgotten Story of Britain and the Great Flu Pandemic of 1918*. London: Macmillan

Horodynski, M., Olson, B., Arndt, M.J., Brophy-Herb, H., Shirer, K. and Shemanski, R. (2007) 'Low-income mothers' decisions regarding when and why to introduce solid foods to their infants: Influencing factors'. *Journal of Community Health Nursing*, 24 (2): 101–18

House of Commons Public Accounts Committee (2009) *The National Programme for IT in the NHS: Progress since 2006, Second Report of Session 2008–09*. London: HMSO

Howes, F., Doyle, J., Jackson, N., and Waters, E. (2004) 'Evidence-based public health: the importance of finding "difficult to locate" public health and health promotion intervention studies for systematic reviews'. *Journal of Public Health*, 26 (10): 101–4

HPA (2006) *Migrant Health: Infectious Diseases in Non-UK Born Population in England, Wales and Northern Ireland. A Baseline Report*. London: HPA.

Online. Available at: **www.hpa.org.uk/web/HPAweb&HPAwebStandard/ HPAweb_C/1201767921328** (accessed 13 March 2009)

HPA (2006a) The public Health Impact of the Buncefield Oil Depot Fire. Online. Available at: **www.hpa.org.uk/web/HPAwebFile/ HPAweb_C/1194947321467** (last accessed 10 September 2009)

HPA (2008a) *Forward Thinking, Future Working. Framework Specification for HPA Local and Regional Service Provision 2008–2010*. Online. Available at: **www.hpa.org.uk** (accessed 6 March 2009)

HPA (2008) *Tuberculosis in the UK: Annual Report on Tuberculosis Surveillance in the UK 2008*. Online. Available at: **www.hpa.org.uk/web/ HPAweb&HPAwebStandard/HPAweb_C/1225268885969** (accessed 13 March 2009)

Huang, J., and Wang, V. (2005) 'Community health development: What is it?'. *International Nursing Review*, 5: 13–7

Hudson, J. and Lowe, S. (2004) *Understanding the Policy Process: Analysing Welfare Policy and Practice*. Bristol: The Policy Press

Human Fertilisation and Embryology Authority (1990) *The Human Fertilisation and Embryology Act*. Online. Available at: **www.hfea.gov.uk/en/1752.html** (accessed 16 March 2009)

Hunter, D. (2007) 'Public Health: Historical Context and Current Agenda' in Scriver, A. and Garman, S. *Public Health: Social Context and Action*, p. 8–19. London: Open University Press McGraw-Hill Education

Information Commissioner's Office (2009a) *Data Protection Guide*. Online. Available at: **www.ico.gov.uk/Home/for_organisations/data_protection_ guide.aspx** (accessed 26 January 2009)

Information Commissioner's Office (2009b) *Freedom of Information Guide*. Online. Available at: **www.ico.gov.uk/Home/for_organisations/freedom_ of_information_guide.aspx** (accessed 26 January 2009)

IPCC (2007) *Climate Change 2007: Synthesis Report. Contribution of Working Groups I, II and III to the Fourth Assessment Report of the Intergovernmental Panel on Climate Change*. Geneva: IPCC

Jeal, N. and Salisbury, C. (2004) 'A health needs assessment of street based prostitutes: cross-sectional survey'. *Journal of Public Health*, 26 (2): 147–51

Jenicek, M. (1997) 'Epidemiology, evidenced-based medicine, and evidence-based public health'. *Journal of Epidemiology*, 7 (4):187–97

Joffe, M. and Mindell, J. (2002) 'A framework for the evidence base to support health impact assessment'. *Journal of Epidemiology and Community Health*, Feb; 56 (2):132–8

Johnstone, M. J. and Kanitsaki, O. (2008) 'The neglect of racism as an ethical issue in health care'. *Journal of Immigrant Minor Health*, 18 (Epub ahead of print)

Jones, B., Kavanagh, D., Moran, M. and Norton, P. (2001) *Politics UK* (4th Ed). London: Pearson Longman

Jones-Devitt and Smith, L. (2007) *Critical Thinking in Health and Social Care*. London: Sage

Kai, J. and Hedges, C. (1999) 'Minority ethnic community participation in needs assessment and service development in primary care: Perceptions of Pakistani and Bangladeshi people about psychological distress'. *Health Expectations*, 2: 7–20

Kanumilli, N. (2006) *NICE Statins Guidance Will Save Lives but Leaves Room for Improvement (NICE Drug overview)*. London: NICE

Kawachi, I., Subramanian, S. V., and Almeidsa-Filho, N. (2002). 'A glossary for health inequalities'. *Journal of Epidemiology and Community Health*, 56: 647–52

Kayani, N. (2003) *Food Deserts – A Practical Guide*. London: Chadwick House Group Ltd

Kayani, N. (2007) 'Recipe for ill health'. *Environmental Health Practitioner*, 5 January 2007. Online. Available at: **www.cieh.org/ehp/ehp3.aspx?id=3014** (accessed 10 January 2009)

Kayani, N. (2006) 'Obsession with food is unhealthy'. *Environmental Health Practitioner*, 2 November 2006. Online. Available at: **www.cieh.org/ehp/ehp3.aspx?id=2620** (accessed 8 January 2009)

Kegler, M., Norton, B. and Aronson, R. (2008) 'Strengthening community leadership: Evaluation findings from the California Healthy Cities and Communities Program'. *Health Promotion Practice*, 9 (2) 170–9

Kemm, J. (2007) *More than a Statement of the Crushingly Obvious: A Critical Guide to HIA, West Midlands Public Health Observatory Version 1*, October 2007. Birmingham: West Midlands Public Health Observatory

Kent Council Council (2008) *The History of Kent*. Online. Available at: **www.kent.gov.uk/Community/kent-and-its-people/history-of-kent/** (accessed 29 December 2008)

Kim, A. (2003) *Social Enterprise Typology*. Online. Available at: **www.virtueventures.com/setypology/index.php?id=PROLOG&lm=1** (accessed 13 February 2009)

Kon, Z. R., and Lukan, N. (2008) 'Ethnic disparities in access to care in post-apartheid South Africa'. *American Journal of Public Health*, 98 (12): 227–7

Kotter, J. (1990) *A Force for Change: How Leadership Differs from Management*. New York: The Free Press

Krieger, J. and Higgins, D. (2002) 'Public health matters: Housing and health: Time again for public health action'. *American Journal of Public Health*, 92 (5): 758–68

Krieger, N. (1987) 'Shades of difference: Theoretical underpinnings of medical controversy on black/white differences in the United States, 1830-1870'. *International Journal of Health Services*, 17 (2): 259–78

Lachmann, P, (1998) 'Public health and bioethics'. *Journal of Medicine and Philosophy*, 23 (3): 297–302

Lake, A and Townshend, T. (2006) 'Obesogenic environments: Built environments and food environments'. *Journal of the Royal Society of Health Promotion*, 126 (6): 262–7. Online. Available at: **www.neoen.org.uk/environment.asp** (accessed 10 January 2009)

Lang, T. (2005) 'Food, trade and health', in Pomerleau, J. and McKee, M. *Issues in Public health*. Maidenhead: Open University Press/McGraw-Hill Education

Lauder. W., Davidson, G., and Anderson, I. (2005) 'Self-neglect: The role of judgements and applied ethics'. *Nursing Standard*, 19 (18): 45–51

Lavalat, M., and Pratt, A. (eds) (2006) *Social Policy Theories, Concepts and Issues*. London: Sage Publications

La Via Campesina (1996) 'Tlaxcala Declaration of the Via Campesina', Mexico: Via Campesina. Online. Available at: **www.viacampesina.org/main_en/index.php?option=com_content&task=view&id=445&Itemid=4** 8 (accessed 31 January 2009)

La Via Campesina (2008) 'Food Sovereignty Now! Unity and Struggle of the People', Fifth international conference of la Via Campesina, Press Kit, 16–23 October 2008, Maputo, Mozambique, La Via Campesina. Online. Available at: **http://viacampesina.org/main_en/index.php** (accessed 8 January 2009)

Lawrence, R. J. (2004) 'Editorial introduction: Housing, health and well-being: Moving forward'. *Reviews on Environmental Health*. Freund Publishing House Ltd 19 (3–4): 161–76

Lee, K. (2000) 'The impact of globalization on public health: implications for the UK Faculty of Public Health'. *Journal of Public Health Medicine*, 22 (3): 253–62

Lee, K. (2005) 'Introduction to global health', in Lee and Collin (eds) *Global Change and Health*. Buckingham: Open University Press

Lewis, A. (2008) 'Let's get radical'. *Environmental Health Practitioner*, 4 December 2008, 116 (12) 24–5

Lewis, O. (1961) *The Children of Sanchez*. New York: Random House

LHC (1999) *Part III Section 6 Models of Health Impact Assessment, a Resource for Health Impact Assessment*. Online. Available at: **www.londonshealth.gov.uk/pdf/r_hia6.pdf** (accessed 19 February 2009)

LHC (2002) *Health Impact Assessment – Draft London Plan*. Online. Available at: **www.london.gov.uk/lhc/docs/publications/hia/mayor/spatial.pdf** (accessed 18 February 2009)

LHC (2003) Evaluation of the Health Impact Assessments on the draft Mayoral Strategies for London. Online. Available at: **www.londonshealth.gov.uk/pdf/hiaeval_sum.pdf** (accessed 18 February 2009)

Lipsky, M. (1980) 'Street-level bureaucracy: An introduction', in Hill, M. (ed) (1997) *The Policy Process: A Reader*, pp. 389–92). London: Prentice Hall Harvester Wheatsheaf

Locker, D. (1997) 'Social determinants of health and disease', in Scambler, G. (ed) *Sociology as Applied to Medicine* (5th Ed). Edinburgh: Saunders

London Borough of Waltham Forest (2008) *Supplementary Planning Document (SPD) – Hot Food Takeaway (Consultation Draft, October 2008)*. Online. Available at: **www.walthamforest.gov.uk/index/environment/envpl-page1/planning-policy/planning-consultations.htm** (accessed 1 November 2008)

London School of Economics (undated) *The Third Way and its Critics*. Online. Available at: **http://old.lse.ac.uk/collections/meetthedirector/third_way_and_its_critics.htm** (accessed 8 December 2006)

Longres, J. F. (1990) *Human Behavior in the Social Environment*. Itasca, Illinois: F.E. Peacock

Loomba, A. (2005) *Colonialism/Postcolonialism* (2nd Ed). London: Routledge

Lukes, S. (1974) *Power: A Radical View*. London: Macmillan

Lupton, D. (1995) *The Imperative of Health: Public Health and the Regulated Body*. London: Sage

Lynch, J. W., Due, P., Muntaner, C. and Davey Smith, G. (2000) 'Social capital: Is it a good investment strategy for public health'. *Journal of Epidemiology and Community Health*, 54: 404–8

Lyon, F. (2007) Social Enterprises in Health and Social Care: Prospects and Challenges, Paper Presented to Social Enterprise Research Conference July 2007, London: South Bank University. Online. Available at: **www.cabinetoffice.gov.uk/third_sector/social_enterprise.aspx** (accessed 8 January 2009)

Mabhala, M. and Lesiamo, P. (2009) 'Sustainable development and public health', in in Wilson, F. and Mabhala, M. (eds) *Key Concepts in Public Health*. London: Sage

MacArthur, I. (1998) 'On the threshold of change. For the common good. 150 years of public health'. *An Environmental Health Journal commemorative issue*. London: CIEH

Macintyre, S. (2003) 'Evidence based policy making: Impact on health inequalities still needs to be assessed'. *British Medical Journal*, 326 (7379): 5–6. Online. Available at: **www.pubmedcentral.nih.gov/articlerender.fcgi?artid=1124938** (accessed 17 November 2006)

Mann, N. (1999) *UK Politics: All aboard the Third Way*. Online. Available at: **http://news.bbc.co.uk/1/hi/uk_politics/298456.stm** (accessed 8 December 2006)

Mant, J. (1999) 'Case control studies', in Dawes *et al.* (1999) *Evidence-Based Practice – A Primer for Health Care Professionals*. London: Churchill Livingstone

Manzano, L. (2003) 'Globalisation and food: Bush meat in the UK', case study cited in Stewart, J., Bushell, F. and Habgood, V. (2005) *Environmental Health as Public Health*. London: CHGL

Marmot, M. and Friel, S. (2008) 'Global Health Equity: Evidence for Action on the Social Determinants of Health'. *Journal of Epidemiology Community Health*, 62: 1095–97

Marmot, M. C., and Wilkinson, R. G. (2006) *Social Determinants of Health*. (2nd Ed). Oxford: Oxford University Press

Maslow, A. H. (1970) *Motivation and Personality*. New York: Harper and Row

Mawson, A. (2008) *The Social Entrepreneur Making Communities Work*. London: Atlantic Books

Mazurek Melnyk, B. and Fineout-Overholt, E. (2005) *Evidence-based Practice in Nursing and Healthcare*. Philadelphia: Lippincott Williams and Wilkins

McCarthy, M. and Ferguson, J. (1999) *Environment and Health in London*. London: Kings Fund

McClean, S. (2003) 'Globalization and health', in Orme *et al.* (eds) *Public Health for the 21st Century: New Perspectives on Policy, Participation and Practice*. Maidenhead: OU Press/McGraw-Hill Education

McDermott, L., Stead, M., Hastings, G., Angus, K., Banerjee, S., Rayner, M. and Kent, R. (2005) *A Systematic Review of the Effectiveness of Social Marketing Nutrition and Food Safety Interventions – Final Report – Prepared for Safefood*.

Stirling: Institute for Social Marketing. Online. Available at: **www.ism.stir. ac.uk/projects_food_description.htm** (accessed 8 January 2009)

McDonnell, J. (MP Hayes and Harlington) (2007) *Orders of the Day. Criminal Justice and Immigration Bill. Order for Second Reading read 8 October 2008.* Online. Available at: **www.publications.parliament.uk/pa/cm200607/ cmhansrd/cm071008/debtext/71008-0019.htm** (accessed 30 December 2008)

McIntosh, P. (1988) *White Privilege and Male Privilege: A Personal Account of Coming to See Correspondences through Work in Women's Studies (Working Paper #89).* Wellesley, MA: Wellesley College Center for Research on Women

McMillan, B., and Conner, M. (2003) 'Using the theory of planned behaviour to understand alcohol and tobacco use in students'. *Psychology, Health and Medicine,* 8: 317–28

Mead, P. (2000) 'Clinical guidelines: promoting clinical effectiveness or a professional minefield?'. *Journal of Advanced Nursing,* 31 (1):110–6.

Medscape (2008) *UK Cancer Experts Deplore NICE Decision on Kidney Cancer Drugs.* Online. Available at: **www.medscape.com/viewarticle/579628** (accessed 16 March 2009)

Meerabeau., E. and Stewart, J. (2007) Franco-British Interreg IIIA European Programme Comparison of Sante/Public Health Project. Health and Health Behaviour in South East England and Northern France: An Investigation of the Views and Perceptions of Residents in Kent, Medway and Nord Pas de Calais of Health Determinants, Health Status and Opportunities for Health Improvement: A Qualitative Study. Document Reporting on the Qualitative Workstream Study Carried out in South East England by the University of Greenwich. Unpublished

Meghani, S. H. and Gallagher, R. M. (2008) 'Disability vs Inequality: Toward reconceptualization of pain treatment disparities'. *Pain Medicine* 9 (5): 613–23

Mezirow, J. (1991) *Transformative Dimensions of Adult Learning.* San Francisco: Josey Bass Inc

Miller, J. N., Colditz, G. A. and Mosteller, F. (1989) 'How study design affects outcomes in comparisons of therapy.II'. *Surgical Statistics in Medicine,* 8: 455–66

Millerson, G. (1964) *The Qualifying Associations: A Study in Professionalism.* London: Routledge Press

Millett, A., Devlin, J., Adams, P. and Gill, B. (1999) 'Patient participation in service improvement; the initial Measures Project experience'. *Health Expectations,* 2: 280–4

Mindell, J. S., Boltang, A. and Forde, I. (2008) 'A review of health impact assessment frameworks'. *Public Health,* 122 (11): 1177–87. Online. Available at: **http://eprints.ucl.ac.uk/5218/1/5218.pdf** (accessed 15 February 2009)

Mindell, J., Hansell, A., Morrison, D., Douglas, M. and Joffe, M. (2001) 'What do we need for robust, quantitative health impact assessment?' *Journal of Public Health Medicine,* 2001 Sep;23(3):173–8

Minton, A. (2005) *Generation Squalor: Shelter's National Investigation into the Housing Crisis.* London: Shelter

Moan, I. S. and Rise, J. (2005). 'Quitting smoking: Applying an extended version of the theory of planned behaviour in predicting intention and behaviour'. *Journal of Applied Biobehavioural Research*, 10: 39–68

Mohan, A., Spiby, J., Leonardi, G. S., Robins, A. and Jeffris, S. (2006) 'Sustainable waste management in the UK: The public health role'. *Public Health*, 120: 908–14

Molnar, S. (1992) *Human Variation: Races, Types and Ethnic Groups* (2nd Ed). New Jersey: Prentice-Hall

Mooney, A., Stathaam, J. and Simon, A. (2002) *The Pivot Generation*. York: The Joseph Rowntree Foundation

Muir Gray, J. A. (1997) *Evidence-based Healthcare – How to Make Health Policy and Management Decisions*. New York: Churchill Livingstone

Muir Gray, J. A. (2000) 'Evidence based public health', in: Trinder, L. and Reynolds, S. (eds) *Evidence-Based Practice: A Critical Appraisal*. Oxford: Blackwell Publishing

Mulrow, C. D. and Oxman, A. D. (1997) *Cochrane Collaboration Handbook*. The Cochrane Library, The Cochrane Collaboration, Oxford: Oxford Updated Software

Murray, H., Packard, C., Shepherd, J., Macfarlane, P. and Cobbe, S. (2007) 'Long Term Follow up of the West of Scotland Coronary Prevention Study'. *New England Journal of Medicine*, 11 October 2007, 357 (15): 1477–86

Naidoo, J. and Wills, J. (2000) *Health Promotion Foundations for Practice* (2nd Ed). London: Balliere Tindall

NAM (2007) *Criminal HIV Transmission*. London: NAM

National Consumer Council (2008) *Cut-price, What Cost? How Supermarkets can Affect your Chances of a Healthy Diet*. Online. Available at: **http://collections.europarchive.org/tna/20080804145057/http://www.ncc.org.uk/research_policy/food/** (accessed 12 December 2008)

Newham, R. and Hawley, G. (2007) 'The relationship of ethics to philosophy'. in Hawley, G. (ed) *Ethics in Clinical Practice, An Interprofessional Approach*, Chapter 5, pp. 76–100. Dorchester: Pearson Education Limited

NGO/CSO Forum for Food Sovereignty (2002) *Food Sovereignty: A Right for All. Political Statement of the NGO/CSO Forum for Food Sovereignty*. Rome: NGO/CSO. Online. Available at: **www.foodsovereignty.org/new/documents.php** (accessed 8 January 2009)

NHMRC (1995) *Guidelines for the Development and Implementation of Clinical Guidelines*. Canberra: Australian Government Publishing Service

NHS Connecting for Health (2009) *Useful Links*. Online. Available at: **www.nhscarerecords.nhs.uk/useful-links/nhs-connecting** (accessed 26 January 2009)

NHS Management Executive (1991) *Assessing Health Care Needs: A DHA Project Discussion Paper May 1991*. London: NHS Management Executive

NHS Trent Regional Office and Sheffield Hallam University (2002) *Determinants of Health Inequalities in the East Midlands, Yorkshire and the Humber*, Trent PHO NHS Wales (last updated 2006); *Introduction to NHS Wales (from the 1989 Welsh Health Planning Forum 'Strategic Intent and Direction for the NHS in Wales'*. Online. Available at: **www.wales.nhs.uk/sites3/page.cfm?orgid=452andpid=11597** (accessed 17 November 2006)

NICE (2006) *HIA Gateway: Demonstrating Health Gain as Added Value.* London: NICE. Online. Available at: **http://hiagateway.org.uk/page. aspx?o=healthgain** (accessed 8 December 2006)

NICE (2008a) *How to put NICE Guidance into Practice to Improve the Health and Well-being of Communities – Practical Steps for Local Authorities.* London: NICE. Online. Available at: **www.nice.org.uk/newsevents/infocus/ infocusarchive/newguideforlocalauthorities.jsp** (accessed 28 January 2009)

NICE (2008) *NHS Evidence Briefing Document October 2008.* Online. Available at: **www.nice.org.uk/media/AA1/CA/NHSEvidenceBriefingDocument. pdf** (accessed 9 January 2009)

Nicholas, S., Povey, D., Walker, A. and Kershaw, C. (2005) Crime in England and Wales 2004/5. Home Office Statistical Bulletin, National Statistics, London in Green, G. and Pugh, P. (2008) *Better Homes, Better Health: Health Impact Assessment of Sheffield Housing Strategy.* Sheffield: Sheffield Hallam University

NMC (2008) *Code of Conduct. Standards of Conduct, Performance and Ethics for Nurses and Midwives.* London: NMC Publishing

NMC (2009) *Guidance for the Care of Older People.* London: NMC Publishing

Noah, N. (2006) *Controlling Communicable Disease.* Maidenhead: Open University Press

Nuland, S. B. (2008) *Doctors: The Illustrated History of Medical Pioneers.* New York: Black Dog and Leventhal Publishers

Northern Ireland Executive (2002) *Investing for Health.* Online. Available at: **www.investingforhealth.com** (accessed 29 July 2009)

North Sheffield PCT (2005) *Parkwood Landfill Site, Sheffield. Health Impact Assessment Study. Volume 2.* Online. Available at: **www.sheffield.nhs.uk/ healthdata/resources/parkwoodreportoct05.pdf** (accessed 6 March 2009)

Nursing Times (2008) *New Social Enterprise Nursing Staff could get Lower Pensions* (25 November 2008). Online. Available at: **www.nursingtimes. net/nursing-practice-clinical-research/new-social-enterprise-nursing-staff- could-get-lower-pensions/1933984.article** (accessed 8 April 2009)

O'Reilly, J., *et al.* (2006) *Cost-benefit Analysis of Health Impact Assessment.* London: Department of Health in WHO (2007)

Obama, B. (2006) *The Audacity of Hope: Thoughts on Reclaiming the American Dream.* New York: Crown Books

ODPM (2002) *More than a Roof: A Report into Tackling Homelessness.* London: ODPM

ODPM (2004a) *The Social Exclusion Unit.* London: ODPM

ODPM (2004b) *The Drivers of Social Exclusion: A Review of the Literature for the Social Exclusion Unit in the Breaking the Cycle Series.* London: ODPM

ODPM (2004c) *Housing Health and Safety Rating System Guidance* (Version 2). London: ODPM

ODPM (2006) *Housing, Planning, Local Government and the Regions Committee: Coastal Towns Session 2005–06, Written Evidence.* London: House of Commons

Ofcom (2007) *The Consumer Experience: Research Report.* Online. Available at: www.ofcom.org.uk/research/tce/ce07/research07.pdf (accessed 24 January 2009)

Office for National Statistics (ONS) (2003) Social Capital: Measuring Networks and Shared Values. Online. Available at: www.statistics.gov.uk/CCI/nugget.asp?ID=314 (accessed 9 September 2009)

Office of Public Sector Information (1929) Infant Life (Preservation) Act. Online. Available at: www.opsi.gov.uk/revisedstatutes/Acts/ukpga/1929/cukpga-1 (accessed 16 March 2009)

Office of Public Sector Information (1861) Offences Against the Person Act. Online. Available at: www.opsi.gov.uk/revisedstatutes/Acts/ukpga/1861/cukpga-1 (accessed 16 March 2009)

Office of the Third Sector and DTI (2005) A Survey of Social Enterprises across the UK: Research Report for Small Business Service. London: IFF Bureau Van DIJK Electronic Publishing

Office of the Third Sector (Cabinet Office) (2008) Social Enterprise Background. Online. Available at: www.cabinetoffice.gov.uk/third_sector/social_enterprise/background.aspx (accessed 7 February 2009)

Ong, B. N. and Humphries, G. (1994) 'Prioritising needs with communities: Rapid appraisal methodologies in health', in Popay and Williams (eds) Researching the People's Health. London: Routledge

Orchard, C., Smillie, C., Meagher-Stewart, D., (2000) 'Community development and health in Canada'. Journal of Nursing Scholarship, 32-2: 205–9

Ormandy, D. (2004) 'Housing conditions and health', in Bassett, W. H. (ed) Clay's Handbook of Environmental Health (19th Ed), Part Five: Housing, Chapter 16: pp. 349–363. London: Spon Press

Orme, J., Powell, J., Taylor, P., Harrison, T. and Grey, M. (2003) Public Health for the 21st Century: New Perspectives on Policy, Participation and Practice. Berkshire: O U Press

Page, R. (2005) 'From democratic socialism to New Labour', in Bochel, H., Bochel, C., Page, R. and Sykes, R. Social Policy: Issues and Developments, pp. 268–91. London: Pearson Prentice Hall

Palmer, A., Marissal J.-P., Poirier, G., Herridge, D., Lee, Y. (2007) Health Inequalities across Northern France and South East England. Conference proceedings. Health and Health Behaviours in Northern France and South East England, 14 June 2007, Unpublished: Lille, France

Palmer, C. A. (1981) Human Cargoes: The British Slave Trade to Spanish America, 1879. Urbana: University of Illinois Press

Palmer, G., MacInnes, T. and Kenway, P. (2006) Monitoring Poverty and Social Exclusion. York: Joseph Rowntree Foundation

Parsons, L. and Day, S. (1992) 'Improving obstetric outcomes in ethnic minorities: an evaluation of health advocacy'. Journal of Public Health, 14: 183–91

Patel, S. P., Jarvelin, M. R. and Little, M. P. (2008) 'Systematic review of worldwide variations of the prevalence of wheezing symptoms in children'. Environmental Health, 7: 57

Patton, R. (2003) Managing and Measuring Social Enterprises. London: SAGE

Paul, R. and Elder, L. (2005) Learn the Tools the Best Thinkers Use. Upper Saddle River, NJ: Prentice Hall

Pearson, A. (2004) *Balancing the evidence: incorporating the synthesis of qualitative data into systematic reviews*. JBI Reports 2: 45–64

Pearson, D. (2005) 'Obesity', in Ewels, L. *Key Topics in Public Health: Essential Briefings on Prevention and Health Promotion*, pp. 79–100. Edinburgh: Elsevier Churchill Livingstone

Peattie, K. and Morley, A. (2008). *Diversity and Dynamics, Contexts and Contributions*. Social Enterprise Coalition and Centre for Business Relationships, Accountability, Sustainability and Society Cardiff University. Online. Available at: **www.socialenterprise.org.uk/data/files/Research/9549_final_web.pdf** (accessed 7 February 2009)

Pember Reeves, M. (1913) (reprinted 1979) *Round About a Pound a Week*. London: Virago Press.

Percy-Smith, J. (1996) 'Assessing community needs', in Percy-Smith, J. (ed) *Needs Assessment in Public Policy*. Buckingham: Open University Press

Peters, T. and Waterman, R. (2004) *In Search of Excellence*. New York: Warner Books Inc.

Petersen, P. E. (2005) 'Socio behavioural risk factors in dental caries – international perspectives'. *Community Dent Oral Epidemiology*, 2005; 33: 274–9. Copenhagen: Blackwell Munksgaard. Online. Available at: **www.who.int/oral_health/publications/CDOE05_aug05/en/** (accessed 3 November 2008)

Pillaye, J. (2004) Health Needs Assessment for Tackling Teenage Pregnancy in Brent (abridged version of report submitted for the Part II Examination for Membership for the Faculty of Public Health Medicine), Unpublished. Online. Available at: **www.shes-site.com/media/files/pages/Tackling_Teenage_Pregnancy_in_Brent.pdf** (accessed 28 January 2009)

Pomerleau, J. and McKee, M. (eds) (2005) *Issues in Public Health*. Maidenhead: OU Press/McGraw-Hill Education

Porter, S. (2003) *The Great Plague*. Stroud: Sutton Publishing

Prince's Trust and The Royal Bank of Scotland Group with the Centre for Economic Performance, London School of Economics (2007) *The Cost of Exclusion: Counting the Cost of Youth Disadvantage in the UK*. Online. Available at: **www.princes-trust.org.uk/main%20site%20v2/downloads/Cost%20of%20Exclusion%20apr07.pdf** (accessed 7 January 2009)

Professor the Lord Darzi of Denham (2008) *High Quality Care for All: Next Stage Review Final Report Summary*. London: NHS. Online. Available at: **www.dh.gov.uk/en/Publicationsandstatistics/Publications/PublicationsPolicyAndGuidance/DH_085825** (accessed 20 March 2009)

Prüss-Üstün, A. and Corvalán, C. (2006) *Preventing Disease Through Healthy Environments. Towards an Estimate of the Environmental Burden of Disease*. Geneva: WHO

Public Health Resource Unit and NHS (2008) *Public Health Skills and Career Framework (PHSCF) – How to Use it: For Public Health Practitioners*. Online. Available at: **www.phru.nhs.uk/Doc_Links/PHSCF04A5_Practitioners-copyrighted.pdf** (accessed 18 January 2009)

Putnam, R. (2000) *Bowling Alone: The Collapse and Revival of American Community*. New Jersey: Princeton University Press

Pye, S., King, K. and Sturman, J. (2006) *Air Quality and Social Deprivation in the*

UK: *An Environmental Inequalities Analysis. Final Report to Defra, Contract RMP/ 2035. AEA Technology*. Online. Available at: **www.airquality.co.uk/archive/reports/cat09/0701110944_AQinequalitiesFNL_AEAT_0506.pdf** (accessed 6 March 2009)

Raine, P. (2003) 'Promoting breast-feeding in a deprived area: the influence of peer support'. Health and Social Care in the Community, 11 (6): 463–9

Randhawa, G. (2007) *Tackling Health Inequalities for Minority Ethnic Groups: Challenges and Opportunities. Better Health Briefing 6*. London: Race Equality Foundation. Online. Available at: **www.reu.org.uk/health/files/health-brief6.pdf** (accessed 23 November 2008)

Raphael, D. (2004) *The Social Determinants of Health: Canadian Perspectives*. Toronto: Canadian Scholars Press

Reynolds, T. (2006) 'Caribbean families, social capital and young people's diasporic identities'. *Ethnic and Racial Studies*, 29 (6):1087–1103

Rhodes, R. and Courneya, K. (2003). 'Investigating multiple components of attitude, subjective norm, and perceived behavioural control: An examination of the theory of planned behaviour in the exercise domain'. *British Journal of Social Psychology*, 42: 129–46

Richman, J. (2003) 'Holding public health up for inspection', in Costello, J. and Haggart, M. (2003) *Public Health and Society*. Basingstoke, Hampshire: Palgrave Macmillan

Rodgers, S (1998) The dissemination and utilisation of research in Roe, B. and Webb, C. (ed) (1998) *Research and Development in Clinical Nursing Practice*. London: Wurr Publishers Ltd

Rodgers, S. E. (2000) The extent of nursing research utilization in general medical and surgical wards. *Journal of Advanced Nursing* 32 (1): 182–93

Rose, D. (2008) 'Parents to face shock tactics in campaign against child obesity', *The Times*, Friday 12 December: 25

Rosen, G. (1993) *A History of Public Health* (Expanded Ed). Baltimore: The John Hopkins University Press

Rowley, J. and Bhuhi, J. (1999) 'Participatory needs assessment: A practical approach in partnerships between local residents and professionals'. *Public Health Medicine*, 1: 27–30

Rowntree, S. (1901) (Reprinted 2000) *Poverty: A Study of Town Life*. Bristol: The Policy Press

Rutter, D. and Quine, L. (2002) *Changing Health Behaviour*. Buckingham: Open University Press

Ryan, C. (2005) *Nurses Say Reform Prostitutes Law*. Online. Available at: **http://news.bbc.co.uk/1/hi/health/4487237.stm** (accessed 30 December 2008)

Sackett, D. L. and Wennberg, J. E. (1997) Choosing the best research design for each question [editorial]. *British Medical Journal*, 315: 1636–7

Sanchez-Martinez, J. A., Ribeiro, C. R. (2008) 'The search for equality: Representation of the Smoking Act among adolescent women'. *Rev Lat Enfermacem*, 16 Spec No: 640–5

Sandelowski, M., Docherty, S. and Emden, C. (1997) Qualitative metasynthesis: issues and techniques. *Res Nurs Health* 20: 365–71

Sarafino, E. P. (2002) *Health Psychology Bio-psychological Interactions* (4th Ed). New York: Wiley

Schneider, M. J. (2000) *Introduction to Public Health*. USA: Aspen Publications

Schon, D. (1987) *Educating the Reflective Practitioner: Towards a New Design for Teaching and Learning in the Professions*. San Fransisco: Josey Bass

Schweigert, F. (2007) 'Learning to lead: Strengthening the practice of community leadership'. *Leadership*, 3 (3): 325–42

Scott, J., Gill, A. and Crowhurst, K. (2008) *Effective Management in Long-term Care Organisations*. Exeter: Reflect Press

Scottish Executive (2003) *Improving Health in Scotland: The Challenge*. Edinburgh: Scottish Executive

Scottish Intercollegiate Group On Alcohol (2009) *There is Strong International Evidence to Suggest that Falling Relative Price of Alcohol has been a Major Factor in Alcohol-related Harm*. Online. Available at: **www.scottish.parliament.uk/business/committees/lg/inquiries/ScottishintercollegiateGrouponAl-2009-02-18** (accessed 16 March 2009)

Scott-Samuel, A. (1998) 'Health impact assessment – theory into practice. *Journal of Epidemiology and Community Health*, 1998; 52: 704–5

Scott-Samuel, A., Birley, M., and Ardern, K., (2001). *The Merseyside Guidelines for Health Impact Assessment*. (2nd Ed), May 2001, Liverpool: International Health Impact Assessment Consortium

Scriven, A. (2007) *Public Health: Social Context and Action*. London: Open University Press McGraw-Hill Education

Seedhouse, D. (2001) *Health – the Foundations for Achievement* (2nd Ed). Chichester: Wiley

Seers, K. (1999) 'Qualitative Research', in Dawes *et al.* (1999) *Evidence Based Practice: A Primer for Health Care Professionals*. London: Churchill Livingstone

SEL London (2008) Social Enterprise London Website. Online. Available at: **www.sel.org.uk** (accessed 10 September 2009)

Senge, P. (2006) The Fifth Discipline: The Art and Practice of the Learning Organisation. Edinburgh: Random House

Sengupta, S. (2009) 'Determinants of Health', in Wilson, F. and Mabhala, M. *Key Concepts Public Health*. London: Sage

Sheeran, P. and Abraham, C. (2003) 'Mediator of moderators. Temporal stability of intention and the intention-behaviour relationship'. *Personality and Social Psychology Bulletin*, 29: 205–15

Sheridan, R. B. (1985) *Doctors and Slaves: A Medical and Demographic History of Slavery in the British West Indies, 1680–1831*. Cambridge/New York: Cambridge University Press

Skills for Health (2004) *National Occupational Standards for the Practice of Public Health Guide*. Bristol: Skills for Health

Skills for Health and Public Health Resource Unit (2008) *Public Health Skills and Careers Framework – Multidisciplinary/Multi-agency Multi-professional*. Bristol: Skills for Health and PHRU

Smedley, B. D., Stith, A. Y. and Nelson, A. R. (2002) *Unequal Treatment: Confronting Racial and Ethnic Disparities in Health Care*. Washington DC: National Academy Press

Sociologyonline (undated) *The Third Way: Searching for a State without Enemies!*

Online. Available at: **www.sociologyonline.co.uk/politics/Giddens_3way. shtml** (accessed 8 December 2006)

Southon, G. and Braithwaite, J. (1998) 'The end of professionalism?'. *Social Science and Medicine*, 46 (1): 23–8

Spear, S. (2008) 'Migrants at risk'. *Environmental Health Practitioner*, 3 April 2008. Online. Available at: **www.cieh.org/ehp/ehp3.aspx?id=9870** (accessed 30 January 2009)

Spigner, C. (2006/2007) 'Race, health and the African diaspora'. *International Quarterly of Community Health Education* 27 (2):161–76

Spring Rice, M. (1939) (reprinted 1981) *Working Class Lives*. London: Virago Press

Stevens, A. (1991) 'Needs assessment needs assessment . . .'. *Health Trends* 23, No 1

Stevens, A. and Raftery, J. (1997) *Health Care Needs Assessment*. Abingdon: Radcliffe Medical Press

Stewart, J. (2005) 'A review of UK housing policy: ideology and public health'. *Public Health*, 119 (06) 525–34

Stewart, J. (2009) 'Homes on the Map'. *Environmental Health Practitioner*, 117 (09): 20–21

Stewart, J., Bushell, F. and Habgood, V. (2005) *Environmental Health as Public Health*. London: Chadwick House Group Ltd

Stewart, J. and Habgood, V. (2008) 'The benefits of a health impact assessment in relation to fuel poverty: Assessing Luton's affordable warmth strategy and the need for a national strategy'. *Journal of the Royal Society for the Promotion of Health*, 128 (03): 124–30

Stewart, J. and Rhoden, M. (2006) 'Children, housing and health'. *International Journal of Sociology and Social Policy*, 26 (7/8): 326–41

Stewart, J., Ruston, A. and Clayton, J. (2006) 'Housing as a health determinant: Is there consensus that public health partnerships are a way forward?'. *Journal of Environmental Health Research*, 5 (02): 87–94

Sullivan, H. (2005) 'Is enabling enough? Tensions and dilemmas in new Labour's strategies for joining up local governance'. *Public Policy and Administration*, 20 (10): 10–24.

Sundquist, K., Maestrom, M., and Johannson, S. E. (2004) 'Neighbourhood deprivation and incidence of coronary heart disease; a multi-level study of 2.6 million women and men in Sweden'. *Journal of Epidemiology and Community Health*, 58: 71–7, in Green, G. and Pugh, P. (2008) *Better Homes, Better Health: Health Impact Assessment of Sheffield Housing Strategy*. Sheffield: Sheffield Hallam University

Sutcliffe, J., Duin, N. (1992) *A History of Medicine*. London: Barnes and Noble Inc/ Morgan Samuel Edition

Swann, C. and Morgan, M. (eds) (2002) *Social Capital: Insights from Qualitative Research*. London: HDA

Syme, S. L. (1994) 'The social environment and health'. *Daedalus*, 123 (4):79–86

Symons Downs, D. and Hausenblas, H. (2005) 'Elicitation studies and the theory of planned behaviour: A systematic review of exercise beliefs'. *Psychology of Sport and Exercise*, 6: 1–31

Tarlov, A. R (1996) 'Social determinants of health: The sociobiological translation', in Blane, D., Brunner, E. and Wilkinson, R. (eds) *Health and Social Organisation*. London: Routledge.

Taske, N., Taylor, L., Mulvihill, C. and Doyle, N. (2005) *Housing and Public Health: A Review of Reviews of Interventions for Improving Health – Evidence Briefing*. London: NICE

Taylor, M. (1995) *Unleashing the Potential: Bringing Residents to the Centre of Regeneration*. York: JRF

TB Alert, TB Alert: The UK's national TB Charity's website. Available at: **www.tbalert.org/** (last accessed 13 March 2009)

Thompson, N. (2004) *Promoting Equality* (2nd Ed). Basingstoke, Hants: Palgrave Macmillan

Thomson, H., Petticrew, M., and Morrison, D. (2001) 'Health effects of housing improvement: systematic review of intervention studies'. *British Medical Journal*, 323:187–90

Thomson, H., Petticrew, M., and Morrison, D. (2002) *Housing Improvement and Health Gain: A Summary and Systematic Review, Medical Research Council Social and Public Health Sciences Unit, Occasional Paper no 5, January 2002*. Glasgow: MRC Social and Public Health Services Unit, University of Glasgow

Timesonline (Feburary 13, 2009) *Alfie Patten Becomes a Father After One Night of Unprotected Sex*. Online. Available at: **http://timesonline.co.uk/tol/news/uk/article5724616.ece** (accessed 16 March 2009)

Tischler, H. L., Whitten, P., Hunter, D. E. K. (1986) *Introduction of Sociology*, (2nd Ed). New York: CBS College Publishing

Tones, B. (1986) 'Health education and the ideology of health promotion: a review of alternative approaches'. *Health Education Research*, 1 (1)1: 3–12

Townsend, P. (1979) *Poverty and Health*. UK: Penguin Books

Trinder, L. (2000) 'Introduction: The Context of Evidence Based Practice', in Trinder, L. with Reynolds, S. (eds). *Evidence-Based Practice: A Critical Appraisal*. Oxford: Blackwell Publishing

TUC (2008) *The Iron Triangle: Women's Poverty, Children's Poverty and in Work Poverty*. London: TUC

Turshen, M. (1989) *The Politics of Public Health*. London: Zed Books

Umble, K. E., Diehl, S. J., Gunn, A. and Haws, S. (2007) *Developing Leaders, Building Networks: An Evaluation of the National Public Health Leadership Institute – 1991–2006*. Chapel Hill, NC: North Carolina Institute for Public Health

UKPHA (2008) *Climates and Change The Urgent Need to Connect Health and Sustainable Development*. Online. Available at: **www.ukpha.org.uk/media/4327/climates%/20and%20change.pdf** (accessed 22 July 2009)

United Nations (1948) Universal Declaration of Human Rights. Geneva: UN. Online. Available at: **www.un.org/Overview/rights.html** (accessed 3 November 2008)

UN (1987) *Report of the World Commission on Economic Development 42/187*. Online. Available at: **www.un-documents.net/a42r187.htm** (accessed 6 March 2009)

UN (1992a) *Report of the United Nations Conference on Environment and*

Development. Annex I: Rio Declaration on Environment and Development. Online. Available at: **www.un.org/documents/ga/conf151/aconf15126-1annex1.htm** (accessed 6 March 2009)

UN. (1992b) *United Nations Framework Convention on Climate Change.* Online. Available at: **http://unfccc.int/resource/docs/convkp/conveng.pdf** (06 March 2009)

UN (1993) *Agenda 21: Earth Summit – The United Nations Programme of Action from Rio.* New York: United Nations Publications

UN (1998) *Kyoto Protocol to the United Nations Framework Convention on Climate Change.* Online. Available at: **http://unfccc.int/resource/docs/convkp/kpeng.pdf** (accessed 6 March 2009)

UNEP/GRID-Arendal. (2008) *Vital Graphics – Vital Climate Graphics: Spread of major tropical vector-borne diseases.* Online. Available at: **www.grida.no/publications/vg/climate/page/3093.aspx** (accessed 6 March 2009)

US Democratic Leadership Council (1999) *The Third Way: Progressive Governance for the 21st Century by Roundtable Discussion (25 April 1999).* Online. Available at: **www.dlc.org/ndol_ci.cfm?kaid=128&subid=185&contendid=880** (accessed December 2006)

US Office of Disease Prevention and Health Promotion (1996) *Healthy People 2000 Midcourse Review and 1995 Revisions.* Washington D.C.: US Office of Disease Prevention and Health Promotion

Van Ryn, M., Burgess, D., Malat, J., Griffin, J. (2006) 'Physicians' perceptions of patients' social and behavioral characteristics and race disparities in treatment recommendations for men with coronary artery disease'. *American Journal of Public Health*, 96: 351–7

Van Ryn, M. M. and Fu, S. S. (2003) 'Paved with good intentions: Do public health and human services providers contribute to racial/ethnic disparities in health?'. *American Journal of Public Health*, 93: 248–55

Wainwright, D. (1994) 'On the waterfront'. *Health Service Journal*, 7 July 1994, 28–9

Walker, A. (2005) 'Quality of life in old age in Europe', in Walker, A. (ed) *Growing Older in Europe*, pp.1 A. 29. Maidenhead: Open University Press

Walker, A. and Walker, C. (2005) 'The UK: quality of life in old age II', in Walker, A. (ed) *Growing Older in Europe*, pp. 233–47. Maidenhead: Open University Press

Walker. G., Mitchell, G., Fairburn, J. and Smith, G. (2005) 'Industrial Pollution and Social Deprivation: Evidence and Complexity in Evaluating and Responding to Environmental Inequality'. *Local Environment*, 10(4): 361–77

Wall, T. (2009) 'Unions protest as Barnet moves to outsource all council services'. Environmental Health News, 30 January 2009, 24 (4)

Walt, G. (1994) *Health Policy: An Introduction to Process and Power.* London: Zed Books Ltd

Wanless, D. (2001) *Securing Our Future Health: Taking a Long Term View.* London: HM Treasury

Wanless, D. (2004) *Securing Good Health for the Whole Population: Final Report.* London: DoH

Watt, S., Norton, D. (2004) 'Culture, ethnicity, race: what's the difference?'. *Paediatric Nursing,* 16 (8) 37–43

Watts, S. (1997) *Epidemic and History: Disease, Power and Imperialism.* New Haven and London: Yale University Press

Webster, C. and French, J. (2002) *'The Cycle of Conflict: The History of The Public Health Promotion Movements',* in Adams, E., Amos, M. and Munro, J. (eds) (2002) *Promoting Health Politics and Practice.* London: Sage

Weinberg, J., (2005) 'The impact of globalization on emerging infectious diseases', in Kelly, L. and Collin, J. (eds) *Global Change and Health,* Chapter 5, pp 53–62, Maidenhead, Open University Press

Welsh Assembly Government (2005) *Designed for Life: Creating World Class Health and Social Care for Wales in the 21st Century.* Cardiff: Welsh Assembly Government

Welsh Assembly Government. (2006 and 2007) *Health Challenge Wales.* Online. Available at: **http://wales.gov.uk/hcwsubsite/healthchallenge/?lang=en** (accessed 18 January 2009)

WHO (1984) *Health Promotion: A Discussion Document on the Concept and Principles.* Copenhagen: WHO Regional Office for Europe

WHO (1986a) 'A discussion document on the concept and principles of health promotion'. *Health promotion,* 1 (1): 73–6

WHO (1986b) *Ottawa Charter for Health Promotion.* Ontario: WHO and Health and Welfare

WHO (1995) *World Health Report 1995: Bridging the Gaps.* Online. Available at: **www.who.int/whr/1995/media_centre/executive_summary1/en/print. html** (accessed 14 September 2005)

WHO (1999) *Gothenburg Consensus Paper. Health Impact Assessment: Main Concepts and Suggested Approach.* Brussels: European Centre for Health Policy, WHO Regional Office for Europe. Online. Available at: **www.who. int/hia/about/defin/en/index.html** (accessed 14 December 2008)

WHO (2002) *Health and Sustainable Development: Key Health Trends.* Online. Available at: **www.who.int/mediacentre/events/HSD_Plaq_02.2_Gb_def1. pdf** (accessed 6 March 2009)

WHO (2004) Health Aspects of Air *Pollution.* Online. Available at: **www.euro.who.int/document/E83080.pdf** (accessed 6 March 2009)

WHO (2006) *Guidelines for Drinking Water Quality. 3rd Edition. Volume 1 Recommendations.* Online. Available at: **www.who.int/water_sanitation_ health/dwq/gdwq3rev/en/** (accessed 6 March 2009)

WHO (2007) *The Effectiveness of Health Impact Assessment; Scope and Limitations of Supporting Decision-making in Europe.* Online. Available at: **http://ec.europa.eu/health/ph_projects/2003/action1/docs/2003_1_20_ book_en.pdf** (accessed 6 April 2009)

WHO (2008) *What is Environmental Health?* Online. Available at: **www.euro. who.int/envhealth/20060609_1** (accessed 6 March 2009)

WHO Commission on the Social Determinants of Health (2008) *Closing the Gap in a Generation – Health Equity through Action on the Social Determinants of Health, Final Report Executive Summary.* Geneva: WHO.

Online. Available at: **http://whqlibdoc.who.int/hq/2008/WHO_IER_ CSDH_08.1_eng.pdf** (accessed 6 March 2009) and full report at **www. who.int/social_determinants/final_report/en/index.html** (accessed 6 March 2009)

WHO-UNEP (2005) *Health and Environment Linkages Initiative. Health and Environment; Tools for Effective Decision-making.* Geneva: WHO Press

Wilkinson, D. (1999) *Poor Housing and Ill Health: A Summary of Research Evidence.* The Scottish Office Central Research Unit

Wilkinson, R. (1996) *Unhealthy Societies: The Afflictions of Inequality.* London: Routledge

Wilkinson, R. and Pickett, K. (2009) *The Spirit Level: Why More Equal Societies Almost Always do Better.* London: Penguin

Wilkinson, R. G. (1997) 'Socioeconomic determinants of health: Health inequalities: relative or absolute material standards?'. *British Medical Journal*, 7080 (314): 591. Online. Available at: www.bmj.com/cgi/content/ extract/314/7080/591 (accessed 27 March 2009)

Williams, C. (2008) 'New deal for migrants'. *Environmental Health News*, 14 November 2008: 7

Williams, D. R. (1997) 'Race and health: Basic questions, emerging directions'. *Annals of Epidemiology*, 7(5): 322–33.

Williams, D. R., Rucker, T. D. (2000) 'Understanding and addressing racial disparities in health care', *Health Care Finance Review*, 21: 75–90

Wilson, W. J. (1988) 'The ghetto underclass and the social transformation of the inner city'. *The Black Scholar* (May/June):10–7

Witzig, R. (1996) 'The medicalization of race: Scientific legitimatization of a flawed social construct'. *Annals of Internal Medicine* 125 (8): 675–9. California: Wadsworth Publishing Company

Wolinsky, F. D. (1988) *The Sociology of Health* (2nd Ed). Belmont, California: Wadsworth Publishing Company

World Bank (2001) *Assessing Globalization, World Bank Briefing Paper, The World Bank Group.* Online. Available at: **www1.worldbank.org/economicpolicy/ globalisation/issueriefs.html** (accessed 5 July 2007)

Zane, N. W. S., Takeuchi, D. T., Young, K. N. J. (1994) *Confronting Critical Health Issues of Asian and Pacific Islander Americans.* London/New Delhi: Sage Publications

Ziegler, J. (2004) *Economic, Social and Cultural Rights: The Right to Food. Report Submitted by the Special Rapporteur on the Right to Food, in Accordance with Commission on Human Rights Resolution 2003/25*, United Nations Economic and Social Council. Online. Available at: **www.unhchr.ch/ Huridocda/Huridoca.nsf/e06a5300f90fa0238025668700518ca4/344 41bf9efe3a9e3c1256e6300510e24/$FILE/G0410777.pdf** (accessed 12 December 2008)

Index